THE AUTONOMIC NERVOUS SYSTEM AND ITS EFFECTORS

THE AUTONOMIC NERVOUS SYSTEM AND ITS EFFECTORS

ALISON BRADING

MA (Oxon), BSc, PhD

Professor of Pharmacology, Department of Pharmacology,
University of Oxford, Mansfield Road, Oxford

Blackwell
Science

Editorial Offices:
Osney Mead, Oxford OX2 0EL
25 John Street, London WC1N 2BL
23 Ainslie Place, Edinburgh EH3 6AJ
350 Main Street, Malden
MA 02148 5018, USA
54 University Street, Carlton
Victoria 3053, Australia
10, rue Casimir Delavigne
75006 Paris, France

Other Editorial Offices:
Blackwell Wissenschafts-Verlag GmbH
Kurfürstendamm 57
10707 Berlin, Germany

Blackwell Science KK
MG Kodenmacho Building
7–10 Kodenmacho Nihombashi
Chuo-ku, Tokyo 104, Japan

First published 1999

Set by Excel Typesetters Co., Hong Kong
Printed and bound in Great Britain by
MPG Books Ltd, Bodmin, Cornwall

For further information on Blackwell Science, visit our website: www.blackwell-science.com

DISTRIBUTORS

Marston Book Services Ltd
PO Box 269
Abingdon, Oxon OX14 4YN
(*Orders*: Tel: 01235 465500
Fax: 01235 465555)

USA
Blackwell Science, Inc.
Commerce Place
350 Main Street
Malden, MA 02148 5018
(*Orders*: Tel: 800 759 6102
781 388 8250
Fax: 781 388 8255)

Canada
Login Brothers Book Company
324 Saulteaux Crescent
Winnipeg, Manitoba R3J 3T2
(*Orders*: Tel: 204 837-2987)

Australia
Blackwell Science Pty Ltd
54 University Street
Carlton, Victoria 3053
(*Orders*: Tel: 3 9347 0300
Fax: 3 9347 5001)

A catalogue record for this title is available from the British Library

ISBN 0-632-02624-3

Library of Congress
Cataloging-in-publication Data

Brading, Alison.
The autonomic nervous system and its effectors / Alison Brading.
p. cm.
Includes bibliographical references and index.
ISBN 0-632-02624-3
1. Autonomic nervous system.
2. Neurotransmitters.
I. Title.
[DNLM: 1. Autonomic Nervous System—physiology. WL 600 B798a 1998]
QP368.B73 1998
612′.8—dc21.
DNLM/DLC
for Library of Congress 97-22696
CIP

Contents

Preface

The stimulus for writing this book has been the striking difference between the fascination that the autonomic nervous system and its effectors has had for me and friends and colleagues working in this area, and the apathy or boredom with which the undergraduates I have had contact with over the years seem to view this part of their syllabus. Uninspired teaching and inadequate coverage in many textbooks must surely take most of the blame here, but the underlying causes may well be historical.

In the second half of the 20th century, the major and exciting advances that attracted the interest of students were initially in understanding the physiology of nerves and striated muscle, the properties of neuromuscular junctions and neuronal synapses. Most of these studies were carried out on relatively large and easily assessible systems. Following this there was a huge development of research into the two extremes of molecular biology and the brain and CNS processing. These are the areas that have excited students and academics alike, and have come to dominate the textbooks. In research into the systems of the body, it is probably only the cardiovascular system that has achieved a comparable status, and the autonomic control of the cardiovascular system is often the only autonomic system that students of medicine, physiology and pharmacology become really familiar with.

Although research into the autonomic nervous system and its effectors has been continuing throughout the century, and was enormously important in the early half, it became distinctly unfashionable in the middle of this century. The cells and systems involved were more complicated and less suitable for the developing technologies to unravel, and it was less likely that major breakthroughs would be made, which discouraged researchers and made it less easy to obtain research funding. However, the techniques have been developed, and more recently the autonomic nervous system is coming into its own as a fascinating system to study. The complex neuronal pathways in the peripheral ganglia and the enteric nervous system are far more available for study than central systems, and lessons can be learnt that throw light on CNS processing. The effectors with their easily recordable contractile or secretory responses provide excellent preparations in which to study pathways involved in cellular control. Our knowledge has grown enormously. Unfortunately, it takes time for such knowledge to filter through into the standard textbooks, the space allocated in most of them to the autonomic nervous system is ridiculously inadequate, and some erroneous early concepts are still being perpetuated. This is particularly unfortunate for medics and scientists, since disorders involving the autonomic systems will provide a major part of clinical practice.

This book is an attempt to improve the balance. It is hoped that it will prove valuable to students in many disciplines, and also to young graduates beginning a research career and clinicians beginning specialist training. It is an attempt to demonstrate just how marvellous and intriguing the autonomic nervous system is, and to provide a more accurate account of our current knowledge.

I am greatly indebted to many friends and colleagues for their help and support. The fact that I only mention a few by name does not detract from the value of all their many contributions. Without Dr Tom Cunnane this book would never have been started; his enthusiasm spurred me on to make the attempt, and his own contribution to research in this field, and in particular to our understanding of transmitter release from autonomic varicosities, has been outstanding, and is reflected in Chapter 4. I am particularly grateful to Dr James Brock for helping with this section. Discussions with Professor Margaret Matthews on the anatomy and physiology of ganglionic transmission have given me insight into this interesting and relevant topic. She has kindly provided micrographs for inclusion. Professor Giorgio Gabella has for years inspired me through his beautiful electron microscopy, and to him I am particularly indebted for his generosity in providing so many new and beautiful micrographs to illustrate the book. Dr Charlotte Slaney spent a long vacation during her undergraduate days painstakingly and intelligently searching the literature for ideas for the illustrations in the book, which proved enormously valuable. Mike Elms converted them into the illustrations, and patiently incorporated my changes and coped with my illegible instructions, with Alice Emmott advising and providing constant help and encouragement in her role as senior production editor. My research group has never been neglected whilst I have been writing this book because Dr Gordon McMurray has stepped in for me, and taken over supervision. Without his help and the understanding of the group, I could not have finished the book; they all have my gratitude. In spite of the help and advice, the book is idiosyncratic, and reflects my views. Any errors and misinterpretations are solely my responsibility.

1 : Historical Background

1.1 Introduction

There is a well-known 'classical' picture of the autonomic nervous system that has been taught for many years to medical students, physiologists and pharmacologists. This encompasses the system's anatomical arrangement, the neuronal organisation (the presence of ganglion cells outside the central nervous system), the cholinergic presynaptic neurones and the predominantly cholinergic and adrenergic postganglionic neurones, and the identification of acetylcholine and noradrenaline as their respective transmitters. Surprisingly, however, the picture was only completed in the late 1940s (see Fig. 2.1, p. 16). A great deal of the important work required to establish these facts was carried out during the life-span of many scientists alive today. In fact, the majority of the most important work on the autonomic nervous system was carried out in the 50 or so years spanning the last decades of the 19th century and the first decades of the 20th century. The time was ripe, and the field attracted some of the very best scientific brains of the time. These early studies had enormous importance in establishing many of the most essential principles in physiology and pharmacology. Consider, for instance, chemical transmission: some 50 years before it was accepted that neuromuscular transmission in skeletal muscles was a chemically mediated event, the scientists working on the involuntary systems had proposed that both the sympathetic nervous system and the parasympathetic nervous system worked by releasing chemical transmitters, and had suggested which chemicals might be involved. The experimental results also led to the concept of receptors and of pharmacological antagonism.

1.2 Availability of techniques

Why was it only so recently that this degree of knowledge was acquired? The understanding of any particular system will always depend very much on the techniques available for its study. The autonomic nervous system is an interesting example of this, and anyone reading the early literature on this fascinating system will be rewarded with intriguing insights into the scientific thinking of that time, and will come across many appealing anecdotes relating to the people carrying out the work. The important techniques that were necessary were: morbid anatomy, histology, general anaesthesia, the ability to stimulate nerves electrically, organic chemistry and the ability to study isolated systems in physiological conditions. Without these various techniques, the quite remarkable achievements of this period would not have been possible.

1.2.1 Morbid anatomy

This was a skill that was perfected many centuries ago, and several outstanding treatises were published in the 16th century, such as that of Andreas Vesalius, who was Professor of Anatomy at the famous Padua University (although he originated from Brussels). The early anatomists were able to describe in detail most of the nerves in the autonomic nervous system. Thus the gross anatomical background was well established. However, they had relatively little evidence of the function of the nerves, apart from their distribution.

1.2.2 Histology

Another technique that was flourishing and available to scientists studying the autonomic system was histology. The compound microscope had been invented by Robert Hooke in 1665, but the lenses suffered from chromatic aberration, and it was only after the development of achromatic lenses and achromatic compound microscopes (the first good one constructed in 1826 by J.J. Lister, father of the antisepsis Lister) that the structure of cells could be made out, and neurones visualised. Although Purkinje in 1837 described the large neurones in the cerebellum that bear his name, and in spite of some other minor advances, improvements in fixing and staining techniques were required before the details of the neuronal structure and the links between neurones and the nerve fibres could be elucidated. The credit for the most marked advances in the histological study of nervous tissue goes to Camillo Golgi, the Italian who perfected a silver staining technique in 1872 that allowed fine details of individual neurones to be studied, and Santiago Ramon y Cajal, a young spaniard, unknown to the scientific community before 1889, whose beautiful and detailed histological works using Golgi's techniques led to them sharing the Nobel prize for medicine in 1906. The early works on neurones and the links between them had split the scientists into two camps: those following the reticular theory, who believed that the nerves formed an interconnecting network, and those following the neurone theory, who believed that the neurones were individual elements.

Even in 1906, the controversy was still apparent; in their speeches at the Nobel prize ceremony, it was clear that Golgi followed the reticular theory and Ramon y Cajal followed the neurone theory.

It is interesting to note that the autonomic physiologists, such as Langley, were at that time mapping the positions of the ganglia in the autonomic nervous system not by histological studies, but by pharmacological ones – they had discovered that when nicotine was applied (with a paintbrush), it would first activate and then inactivate the neuronal pathway under study, but only if applied to the ganglia. Thus activation by nicotine implied the presence of neurones in the pathway. Incidentally, the fact that nicotine then blocked transmission through the pathway was possible evidence against the reticular theory, and the autonomic physiologists were already speculating that chemical transmission occurred between neurones.

1.2.3 General anaesthesia

Analysis of the functional aspects of the system depended largely on the advent of general anaesthesia, which only began to be used with tooth extraction under ether by Henry Morton in 1846, and for the relief of the pain of childbirth by James Simpson with chloroform in 1847. General anaesthetics, combined with the skilled surgical and observational techniques and the curiosity of the anatomists and physiologists in the second half of the 19th century, greatly furthered understanding of the autonomic nervous system.

In anaesthetised animals, the parts of the body that were obviously working were of course the involuntary systems, and it was comparatively easy for physiologists to record such things as heart rate, blood pressure, gastrointestinal motility, pupil diameter, piloerection, and the production of various secretions.

1.2.4 Electrical stimulation

As we have seen, the anatomy of the nerves to the involuntary systems was known, but to discover their individual functions it was necessary to stimulate the nerves electrically and monitor their effects. An interesting sideline to follow is the history of animal electricity (Box 1.1).

Machines that could be used for generating electric shocks were available from 1745. Faraday's discovery of electromagnetic induction in 1831 allowed the manufacture of machines that could produce more precise stimuli, and the possibility of arranging repetitive activation of nerves. Several methods of applying electricity to nerves were thus available to the autonomic physiologists to study the roles of the particular autonomic outflows controlling the involuntary systems of the body. This allowed them to appreciate their functional significance.

Box 1.1 Animal electricity

An early theory of nervous activity was that the nerve axons were tiny tubes full of 'animal spirits', which on activation flowed down the nerves from the brain, and caused activation of the end organs. Early scientists in the 17th and 18th centuries were aware of electricity, and knew that it interacted with animals in some way. Natural electricity was known in the form of lightning, and experiments were carried out on its effects on animals (with one reported death of an experimenter). Several machines were invented in which static electricity could be produced or stored, such as the 'electric influence machine' (a globe of sulphur mounted on a spindle and rotated by hand) invented by Otto von Guericke in 1672, and the Leyden jar, which was invented in 1745.

Galvani was a keen investigator, and worked extensively on electricity beginning in 1771. His famous book on animal electricity was published in 1791. He noticed that when electricity was applied to dissected frog muscles they would twitch. He also harnessed natural electricity from thunderstorms and clouds using a long insulated conductor installed on his roof; he could connect the conductor to the frog muscles. Galvani then made the important discovery that if freshly dissected (and thus moist) muscles were contacted by metals – particularly two different metals – and included in a circuit, they would twitch. Galvani interpreted this discovery as a method of harnessing animal electricity, but Volta regarded it more accurately as a way of generating electricity. This culminated in the invention by Volta of his voltaic pile in 1799, made from discs of dissimilar metals separated by acid-moistened pads – the first man-made batteries. All this demonstration and investigation of animal electricity led to the hypothesis that the 'animal spirits' of the nerves were in fact just electrical currents. However, this was disproved by Helmholtz in 1850 by measuring the speed of conduction of nerves, which was much slower than the conduction of electricity in a wire.

1.2.5 Organic chemistry

Another important arm of this story is that of the development of organic chemistry, and it may perhaps surprise modern students to realise just how skilled 19th century chemists were. In the 1820s, techniques were developed that allowed the isolation of organic molecules, and their elemental structure could therefore be determined. During the 1850s and 1860s, organic analysis and synthesis progressed rapidly. It was soon possible to isolate the active principles in many plant and animal extracts, and if enough material was available, to establish the composition of the less complicated molecules. These skills became increasingly useful, particularly in the first half of the 20th century. Once the structure of a bioactive molecule had been established, it became possible to synthesise variants of simpler molecules and test them on living systems.

However, Sir William Paton (Professor of Pharmacology at Oxford from 1959 to 1984), when attempting to determine when pharmacology developed into an independent and flourishing discipline (he dates this in the 1930s), observed that the first *British Pharmacopoeia*, printed in 1864, gives the chemical structure of water as HO, silver nitrate as $AgNO_6$ and atropine as $C_{34}H_{23}NO_6$ (more carbon atoms than all the other atoms put together!). This was explained by the list of atomic weights, in which oxygen was given as 8 and carbon as 6, with N and H near our present values. It was only in 1885 that the *British Pharmacopoeia* adopted the currently used values. It is probable that the use of the 'old' notation for atomic weight hindered the development of chemistry for more than 50 years.

1.2.6 The study of isolated systems

The development of suitable physiological saline solutions that allowed organs to function outside the body might be said to start with Ringer, who investigated the effect of various ions on the frog heart in the early 1880s, and Locke's work on mammalian tissues towards the end of the century. This work resulted in the design of various physiological saline solutions that could maintain the viability of tissues *in vitro*.

1.3 Nomenclature

Through the use of these various techniques, the autonomic physiologists were able to appreciate the design and overall functions of the autonomic nervous system. For many years, the whole system was called the 'sympathetic nervous system', with the word 'sympathetic' coming from 'sympathy', suggesting the co-ordinated action of the system. The vertebral chains were called the 'great sympathetic nerves', and were clearly involved in co-ordinating activity, and many of the autonomic responses of the body could be observed to activate together, such as the famous set of 'flight or fight' responses, which included aspects as diverse as dilation of the pupil, increase in the heart rate, redistribution of blood flow to the muscles, suppression of activity in the gut, etc., all co-operating in preparing the body for activity.

The two scientists most responsible for establishing our basic knowledge of the system were Gaskell (Box 1.2) and Langley (Box 1.3). By 1866, Gaskell had given the first clear account of the overall structure of the system, with its origin in the cranial, thoracolumbar and sacral outflows from the brainstem and spinal cord. From 1875, Langley and Gaskell were close colleagues both working in Cambridge, with Langley's functional and Gaskell's anatomical studies allowing cross-fertilisation of ideas. The

Box 1.2 Walter Holbrook Gaskell (1847–1914)

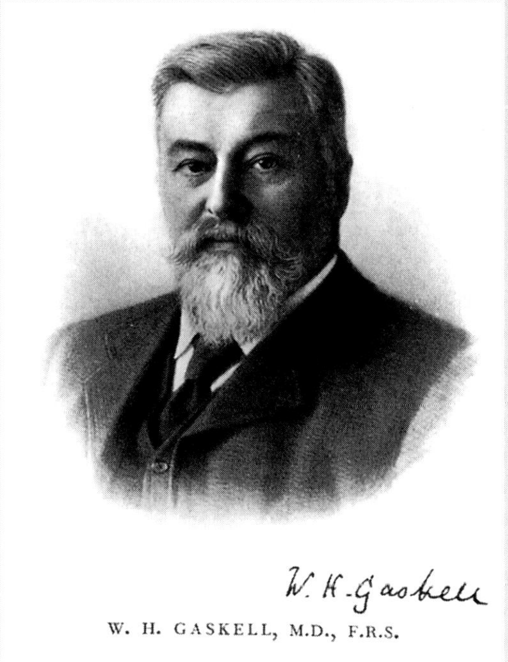

Gaskell was born in Naples. He studied mathematics at Trinity College, Cambridge, and then transferred to the Physiology Department. He qualified in medicine at University College, London. He returned to Cambridge in 1875 as a research scientist in the Physiological Laboratory with private means. He became a University Lecturer in 1883 and a fellow of Trinity College, Cambridge in 1889. Working initially on the control of the cardiovascular system, he widened his interests to undertake an extensive examination of the anatomy and physiology of the autonomic nervous system. He revealed the presence of the complementary sympathetic and parasympathetic divisions.

overall term 'autonomic nervous system' was first suggested by Langley in 1898, but did not gain general acceptance at the time. In his textbook in 1916, Gaskell called it 'the involuntary nervous system'. In 1921, Langley published his book, *The Autonomic Nervous System,* in which he proposed that the system could be divided on functional and anatomical grounds into three components: the sympathetic nervous system, producing co-ordinated activity using the thoracolumbar outflow; the parasympathetic nervous system, producing more individual actions often opposing the sympathetic and using the cranial and sacral outflows; and the enteric nervous system. The rationale for treating the enteric nervous system as a separate system came from his estimation that it could not be classified as

Box 1.3 John Newport Langley (1852–1925)

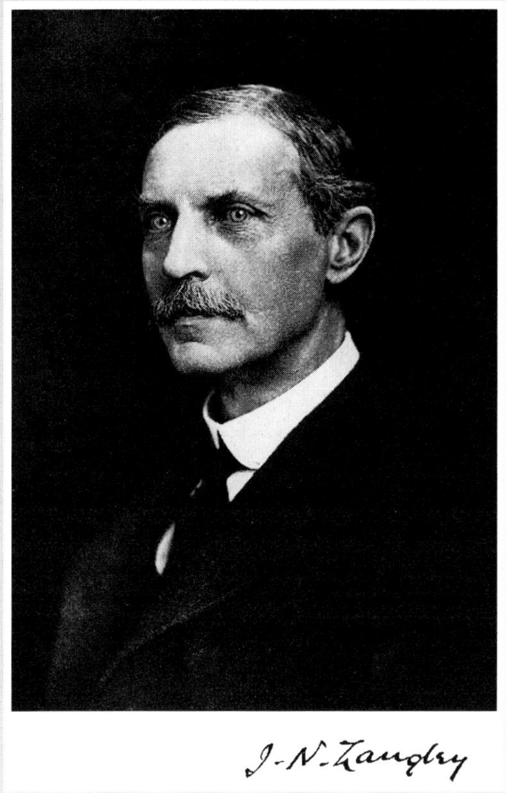

Langley was born in Newbury. He studied mathematics at St John's College, Cambridge, later transferring to natural science. He spent his entire scientific career in the Physiological Laboratory, initially as a demonstrator in 1875, then as University Lecturer in histology in 1884, and as Professor of Physiology from 1903 to 1925. With Gaskell, he determined the anatomical and principal physiological functions of the autonomic nervous system. He was also the owner and editor of the *Journal of Physiology* from 1894 until his death, and through this played a major role in shaping British physiology. He was a keen sportsman and member of the National Skating Association, and a judge of international skating competitions.

parasympathetic, since the number of vagal fibres innervating the gut was far less than the number of neurones in the gut wall, and also from the demonstration that the reflex activity of the gut (e.g. peristalsis) did not alter when its extrinsic innervation was cut and no connection remained with the central nervous system.

Although in retrospect Langley's classification was the most sensible one, and one that is accepted today, for many years the enteric system was largely ignored, and the main focus was on the sympathetic and parasympathetic systems. However, the term 'sympathetic nervous system' for the whole autonomic system was retained by many, particularly in Europe, and even as late as the 1950s there were still arguments over terminology, since it was illogical for many physiologists to refer to the parasympathetic system as part of the sympathetic nervous system, since 'para' means 'alongside'. At a Physiological Society Meeting in 1954, it was proposed that if the whole thing was to be the 'sympathetic' nervous system, then the two main divisions might be the 'parasympathetic' and 'orthosympathetic' systems (a light-hearted alternative put forward by Bernard Katz at that meeting was 'unsympathetic'!).

1.4 Chemical transmission

The development of the idea that chemicals were involved in the functioning of the autonomic nervous system depended very much on the considerable curiosity there was about the actions of plant alkaloids and various toxins. There was a great deal of folk knowledge of the medicinal and toxic properties of plants and fungi, and many explorers were bringing back interesting chemicals of plant and animal origin from all over the world that had marked effects on living tissues, such as arrow poisons. It was a relatively simple matter for the physiologists to apply extracts of such substances to the body and observe their effects.

Even with the availability of these techniques, how did scientists conclude that acetylcholine and noradrenaline were the main transmitters in the autonomic nervous system? It was certainly not possible to obtain enough of the chemicals from the nerve endings to identify them chemically. Most of the work consisted of comparing the effect of adding chemicals with that of stimulating nerves, and of looking at the way various chemicals modified the effects of nerve activation.

One fairly early source of biologically active material was the adrenal glands (glands as conspicuous and highly coloured as these were obvious targets for extraction). A difference between the cortex and the medulla was apparent, and it was soon shown that extracts of the adrenal medulla mimicked to a considerable extent the effects of sympathetic nerves on their target organs. The adrenal extracts were rich enough to allow the early identification of adrenaline as the active principle, and in 1904, after comparing the effect of nerve stimulation to that of application of adrenaline, Elliott proposed that it was released from the sympathetic nerves. Other important sources of biological materials were the poisonous fungi – such as fly agaric, *Amanita muscaria* (the red and white spotted toadstool). When applied to organs innervated by the parasympathetic nervous system, extracts of fly agaric were shown to mimic the effects of activating these nerves. The active principle was called muscarine, and after performing experiments in 1906, Dixon proposed that it was released from the nerves. At this stage in the story, neither suggestion was in fact correct. Further experimental results involved the discovery and use of substances that blocked the effects of nerves and applied extracts, and of substances that enhanced these effects.

Ergot of rye (*Claviceps purpurea*) was important here. Ergot is a fungus that grows on cereal crops, particularly in cool, damp climates. If rye was badly contaminated, ergot could get into flour and thus into rye bread, and was responsible for a disease called St Anthony's fire – prevalent at one time in the Low Countries. This caused burning feelings and ulceration of the legs (to cure this required a visit to St Anthony's shrine, fortuitously in an ergot-free region of France!). It was soon found that an extract of ergot could have powerful effects on the actions of sympathetic nerves and adrenaline. After an initial sympathomimetic effect (which probably accounts for the vasoconstriction responsible for the symptoms), the extract inhibited the excitatory actions of adrenaline and of sympathetic stimulation, but did not affect (and in fact would often reveal) the inhibitory effects. Extracts from the berries of deadly nightshade (*Atropa belladonna* – so called because when the juice was squeezed into the eye by fashionable ladies, the resultant dilated pupils were thought to add a beautiful dark, lustrous appearance to the eyes) turned out to block the effects of muscarine and of stimulating parasympathetic nerves. Another plant alkaloid was extracted from the Calabar bean (once used in ordeal by poison to establish guilt or innocence – death implying guilt). The extract from this was physostigmine, which markedly potentiated the effects of stimulating parasympathetic nerves.

Although many autonomic physiologists were beginning to suspect that the nerves were releasing chemicals, the first demonstration that autonomic nerves actually did release chemicals that could reproduce the effects of nerve stimulation was in 1921, in the frog heart. This was the famous experiment by Otto Loewi. He stimulated the vagus nerve to a beating frog's heart while perfusing the organ, demonstrating the classical slowing effect on the heart rate; he then showed that the perfusate itself could slow another heart that was not stimulated. There is a story that the idea of this experiment came to him in a dream. He was in the habit of writing notes on his dreams on paper he kept for the purpose by his bed. On this occasion he woke in the middle of the night, realised the importance of the dream and wrote notes, only to find that he couldn't read or remember them next morning. Luckily he dreamt the dream again the next night, and as he slept next door to his laboratory, he decided to get up and do the experiment there and then.

It was subsequently found difficult for others to repeat his experiment. The sympathetic nerves that accelerate the heartbeat run with the vagus nerve into the frog heart, and Loewi had to stimulate the mixed nerve. It turns out that the activity of the sympathetic system in the frog has a marked seasonal variation in potency, and was probably in a phase of low activity when the experiment was initially performed. Loewi may also have been lucky to have a type of frog with enzymes that did not rapidly break down the active substance released from the vagus (which he called *Vagusstoff*). Later he showed that the effect of the perfusate, but not its release, was blocked by atropine and potentiated by a cholinesterase inhibitor, and that the active principle was destroyed on contact with ground-up heart tissue. He also repeated the experiments with atropine added to the perfusate, and showed that the nerves could produce an excitatory substance (*Acceleransstoff*), which turned out to be adrenaline (this is actually the transmitter in the frog, not noradrenaline).

Although Dixon had proposed that muscarine was the parasympathetic transmitter, one argument against muscarine was that it had not been shown to be present in animals. The man most responsible for establishing the identity of the actual transmitter (acetylcholine) was Sir Henry Dale (Box 1.4), for which he shared the 1936 Nobel Prize for Physiology and Medicine with Otto Loewi. In 1914, Dale was working with an extract of ergot that had the unexpected effect of causing a profound drop in blood pressure, like muscarine. Unlike muscarine, the contaminant proved to be very unstable. Dale remembered earlier work of Hunt and Taveau, who had synthesised the acetic ester of choline (in fact acetylcholine), and had shown it to be extremely powerful in causing a drop in blood pressure. He asked his colleague Ewins to synthesise acetylcholine, and by a careful comparison with the ergot extract, provided clear evidence that acetylcholine was the contaminant present (it was later discovered that this was due to bacterial degradation of the ergot). This led to the thought that acetylcholine might be the compound secreted. Its presence in animals was also established by Dale, but only in 1929, when Dale and Dudley demonstrated it in the spleen of horses and oxen.

Careful studies on the distribution of the autonomic nerves containing acetylcholine or an adrenaline-like substance had shown that they did not precisely correspond to the anatomically defined parasympathetic and sympathetic divisions, and in 1933 Dale suggested that the autonomic nerves should be called cholinergic and adrenergic, on the grounds that they acted by secreting acetylcholine-like and adrenaline-like chemicals. The evanescence of acetylcholine, particularly in the blood or when exposed to minced tissue, suggested the presence of an esterase enzyme (enzymes of various sorts had been discovered and studied by biochemists since fairly early on in the 19th century). The ability of the enzyme in tissues to break down acetylcholine was soon shown to be inhibited by physostigmine, and after that several cross-perfusion experiments were carried out in the presence of physostigmine, and bioassays (Box 1.5) indicated the presence of acetylcholine.

The establishment of noradrenaline as the normal transmitter from the adrenergic nerve endings was longer in coming. One reason for this was that, like acetylcholine, noradrenaline was initially only known as a

Box 1.4 Sir Henry Hallett Dale (1875–1968)

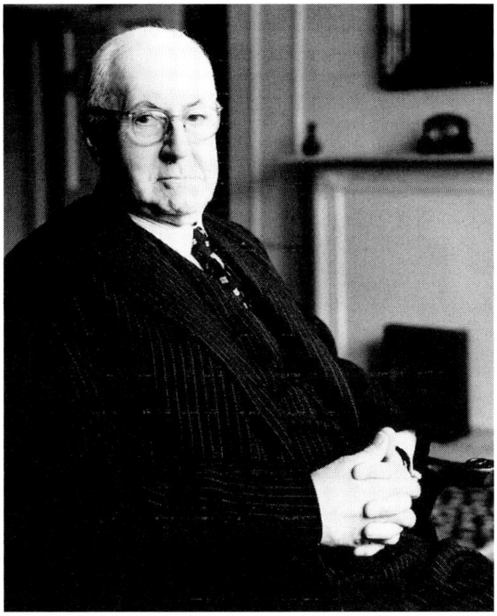

Dale was born in London, and studied natural sciences at Trinity College, Cambridge. He spent a brief period of research with John Langley, and then qualified in medicine at St Bartholomew's Hospital Medical School in 1902. He then returned to research, working initially with Bayliss and Starling at University College, London, and went on to become Staff Pharmacologist at the Wellcome Physiological Research Laboratories. In 1914, he became head of the Department of Biochemistry at the newly created National Institute of Medical Research, and was appointed its first director in 1928. His work focused on the physiology and pharmacology of naturally occurring chemicals. He played an important part in establishing the role of acetylcholine as a transmitter, and shared the 1936 Nobel Prize for Physiology and Medicine with Otto Loewi.

synthetic compound, and had not been shown to occur in the body. Also, the commercially available preparations of adrenaline that were often used in bioassays were later all shown to be contaminated with noradrenaline. Nevertheless, many keen observers were not satisfied that adrenaline could exactly mimic the activity of the adrenergic neurones, and for this reason the adrenergic transmitter was commonly called 'sympathin'. This term was introduced by the American physiologist, Cannon, from whose laboratory at Harvard much of the work leading to the identification of

Box 1.5 Bioassay

Demonstration of the presence of suspected transmitters in perfusates was done by bioassay – this was, and often still is, the only way of checking whether a putative transmitter is actually being secreted, since the amount of transmitter released is usually far too small to allow chemical detection. In order to go beyond the detection of a putative transmitter or other naturally produced substance and identify what it is, Gaddum developed the important technique of parallel assay. In this, a sample of perfusate or a tissue extract is prepared and tested on a series of different assay tissues, which respond in different ways to the sample. The responses are carefully compared both qualitatively and quantitatively with the response of the same tissues to the suspected substance.

This has to be done with a sound statistical design, so that the natural variability of the response is taken into account. If the response of each of the assays to the perfusate matches the response to the same concentration of the known sample in each of the assays, i.e. if the relative potency of the sample to the known drug is the same for each assay, then it can be increasingly safely assumed that they are the same. In fact, it is really only necessary for the sample to have the same relative potency for four different assay tissues before an extremely high probability is reached that they are the same. Other obvious tests are equal susceptibility to blocking and potentiating drugs, and identical ability to be denatured by various chemical or physical procedures.

noradrenaline as the transmitter originated. In 1933, Bacq was able to obtain sympathin from the aqueous humour of the eye, where it appears after stimulation of the adrenergic cervical sympathetic nerve. Chemical and spectrographic tests led him to believe it was a catechol derivative with an aminated side chain, and in 1934 he suggested that sympathin might be noradrenaline, but it had to wait until 1946 for von Euler to demonstrate unequivocally that this was, in fact, the case.

An additional complexity in the adrenergic division of the autonomic nervous system was the fact that its stimulation could produce excitation or inhibition of a tissue. Applications of adrenaline could likewise have two actions, although not always in the same proportions as adrenergic nerve stimulation. An early explanation for the dual effects of adrenergic nerve stimulation was proposed by Cannon, who suggested that there might be two receptive substances in the target organ that could combine with the released transmitter and produce new compounds (sympathin E and sympathin I) which were responsible for the excitatory and inhibitory effects respectively. An explanation for the different proportions of excitation and inhibition that adrenaline and sympathetic nerve stimulation could induce in a tissue required the demonstration that sympathin and adrenaline were in fact different substances. This knowledge allowed Ahlquist, an American pharmacologist, to study the relative sensitivity of tissues to noradrenaline and adrenaline, and led him in 1948 to the proposal (then controversial) that there were two populations of receptors with differential sensitivities to the two principal catecholamines. The response of the tissue to activation of a receptor was specific to the tissue and could be excitatory or inhibitory. This made sense of many of the earlier results, although it took some time to be accepted. Leading on from this was the synthesis and development of synthetic chemicals, both activating and blocking specific receptors. Worth mentioning here is the work of Sir James Black, who developed drugs specifically blocking Ahlquist's β-receptors – an advance of considerable clinical significance – and later developed specific blockers of a class of histamine receptors. He was recently awarded the Nobel Prize for this work.

1.5 Further advances

After the main divisions and transmitters in the autonomic nervous system had been established, advances in our knowledge blossomed in many areas, due to the work of physiologists and pharmacologists far more numerous than would be appropriate to mention in this book. Two areas of advance are, however, particularly relevant.

The invention of microelectrodes, and the increasing interest in electrophysiology, switched the emphasis away from the autonomic nervous system in the middle of this century, since the nerves and the tissues they innervated were small and not easily studied by electrophysiological techniques. However, when considering increases in our understanding of the mechanisms involved in the action of autonomic nerves on target tissues, considerable advances stemmed from the work of Edith Bülbring and her colleagues in Oxford, beginning in the 1950s. She was instrumental in applying the new techniques, in particular to smooth muscles. Through her influence, considerable progress was made in understanding the behaviour of smooth muscles and the effects of autonomic nerves on them.

After the synthesis of specific blocking drugs for the receptors involved in adrenergic and cholinergic transmission, physiological and pharmacological studies of many organs led to the discovery of non-adrenergic, non-cholinergic nerves, and in this field Geoffrey Burnstock and his colleagues have made important advances, particularly with the concept of co-transmission and the identification of many other transmitters, the most controversial of which was the purine, ATP.

Further reading

Bolton, T.B. & Brading, A.F. (1992) Edith Bülbring. *Biographical Memoirs of the Royal Society* **38**, 69–95.

Campbell, G. (1970) Autonomic nervous supply to effector tissues. In: *Smooth Muscle* (eds E. Bülbring, A.F. Brading, A. Jones & T. Tomita), pp. 451–95. Edward Arnold, London.

Dale, H.H. (1953) *Adventures in Physiology.* Pergamon Press, Oxford.

Gershon, M.D. (1970) The identification of neurotransmitters to smooth muscle. In: *Smooth Muscle* (eds E. Bülbring, A.F. Brading, A. Jones & T. Tomita), pp. 496–524. Edward Arnold, London.

Paton, W.D.M. (1962) The growth of pharmacology with special reference to its dependence on the advance in chemical knowledge. *Ithaca* **26VIII–21X**, 895–7.

Tansey, E.M. (1991) Chemical neurotransmission in the autonomic nervous system: Sir Henry Dale and the discovery of acetylcholine. *Clinical Autonomic Research* **1**, 63–72.

Tansey, E.M. (1995) What's in a name: Henry Dale and adrenaline. *1906 Medical History* **39**, 459–76.

2 : The Anatomy of the Autonomic Nervous System

2.1 Introduction

The autonomic nervous system comprises all of the nervous pathways leaving the central nervous system (efferent nerves) that have a ganglionic synapse situated outside the central nervous system. *Ganglia* are simply groups of neuronal cell bodies; the nerves that synapse onto cells in a ganglion are called *preganglionic,* and those leaving it, and thus having their cell bodies in the ganglion, are called *postganglionic*. There are three distinct anatomical divisions: the *sympathetic*, the *parasympathetic*, and the *enteric* nervous systems. It is worth pointing out that, although there may be similarities within each division other than anatomical ones, the classification of a particular autonomic nerve is made on strictly anatomical grounds. As will be seen later, this leads to problems in classifying nerves when their presence has only been demonstrated experimentally in isolated organs, and their origins are unknown.

The sympathetic and parasympathetic nervous systems are normally described as being made up of preganglionic and postganglionic neurones, the preganglionic neurones having their cell bodies in the brain and spinal cord, and the postganglionic neurones being outside the central nervous system (Fig. 2.1). Thus the activity in these divisions is generated in the central nervous system. The enteric nervous system, on the other hand, is contained within the walls of the gut. It is thus entirely outside the central

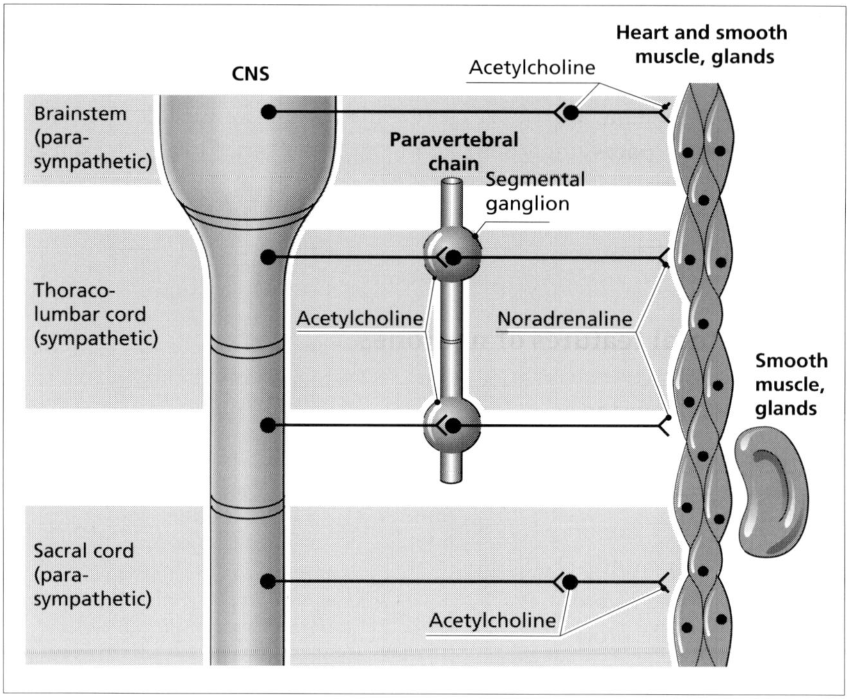

Fig. 2.1 A diagrammatic representation of the classically described arrangement of neurones in the parasympathetic and sympathetic nervous systems. Preganglionic neurones have their cell bodies in the brainstem and spinal cord, and they use acetylcholine as their transmitter. They synapse with postganglionic neurones outside the central nervous system. The preganglionic parasympathetic neurones are in the brainstem and sacral cord, and synapse with postganglionic neurones near the organs they innervate. The transmitter of these neurones is also acetylcholine. The preganglionic sympathetic neurones are in the thoracolumbar cord, and they synapse with postganglionic neurones that are usually more remote from their end organs, being located in paravertebral chains or prevertebral ganglia. These postganglionic neurones use noradrenaline as their transmitter.

nervous system, and can function in isolation from it, although it can be controlled by input from the sympathetic and parasympathetic nervous systems.

In practice, the systems are not always as clearly defined and anatomically distinct as would be convenient. For instance, the preganglionic neurones in the parasympathetic system that supply the gut synapse onto neurones in the gut wall, which are part of the enteric nervous system (see p. 36). They are therefore not just postganglionic parasympathetic neurones, but an important element of a much more complex system. Also, many of the postganglionic neurones involved in the sympathetic control of the gut synapse onto neurones in the enteric plexus. Similar complexities occur in the prevertebral plexuses (particularly the coeliac and hypogastric), where the sympathetic and parasympathetic systems converge.

In this chapter, we will first look at the structure of the neuronal components of the system, and then describe the features of the three divisions: the sympathetic, parasympathetic and enteric systems. Finally, the sensory (afferent) pathways taking information back to the central nervous system will be outlined, and the interactions between the autonomic and somatic systems will be discussed.

2.2 Structural features of neurones

2.2.1 Types of neurone

Neurones are often structurally identified by the number of processes emanating from the cell body; they may be *unipolar, bipolar,* or *multipolar.* Sensory neurones are often unipolar, and the motor and interneurones are often bipolar or multipolar. Bipolar and multipolar neurones give rise to two distinct types of processes, *dendrites* and *axons.* In the unipolar sensory neurones, a single process leaves the neurone and branches into two, one branch carrying incoming sensory information from the periphery, and the other transmitting the information towards the interneurones or motor neurones in the circuitry. These features are best illustrated by reference to Fig. 2.2.

2.2.2 Neuronal structure

The cell body

The cell body can be thought of as the 'factory' of the neurone, containing the nucleus and most of the machinery required to manufacture neuronal macromolecules and membranes – ribosomes, endoplasmic reticulum, Golgi apparatus, mitochondria (Fig. 2.3). The nucleus and cell body are essential to the growth and continued existence of nerve fibres, but not for the conduction of nerve impulses. Axons do not contain ribosomes and thus cannot synthesise proteins. When the axon is severed from the cell body it usually degenerates. However, nerve axons can conduct impulses for some time after being separated from their cell bodies, and this property has been used to advantage by physiologists in studying the properties of isolated nerve axons *in vitro.*

The dendrites

Dendrites are usually relatively short, elaborately branched processes that emerge from the cell body of the neurone, often from several sites. The dis-

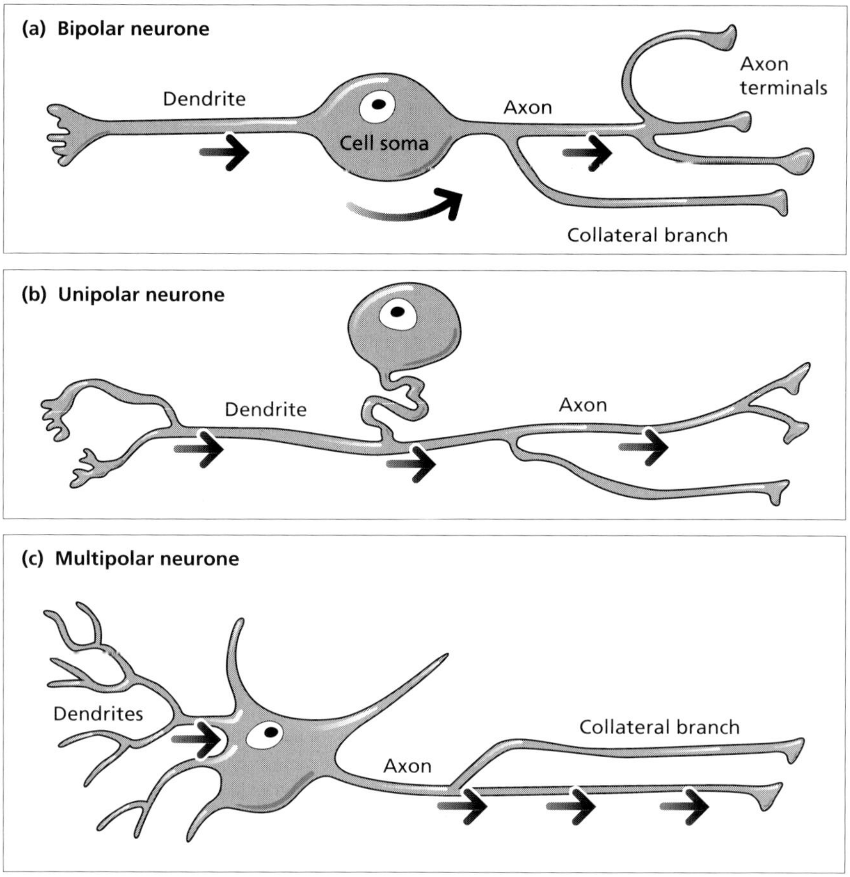

Fig. 2.2 Types of neurone. (a) Bipolar neurone. The soma has two processes arising from it. The single dendritic shaft may receive input from an extensive dendritic tree, and the single axon may give off collaterals and terminate in an extensive terminal arborisation. Interneurones and motor neurones are often of this type. (b) Unipolar neurone. A single process leaves the cell body and branches into two. Sensory neurones are of this type. The cell body does not receive synaptic input, and is often in a dorsal root ganglion. (c) Multipolar neurone. The soma gives rise to multiple dendritic processes and a single axon. Again interneurones and motor neurones may have this form.

tinction between an axon and a dendrite is made on both morphological and functional grounds, but the picture is far from clear due to the bewildering variety of processes that arise from different neurones. A simple definition is that a dendrite is a process that is not an axon, but there are many exceptions to this rule. Functionally, dendrites can be defined as those processes that conduct graded electrical signals, or occasionally action potentials, towards the cell body. Most neurones have a complex network of dendrites (*dendritic tree*) whose role, therefore, is to receive information from connections made with the axons of other nerve fibres. Dendrites receive and integrate a variety of incoming signals, and function as the 'receptive apparatus' of the neurone.

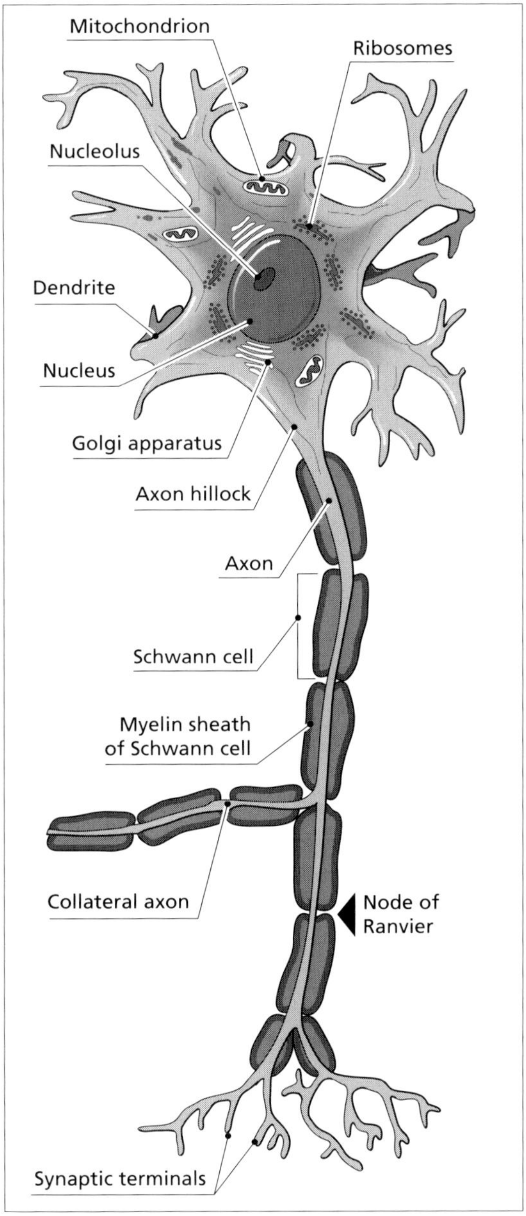

Fig. 2.3 Features of a neurone. This is a multipolar neurone, with many dendrites leaving the cell body. The cell body contains rough endoplasmic reticulum with ribosomes, Golgi apparatus and mitochondria.

The axon

Although dendrites may arise from many sites on each neuronal cell body (or soma), the axon arises from a single site, the *axon hillock.* The axon hillock leads into the *initial segment,* and it is in this region that converging electrical signals from the dendrites and cell body initiate nerve action potentials. The axon itself is specialised for the conduction of the action potentials from the cell body to the secretory nerve terminals. The axoplasm contains many of

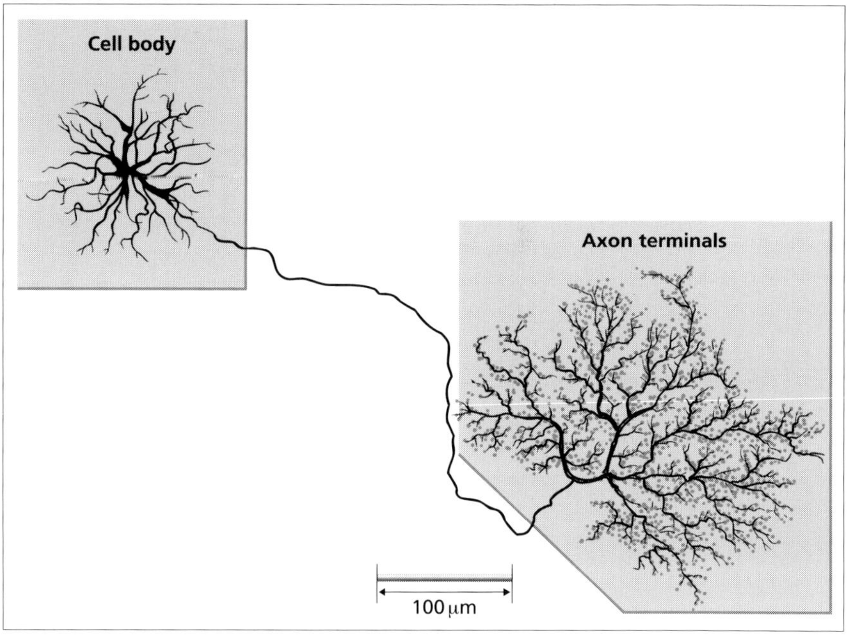

Fig. 2.4 A drawing of a single neurone stained by the Golgi method. This is a horizontal cell from a cat retina. Note the dendritic tree and the extensive axonal arborisation. From Dowling (1992).

the normal organelles, such as mitochondria and smooth endoplasmic reticulum, although it contains no ribosomes or rough endoplasmic reticulum. Also characteristic of axoplasm is the presence of neurofilaments and neurotubules, which are involved in transporting material from the nucleus to the terminals. Axons may have branches that carry action potentials to more than one destination. An axon may simply divide into two smaller branches of equal diameter, or give off a larger branch known as a *collateral.* The collateral may run for quite long distances, or collaterals may arise close to the cell body and have a generally lateral orientation. Collaterals that run backwards within the region are termed *recurrent collaterals.* Axons usually divide profusely at their ends, to form many-branched terminal arborisations (Fig. 2.4).

Secretory terminals (boutons or varicosities)

The axon terminals secrete the transmitters that link the presynaptic and postsynaptic systems. The shapes and sizes of the endings vary widely. In mammalian neuromuscular junctions, a single axon may contact multiple muscle fibres, ranging from tens to a few hundred, depending on the size of the axon. At each junction, several branches of the axon terminate, indenting the surface of a single muscle fibre, and thus provide a large contact area

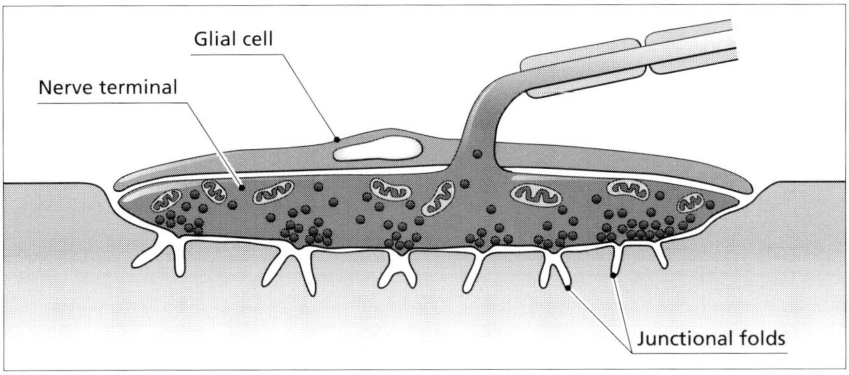

Fig. 2.5 A neuromuscular junction. The myelinated axon loses its myelin sheath and indents the surface of a striated muscle fibre, forming a large contact area. The terminal contains mitochondria and synaptic vesicles that cluster at release sites. The postjunctional membrane is specialised. Junctional folds occur at regular intervals under the release sites.

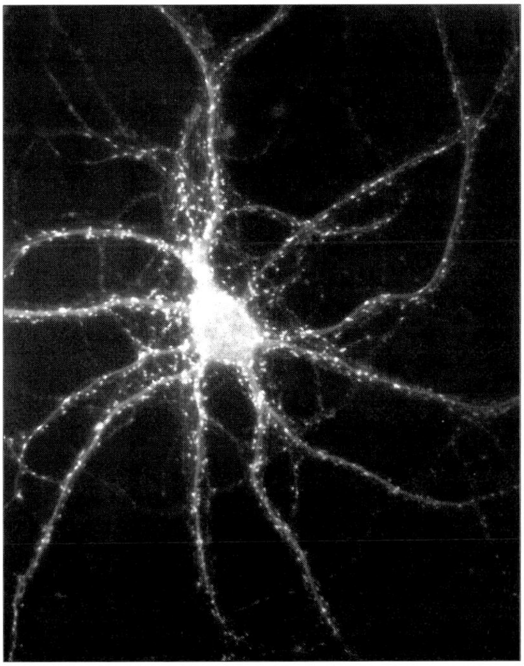

Fig. 2.6 The synaptic input to a neurone. The neurone is from the hippocampus, grown in primary culture, and is receiving synaptic input from other neurones. The synaptic boutons are stained with a fluorescent antibody against a specific presynaptic protein. Note the very large number of synapses, each of which provides only a small contribution to the synaptic input. Courtesy of Matteoli *et al.* (1993), Cover image, *Neuron* **10** (Suppl.).

and powerful effect (Fig. 2.5). In contrast, in some nerve-to-nerve synapses (particularly in the central nervous system), a single axon may innervate many hundreds of postsynaptic neurones, with only one or a few contacts on each. Each terminal ends in a synaptic bouton, which provides a very small area of contact and thus a weak input, so that co-operative action of many synapses is required to influence the postsynaptic neurone (Fig. 2.6). Terminals of a single presynaptic neurone in the autonomic nervous system

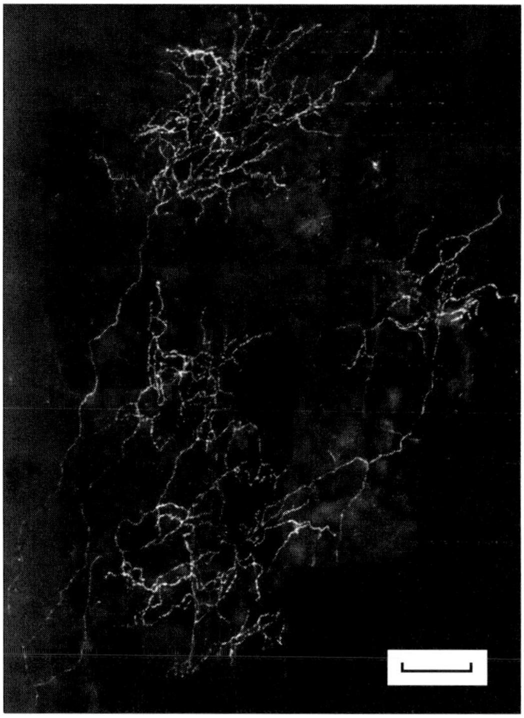

Fig. 2.7 The termination of a single postganglionic sympathetic nerve fibre in a smooth muscle. One axon (lower left-hand corner) branches twice to give rise to several systems of varicose nerve terminals. The preparation has been stained by the Falck–Hillarp technique for localisation of catecholamines. Calibration bar 100 μm. From Olson & Malmfors (1970).

again may innervate many peripheral ganglion cells, although the number of terminals that a postganglionic neurone receives will vary. In prevertebral ganglia, activation of the postganglionic neurone may be achieved through activation of only a few preganglionic axons. Terminals of the postganglionic neurones in the autonomic system branch extensively through the tissues they innervate (smooth and cardiac muscle, glands) and the branches have a beaded or varicose appearance (Fig. 2.7), each varicosity being a site for the release of transmitter, possibly equivalent to a single synaptic bouton.

2.2.3 Nerve fibres

The axon and its outer layers together constitute a nerve fibre, and groups of nerve fibres bound together by connective tissue constitute the nerves. Each axon is enveloped in a sheath derived from the non-neural Schwann cells. Each Schwann cell runs for 0.2–1 mm or more along the axon. A single Schwann cell may surround many small axons (diameter 0.1–1 μm), in which case the axons will be unmyelinated, or a series of cells can form a more complicated relationship with a single axon (diameter greater than 1 μm), and develop into a myelin sheath (Fig. 2.8).

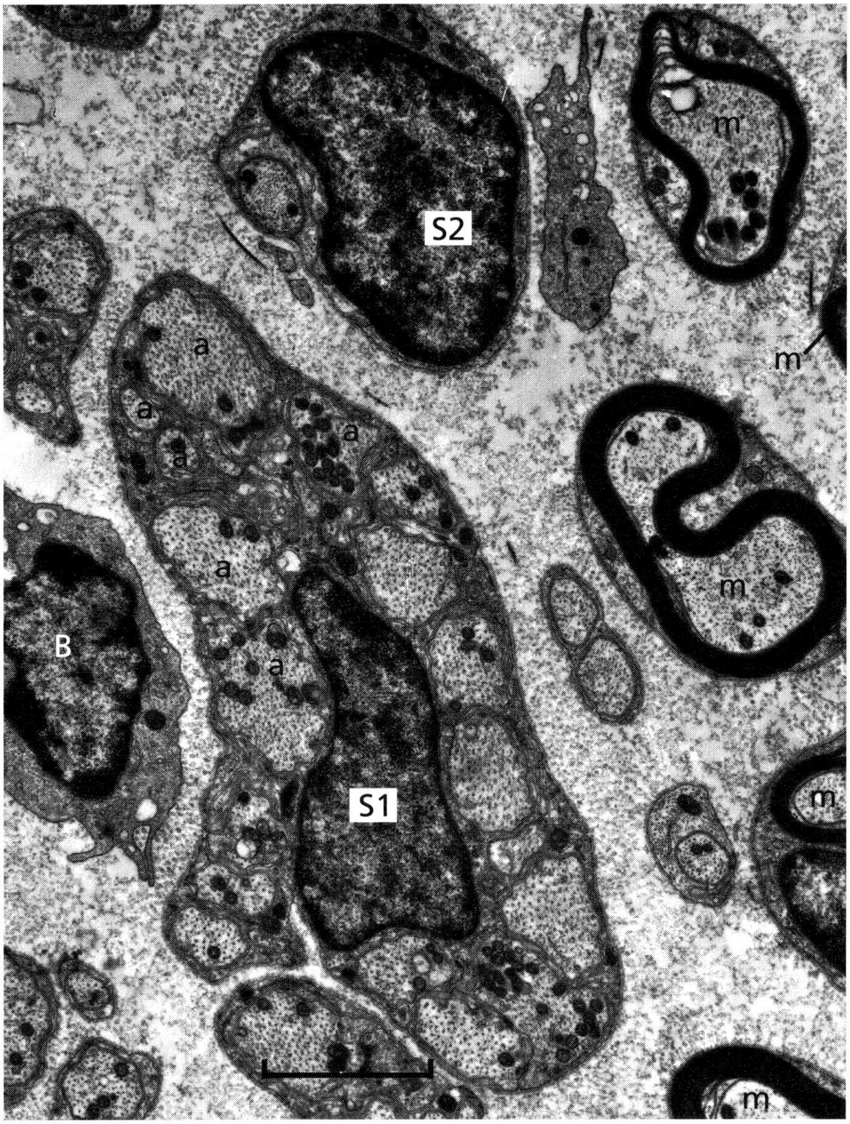

Fig. 2.8 In this electron micrograph of a sympathetic ganglion, some nerve bundles appear in transverse section. To the right, parts of five myelinated axons are visible (m). The myelin sheaths, being intensely osmiophilic, appear as dark bands at this magnification, each surrounding an axon or irregular shape. A large Schwann cell (S1), with its nucleus in the middle, is associated with about twenty unmyelinated axons (some labelled (a)). Another Schwann cell (S2), also nucleated, is associated with a single unmyelinated axon. Other unmyelinated axons, either single or in small bundles, are seen elsewhere in this microscopic field. To the left is a blood-borne extravasated cell (B). Scale bar: 2 μm. Micrograph kindly supplied by G. Gabella.

Box 2.1 Myelination

During myelination, the axon indents its surrounding Schwann cells early in development, and comes to lie in an elongated furrow. The walls of the furrow come into apposition, and the sheath cells rotate around the axon, laying down concentric double layers of plasma membrane (Fig. B2.1.1). The outcome is a myelinated nerve fibre, which may have the major part of its diameter composed of myelin. The number of layers depends on the diameter of the axon, axons of 5 μm having about 20 layers and those of 10 μm about 50 layers. The largest axons (20–30 μm) may have several hundred layers. The myelin sheath is interrupted at regular intervals at a junction between the Schwann cells by a node – the node of Ranvier. The nodes occur at intervals determined by the

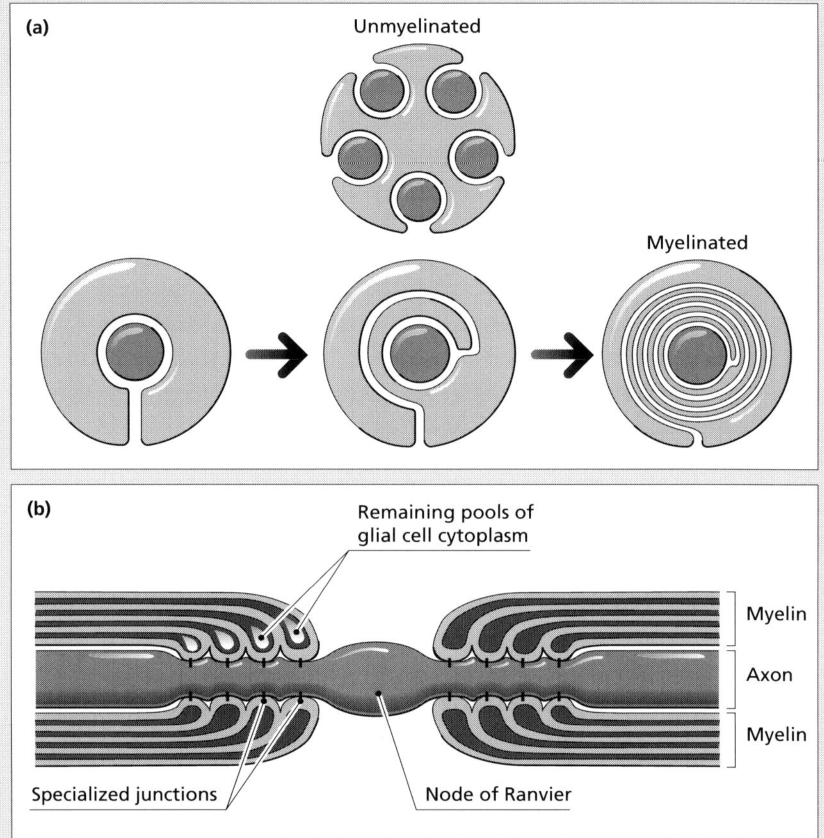

Fig. B2.1.1 Schwann cells and nerves. (a) A single Schwann cell is shown surrounding five unmyelinated axons above, and below is a diagram of a Schwann cell generating a myelin sheath around a single axon. (b) Diagram of a longitudinal section of a node of Ranvier.

Continued

Box 2.1 *Continued*

diameter of the axon, about every 1 mm in large human motor neurones. These nodes were discovered by and named after the French neuroanatomist Louis Ranvier, working in Paris in the 19th century.

Box 2.2 Classification of nerve fibres

When a nerve is stimulated at one end, the action potentials arriving some distance away can be recorded by a pair of extracellular electrodes. The velocity of the action potentials in individual nerve fibres varies with the size and degree of myelination of the axons, and thus action potentials do not all arrive at the recording electrode simultaneously. However, after a single supramaximal stimulus to a nerve, the action potential volley arrives as a series of discrete peaks, suggesting that the axons can be grouped into classes (Fig. B2.2.1). Thus, the fibres in mammalian nerves have been classified into three groups, termed A, B and C (Table B2.2.1). Group A has been shown to consist of the large-diameter, rapidly conducting myelinated fibres of the somatic system. Group B contains the smaller myelinated fibres of the preganglionic autonomic system, and Group C contains small unmyelinated fibres, including the postganglionic autonomic axons and many slowly

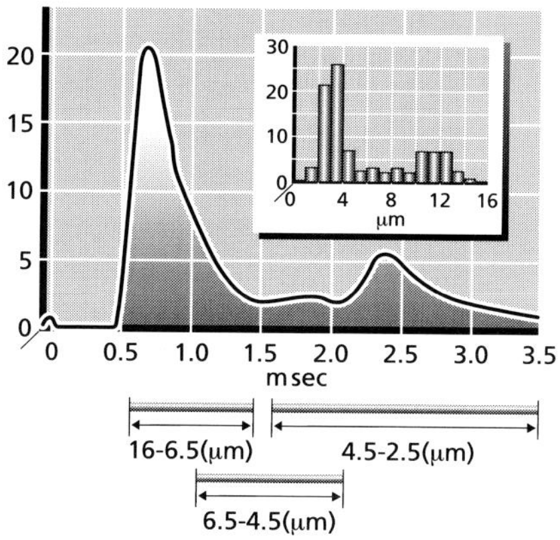

Fig. B2.2.1 A compound action potential recorded with extracellular electrodes from a human nerve after stimulation some distance from the recording site. The first peak arrives within 1 ms, and is the sum of the currents flowing in the large-diameter, rapidly conducting fibres. A small second peak is seen between 1.5 and 2 ms, and a third peak at about 2.4 ms. The ordinate is in arbitrary units. Under the time scale the ranges of the fibre diameter giving rise to each peak are shown. The inset shows a histogram of the diameters of the nerve fibres in this nerve.

Continued on p. 26

Box 2.2 *Continued*

conducting sensory fibres. Group A fibres have been subdivided into four separate classes, termed α, β, γ and δ, in order of decreasing conduction velocity. Sensory nerves were later reclassified according to a different convention as group I, group II and group III. Group I corresponds to Aα, group II corresponds to Aβ and group III corresponds to C.

Table B2.2.1 Nerve fibre types in mammalian nerves.

Fibre type*	Function	Fibre diameter (μm)	Conduction velocity (m/s)
A			
α	Proprioception; somatic motor	12–20	70–120
β	Touch, pressure	5–12	30–70
γ	Motor to muscle spindle	3–6	15–30
δ	Pain, cold, touch	2–5	12–30
B	Preganglionic autonomic	<3	3–15
C			
Dorsal root	Pain, temperature, some mechanoreceptors	0.4–1.2	0.5–2.0
Autonomic	Postganglionic autonomic	0.3–1.3	0.7–2.3

* A and B fibres are myelinated, C fibres are unmyelinated.

2.3 The sympathetic nervous system

The sympathetic system is defined as that which consists of the autonomic outflow from the thoracolumbar cord, and which passes through the paravertebral chains to synapse with postganglionic neurones that are normally situated in the paravertebral or prevertebral ganglia (Fig. 2.9). Thus, the ganglionic synapse is often more remote from the organ innervated than is the case in the parasympathetic system.

Preganglionic axons have their cell bodies in the lateral columns of grey matter in the spinal cord between the first thoracic and second lumbar segments, and emerge through the ventral roots (T1–L2) with the axons of the somatic motor neurones. The preganglionic axons vary in size and myelination, but are predominantly myelinated. Most are B fibres (about 3 μm in diameter), although some may be as large as 15 μm in diameter. On leaving the spinal cord, the axons leave the spinal nerves in the white rami communicantes, which link with the sympathetic chains (Fig. 2.10).

2.3.1 Paravertebral ganglia

The sympathetic chains in humans are normally composed of 24 pairs of paravertebral ganglia and their connecting trunks. The chains extend

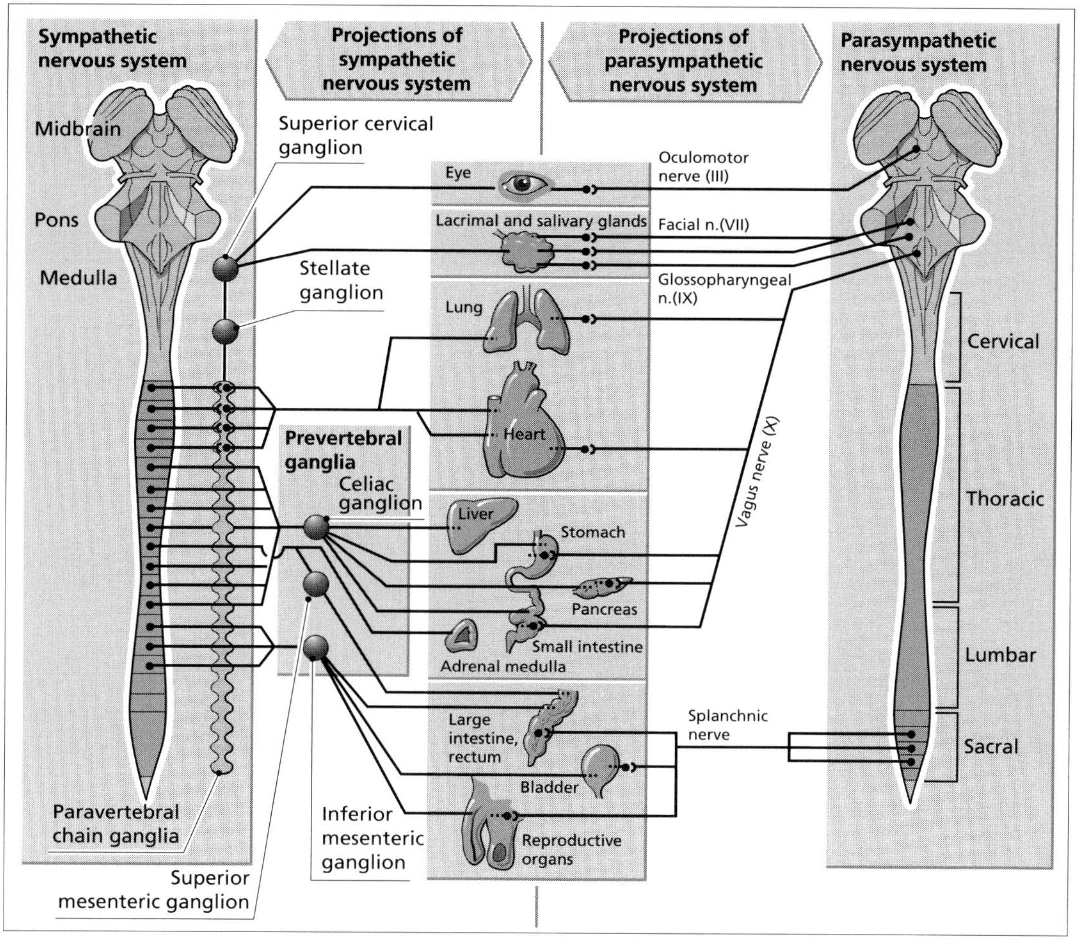

Fig. 2.9 The sympathetic (left) and parasympathetic (right) divisions of the autonomic nervous system. The preganglionic neurones in the sympathetic system are located in the spinal cord from the first thoracic segment to the second lumbar segment. They synapse with postganglionic neurones located either in the paravertebral chains on each side of the spinal cord, or in the unpaired prevertebral ganglia. The parasympathetic outflow is from the brainstem and the sacral spinal cord. The postganglionic neurones lie in ganglia closer to their target organs. From Kandel *et al.* (1991).

cranially in the cervical chain to the base of the skull, and caudally to the sacrum. In humans, there is normally one pair of ganglia for each segment in the thoracic and lumbar regions, but in the cervical region the ganglia are fused, and on each side there is normally a superior cervical ganglion (originating from the ganglia of C1–C4), a middle cervical ganglion (C5 and C6) and an inferior cervical ganglion (C7 and C8). The inferior cervical ganglion is often fused with the first thoracic ganglion (or with the first and second thoracic ganglia) to form the stellate ganglion. In the sacrum, there are four

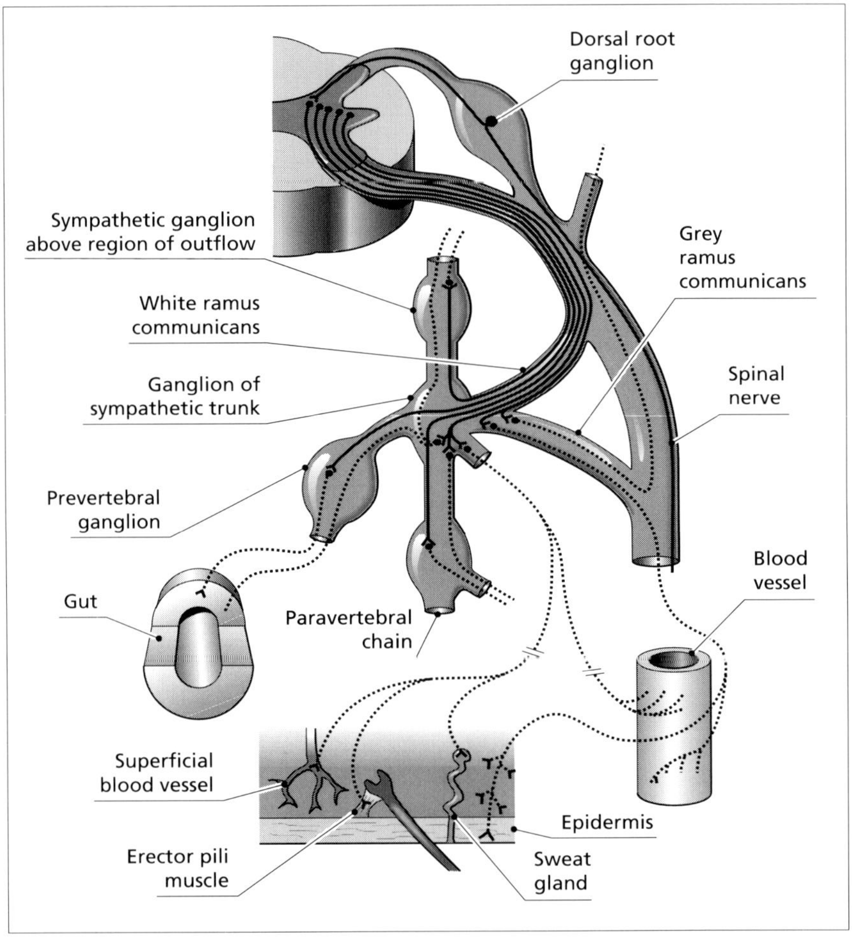

Fig. 2.10 Diagram of the sympathetic outflow from the spinal cord, and the distribution through ganglia of the sympathetic fibres to peripheral structures. The preganglionic axons (solid lines) leave the cord with the spinal nerves, and then enter the paravertebral chains through the white rami communicantes. Preganglionic and postganglionic (dotted lines) axons may run up and down the paravertebral chain before leaving it to run to prevertebral ganglia. Postganglionic axons may go directly from the paravertebral ganglia to end organs via visceral nerves, or rejoin the spinal nerves through the grey rami communicantes. Arteries also provide major routes for distribution of postganglionic axons. From Hamilton (1976).

pairs of ganglia, and the chains then usually unite in front of the coccyx and end in a small unpaired ganglion (the ganglion impar) (Fig. 2.11).

2.3.2 Prevertebral ganglia

These occur in the unpaired autonomic plexuses which lie in front of the vertebral column. The major plexuses are the cardiac and pulmonary

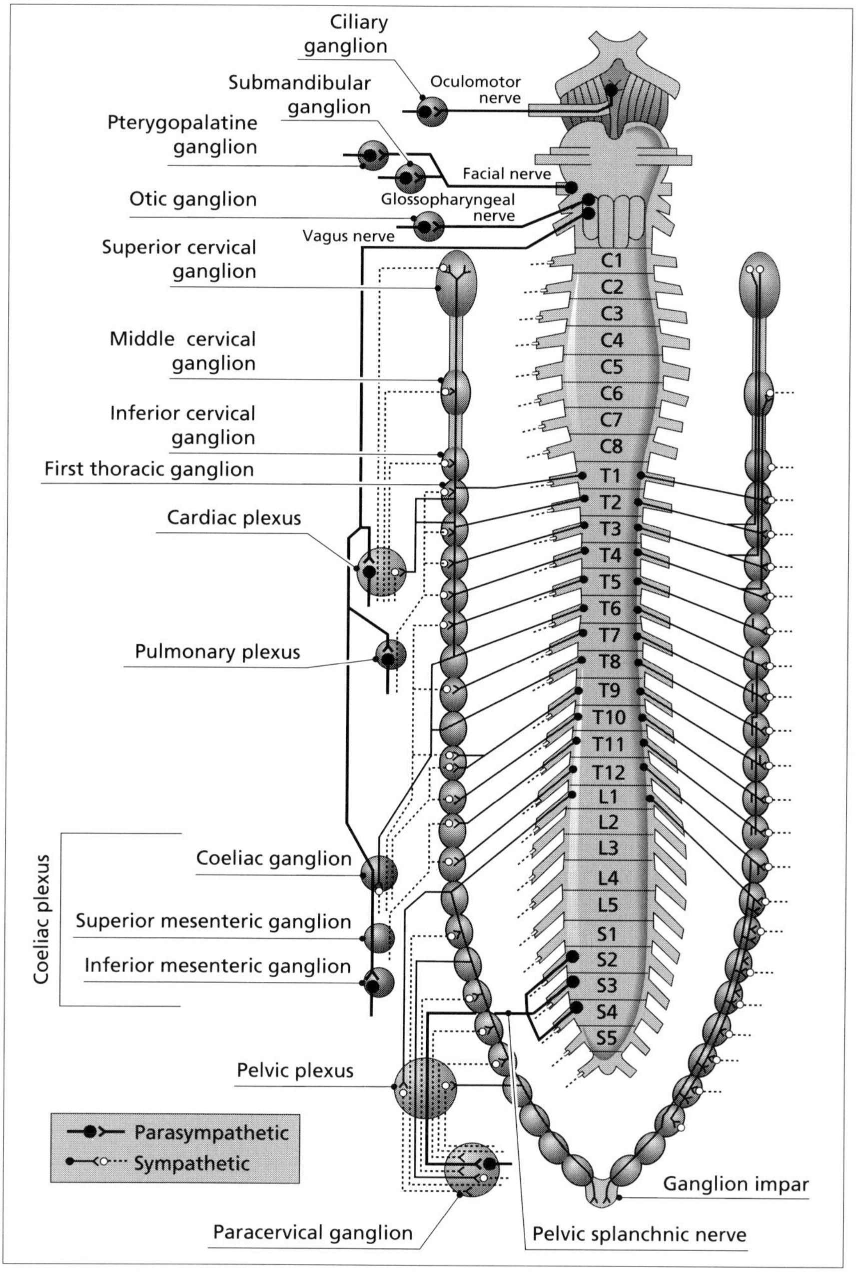

Fig. 2.11 The arrangement of the sympathetic and parasympathetic nervous systems in humans. From Hamilton (1976).

plexuses in the thorax; the coeliac plexus (containing the coeliac, superior mesenteric and inferior mesenteric ganglia) in the abdomen; and the pelvic plexus, containing the superior and inferior hypogastric plexuses (Figs 2.11 & 2.12). These plexuses are complicated structures, involved in both

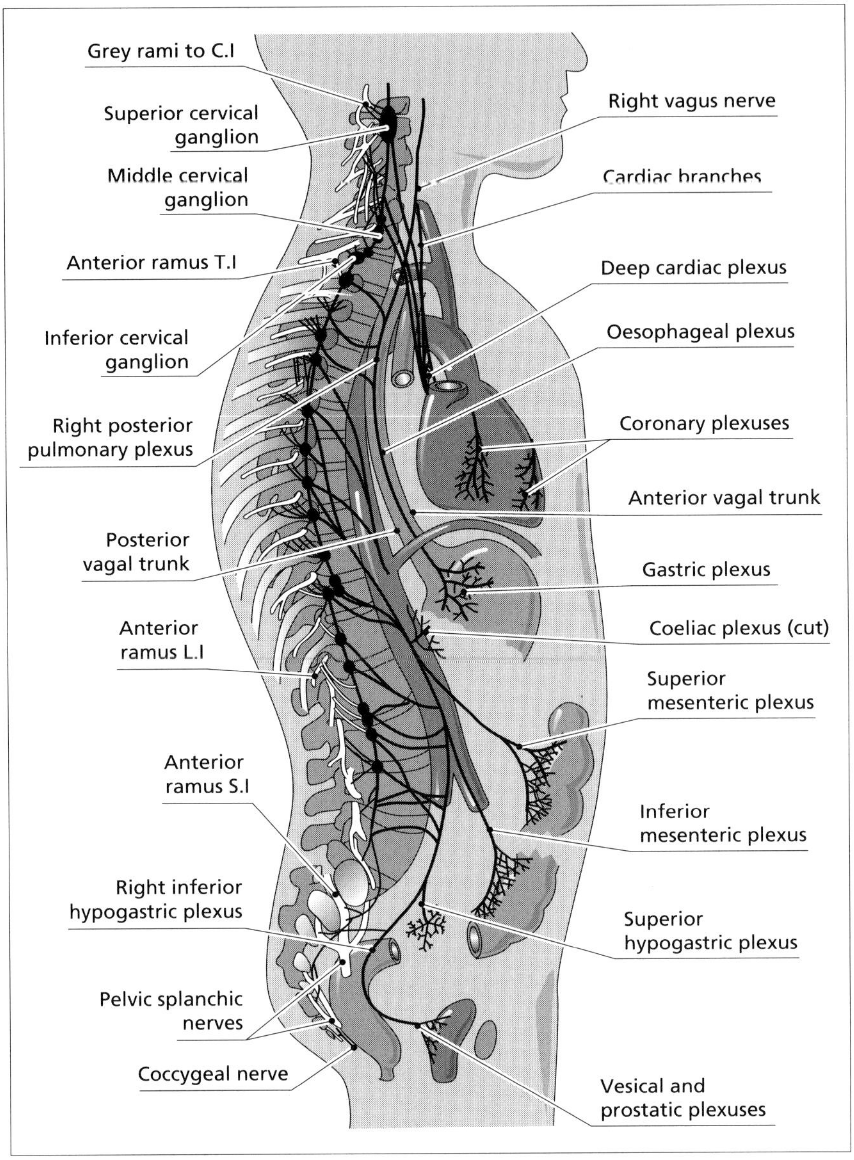

Fig. 2.12 The right sympathetic trunk and its connections with the thoracic and pelvic plexuses (From *Gray's Anatomy*).

parasympathetic and sympathetic pathways and receiving input from preganglionic and postganglionic fibres, as well as visceral afferents.

2.3.3 Distribution of preganglionic fibres

The pathways taken by the preganglionic sympathetic nerves and their connections may be complex (Fig. 2.10). There are many more ganglionic neurones than preganglionic neurones (up to 200 : 1 in some examples), suggesting extensive divergence of presynaptic input. The neurones may synapse in the paravertebral ganglion of their own segment, pass up or down the sympathetic chain and synapse with neurones in other ganglia, or pass through the chain without synapsing, to synapse with ganglia in the prevertebral plexuses. Some neurones have axons that divide and take all three routes.

2.3.4 Distribution of postganglionic fibres

These are small, unmyelinated C fibres. From the sympathetic chains there are four routes of distribution, firstly via the spinal nerves, secondly via the cranial nerves, thirdly via arteries, and fourthly via direct visceral nerves. The *spinal nerves* are entered from the paravertebral chains through the grey rami communicantes (Fig. 2.10). They distribute the fibres to their termination in blood vessels, sweat glands and erector pili muscles of the hair follicles. Fibres distributed with the *cranial nerves* come from the superior cervical ganglion, which contributes fibres directly to the glossopharyngeal, vagus, accessory and hypoglossal nerves, again to terminate in sweat glands, blood vessels and erector pili muscles, and also indirectly via arteries to the parasympathetic cervical ganglia, which they pass through without synapsing, and innervate the eye (ciliary ganglion), tear glands and nasal glands (pterygopalatine ganglion) and salivary glands (submandibular and otic ganglia). Fibres distributed via the *arteries* enter the arterial walls, which provide a major route of distribution of sympathetic fibres around the body. The *direct visceral nerves* arise from the sympathetic trunk, and contain both presynaptic and postsynaptic fibres and also scattered cell bodies of postganglionic neurones. From the cervical part of each trunk arises a laryngopharyngeal nerve and three cardiac nerves (one from each of the cervical ganglia), which connect the sympathetic chain with the cardiac plexus. From the thoracic part, three splanchnic nerves pass down through the diaphragm to the abdominal plexus. From the lumbar part, several lumbar splanchnic nerves arise, one from each lumbar ganglion, and pass down to the plexuses in the pelvis. From the sacral part, sacral splanchnic nerves also run to the pelvic plexus (Fig. 2.11). Postganglionic fibres from neurones in the prevertebral ganglia are distributed to their destination largely in the walls of the arteries supplying the various organs.

2.3.5 Adrenal medulla

The central cores of the adrenal glands, the adrenal medullae, contain chromaffin cells which are homologous with the sympathetic ganglion cells (see Fig. 2.20) and the medullae can be thought of as transformed sympathetic ganglia. Each medulla is innervated by preganglionic sympathetic fibres, which are distributed to it via the splanchnic nerves and pass to the gland through the periarterial nerves of the coeliac plexus.

2.4 The parasympathetic nervous system

The parasympathetic nervous system is defined as that which consists of autonomic pathways in the cranial and sacral nerves, which run to their destinations without passing through the paravertebral chains and have ganglion cells in, or close to, the organs they innervate (Fig. 2.11). The preganglionic fibres are thus often long, and the postganglionic fibres short. Preganglionic nerves may be small and myelinated (group B, about 3 μm in diameter) or unmyelinated. Postganglionic nerves are unmyelinated.

2.4.1 Cranial outflow

The cranial nerves that carry autonomic fibres are the oculomotor (III), the facial (VII), the glossopharyngeal (IX) and the vagus (X). The first three supply organs in the head, while the vagus supplies organs in the thorax and abdomen. The cell bodies of the preganglionic fibres lie in nuclei in the brainstem – the Edinger–Westphal, superior and inferior salivary and dorsal vagal nuclei. The ganglion cells of the first three cranial nerves lie in four pairs of ganglia, namely the ciliary, pterygopalatine, submandibular and otic ganglia (Fig. 2.11).

The *ciliary ganglia* are situated near the back of the orbit, with preganglionic fibres running to them from the Edinger–Westphal nucleus in the brainstem in the oculomotor nerves. The postganglionic fibres innervate the ciliary muscle and the sphincter pupillae muscle in the eyeball (Fig. 2.13). The *pterygopalatine ganglia* are in the pterygopalatine fossae, with preganglionic fibres from the superior salivary nucleus running to them in the facial nerve. Their postganglionic fibres innervate glands in the mucosa of the nose and palate, and the tear glands. The *submandibular ganglia* are on the surface of the hyoglossus muscles, and their preganglionic fibres also come from the superior salivary nucleus via the facial nerve. Postganglionic fibres leave them to innervate the submandibular and sublingual salivary glands. The *otic ganglia* are situated just below the foramen ovale, and their preganglionic fibres come from the inferior salivary nucleus via the glossopharyngeal nerve. The postganglionic fibres innervate the parotid salivary glands (Fig. 2.14).

The preganglionic parasympathetic neurones running in the vagus have their cell bodies in the dorsal vagal nuclei, which lie in the floor of the fourth ventricle lateral to the hypoglossal nuclei (Fig. 2.14). Fibres pass to the heart, lungs, liver and pancreas, as well as those parts of the gut that are supplied by the coeliac and superior mesenteric arteries (the oesophagus to the splenic flexure of the colon). They synapse with neurones on or near the organs they innervate, for the heart in the cardiac plexus, for the lungs in the pulmonary plexuses and ganglion cells alongside the bronchi, and for the gut in the intrinsic nerve plexuses of the gut wall.

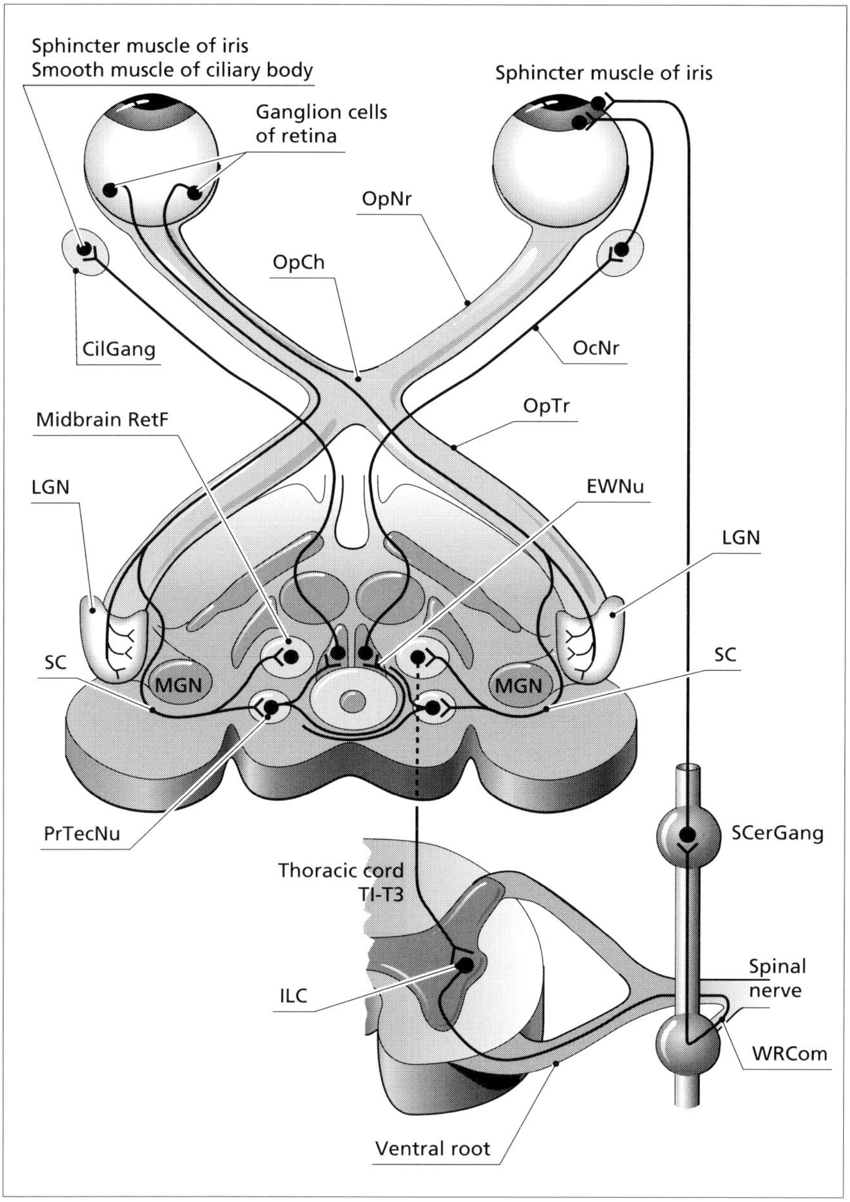

Fig. 2.13 Arrangement of the midbrain nuclei and the autonomic innervation of the eye. Information from the retina passes up the optic nerves (OpNr) through the optic chiasm (OpCh) via the superior colliculus (SC) to the pretectal nucleus (PrTecNu) and midbrain reticular formation (Midbrain RetF). From the pretectal nucleus, the preganglionic parasympathetic neurones in the Edinger–Westphal nucleus (EWNu) are activated, which travel in the oculomotor nerves (OcNr) to synapse on postganglionic neurones in the ciliary ganglia (CilGang) that innervate the constrictor smooth muscles of the iris and the ciliary body that controls the lens. From the midbrain, reticular formation neurones project to the preganglionic sympathetic neurones in the intermediolateral columns (ILC) of the spinal cord. These leave the spinal nerves through the white rami communicantes (WRCom), enter the paravertebral chains and pass to the superior cervical ganglion (SCerGang), where they synapse with the postganglionic neurones that innervate the dilator smooth muscles of the iris. LGN lateral geniculate nucleus, MGN median geniculate nucleus. From Haines (1985).

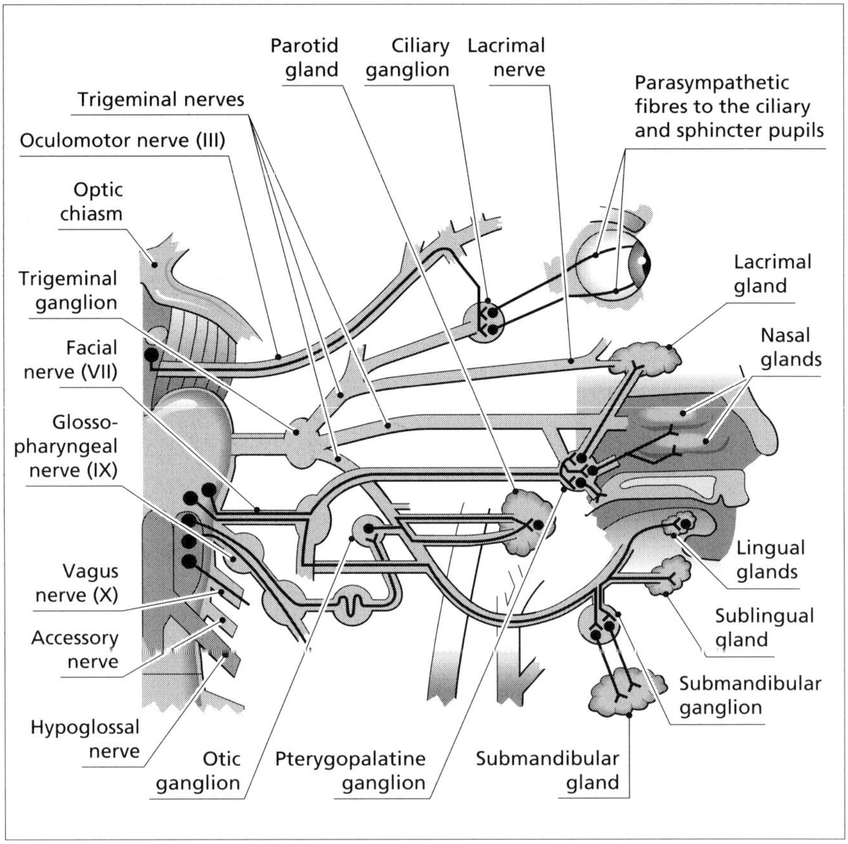

Fig. 2.14 Diagram to show the details of the parasympathetic innervation of the head and neck. From Hamilton (1976).

2.4.2 Sacral outflow

The sacral division of the parasympathetic nervous system arises from preganglionic neurones in the sacral cord, whose axons leave in the second, third and fourth sacral roots and form the pelvic splanchnic nerves. These nerves pass to the pelvic plexus, and may continue through to synapse with ganglion cells in the gut wall (from the splenic flexure of the colon to the anus) and in the wall of the bladder, as well as in the ganglia of the pelvic plexus. Postganglionic neurones innervate the lower gut, the urinary tract and the male and female genital tracts (Figs 2.9 & 2.11).

2.5 The enteric nervous system

In humans, there are between 10 and 100 million neurones in the enteric nervous system embedded in the wall of the gut, probably as many neurones as in the spinal cord. The nerve cells may be sensory, motor (and

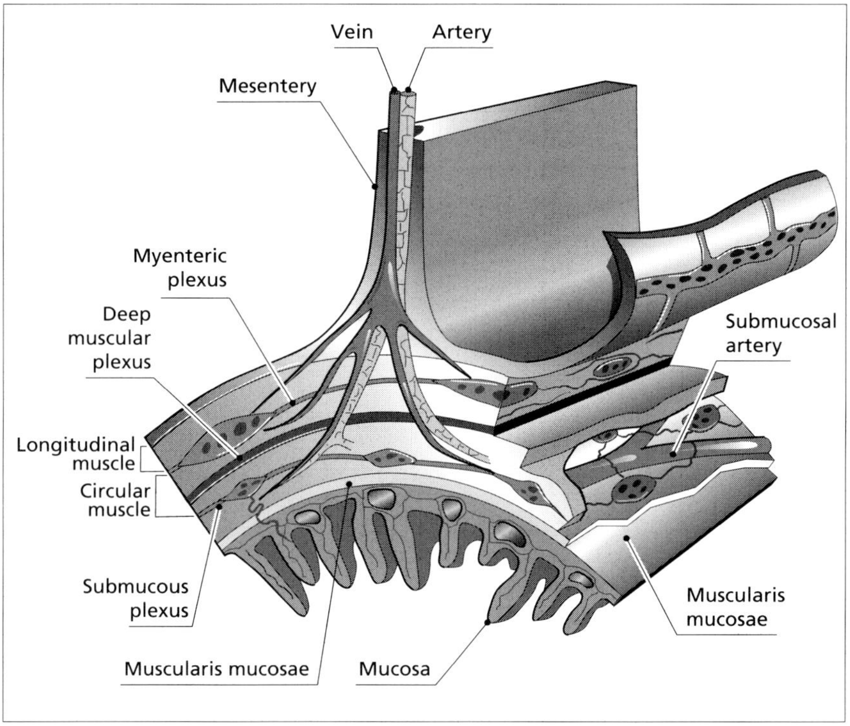

Fig. 2.15 Diagram to show the arrangement of the enteric nervous system in the gut wall. The cell bodies of the neurones lie in the myenteric or Auerbach's plexus and the submucous or Meissner's plexus. The myenteric plexus lies between the longitudinal and circular smooth muscle layers, and the submucous plexus lies between the circular smooth muscle and the muscularis mucosae. Nerve fibres run between the two plexuses, and there is a deep muscular plexus of fibres in the middle of the circular smooth muscle layer. A plexus of fibres also runs in the mucosa. From Furness & Costa (1987).

secretomotor) or interneurones. The sensory nerves may be restricted to the gut, or project to the prevertebral or paravertebral ganglia. The nerve cell bodies are clustered together in ganglia, and these are arranged predominantly in two major plexuses (Fig. 2.15) – the myenteric plexus (Auerbach's plexus) and the submucous plexus (Meissner's plexus). The ganglia within each plexus are interconnected with nerve bundles to form a meshwork, the pattern of which is characteristic of the various parts of the alimentary canal and varies from species to species. Interconnections also occur between the two plexuses. Non-ganglionated nerve fibres run in bundles throughout the thickness of the various muscle layers (longitudinal, circular and muscularis mucosae) and in the mucosa. In the small intestine, where the circular muscle is specialised into two layers, a thick outer layer and a thin inner layer, there is a dense network of nerve fibres between these layers called the deep muscular plexus (Fig. 2.15).

Although the enteric nervous system can function on its own, it can be regulated by the CNS through the parasympathetic and sympathetic

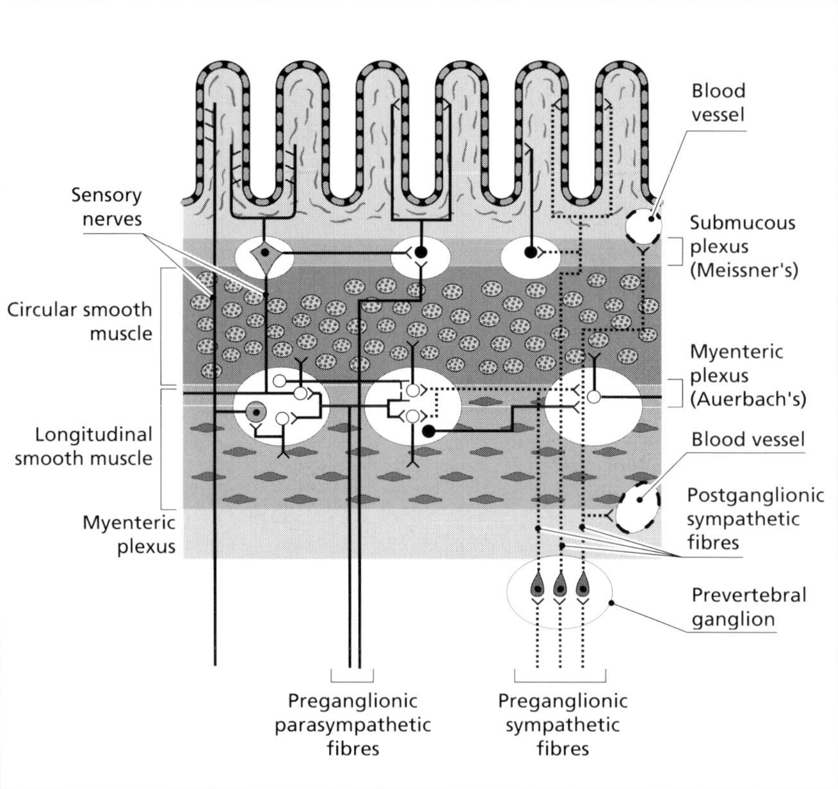

Fig. 2.16 Diagram showing the parasympathetic and sympathetic input to the enteric nervous system. Postganglionic sympathetic fibres innervate blood vessels and glands in the gut wall, and also provide a modulatory innervate to the motor neurones in the myenteric plexus. Preganglionic parasympathetic fibres synapse with ganglion cells in the two plexuses.

nervous systems. The sympathetic input is postganglionic, and is predominantly used for reducing activity in the gut when energy expenditure in the body is needed immediately, for example in 'flight and fight' situations. In contrast, the parasympathetic input to most of the gut wall is preganglionic, the neurones synapsing with the motor neurones in the enteric plexuses. Parasympathetic input enhances the activity of the gut during periods when the rest of the body is resting. The input is illustrated in Fig. 2.16.

2.5.1 The myenteric plexus (Auerbach's plexus)

This lies between the longitudinal and circular smooth muscle layers of the external muscle coat, and forms a continuous network throughout the length of the gut from the upper oesophagus to the internal anal sphincter (Figs 2.17 & 2.18). The ganglia are flattened in the plane of the plexus, and

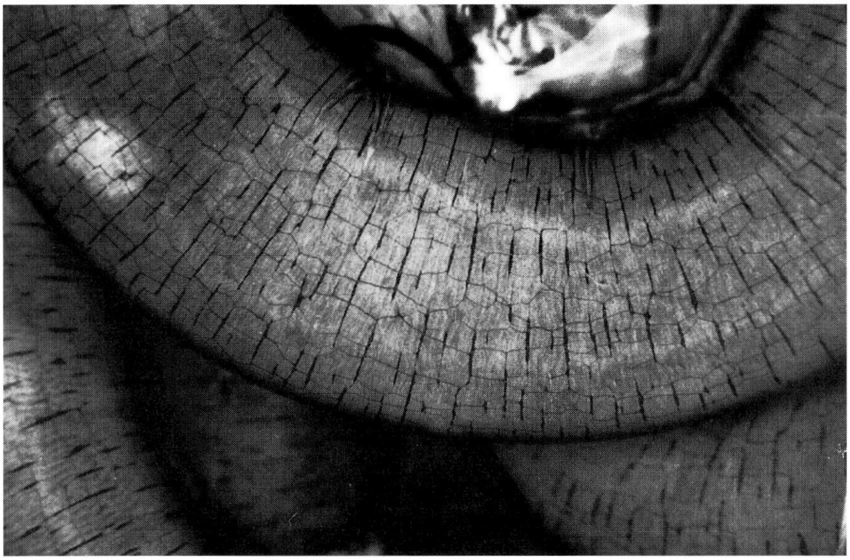

Fig. 2.17 A photograph of a preparation of guinea-pig ileum, with the serosa and longitudinal smooth muscle layers removed, stained to show the myenteric plexus. Kindly provided by G. Gabella.

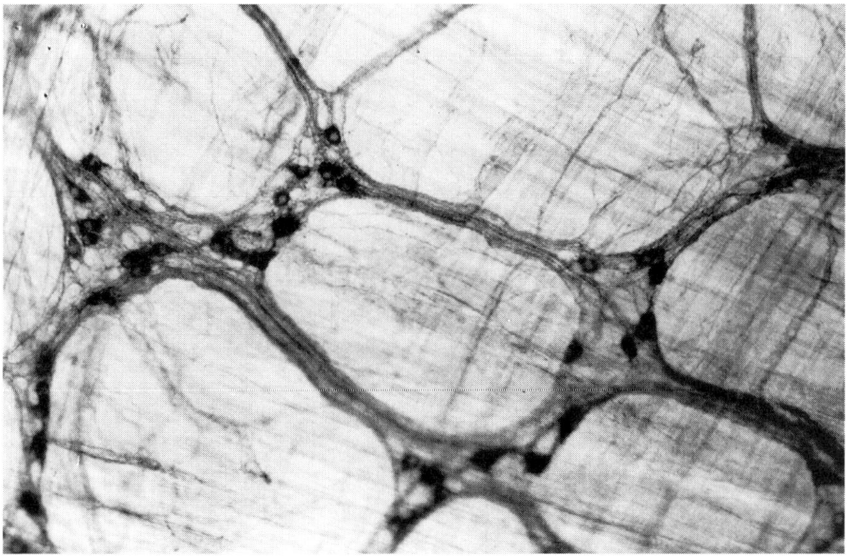

Fig. 2.18 Part of the myenteric plexus of the guinea-pig ileum at a higher magnification. A whole mount preparation has been made, and stained for the presence of nitric oxide synthase. This stains a subpopulation of the ganglion cells. Kindly provided by J. Stebbing.

vary in size, containing from a few to more than a hundred neurones. The primary component of the plexus consists of the ganglia and the internodal strands. There are other nerve strands joining with the primary plexus, which run circumferentially to constitute the secondary component of the plexus. Other branches from the primary and secondary components run straight through the circular muscle to connect with the submucous plexus when this is present.

2.5.2 The submucous plexus (Meissner's plexus)

This is found as a continuous network of small ganglia and internodal strands running throughout the small and large intestine. It is absent from the stomach. The submucous plexus may contain two layers of ganglia, one lying close to the circular muscle and the other nearer the mucosa.

2.6 Neuroanatomy of ganglia

The internal structure and connections of the individual ganglia in the autonomic nervous system vary according to the functional subdivision to which the ganglion belongs. Ganglia in the sympathetic pathway tend to be larger than in the parasympathetic system, and are often more discrete, since many of the parasympathetic ganglia are embedded in the walls of the organs they innervate. Nevertheless, these ganglia are similar in overall structure. They are surrounded by a continuous connective tissue capsule, the neurones are individually sheathed in satellite (glial) cells (Fig. 2.19), and the ganglia contain blood vessels and connective tissue elements. Enteric ganglia, on the other hand, do not have a connective tissue capsule, and the neurones do not have a complete satellite cell sheath, although the spaces between them are filled with glial cells. In addition, they do not contain blood vessels or connective tissue. The parasympathetic ganglia, and particularly the sympathetic ganglia, contain small intensely fluorescent cells (SIF cells), which may act as interneurones, or have a paracrine function (Fig. 2.20). Figure 2.20 compares the structures of neurones, SIF cells and the adrenal medullary enterochromaffin cells. In the enteric ganglia, neurones with distinct morphologies can be identified, and in the late 19th century these were classified by the anatomist A.S. Dogiel, who suggested that his 'Type-I' neurones were motor neurones, and his 'Type-II' neurones sensory. Other classes of neurones are being identified in all ganglia by the use of specific histochemical and immunohistochemical markers. It is becoming apparent that groups of neurones that can be identified by their common expression of certain markers also share the same function.

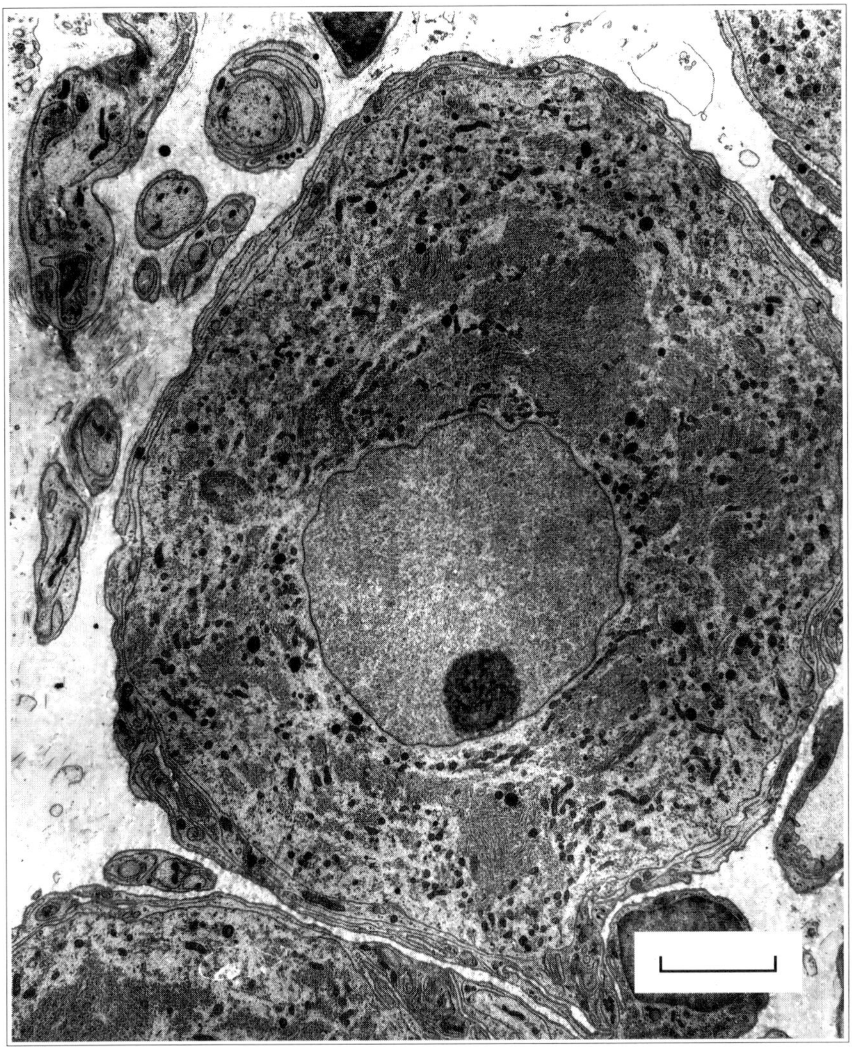

Fig. 2.19 Photomicrograph of a cell body of a sympathetic neurone in the superior cervical ganglion of a rat. The neurone is ensheathed by a layer of satellite cell processes, which separates it from the intraganglionic tissue space, and also contains a few small nerve profiles. The cell body and nucleus of a satellite cell are seen just below and to the right of the neurone, and there is a nearby capillary. Within the neurone note the large centrally placed nucleus and its nucleolus. Masses of granular endoplasmic reticulum lie in the cytoplasm, and numerous profiles of Golgi apparatus are also seen. The cytoplasm contains many mitochondria (seen as dark circular or elongated profiles) and a number of cytoplasmic dense bodies. Scale bar: 2 μm. Kindly provided by M. Matthews.

2.7 Visceral afferents

Although not strictly part of the autonomic nervous system, the axons of sensory neurones often run with the autonomic nerves. Their cell bodies are in the dorsal root ganglia, and they carry information from sense organs in

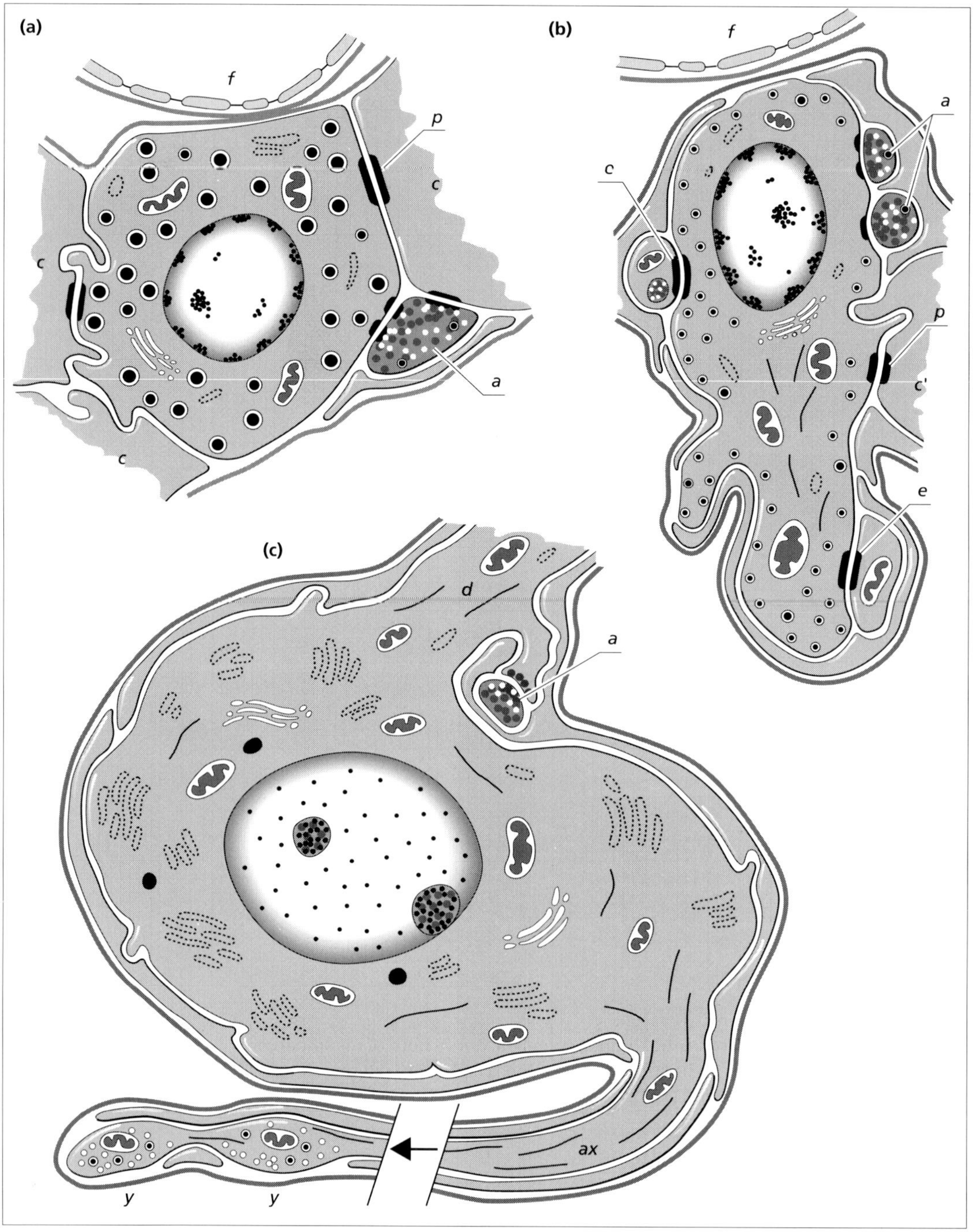

Fig. 2.20 A comparison of the structures of adrenal medullary enterochromaffin cells, SIF cells and sympathetic neurones. (A) Adrenal medullary chromaffin cell. Note afferent synapse (a), many dense cored vesicles and close connection to fenestrated capillary (f). Transmitter is released into the blood stream. Adjacent chromaffin cells (c) are held together through attachment plaques (p). (B) SIF cell (small granule containing cell).

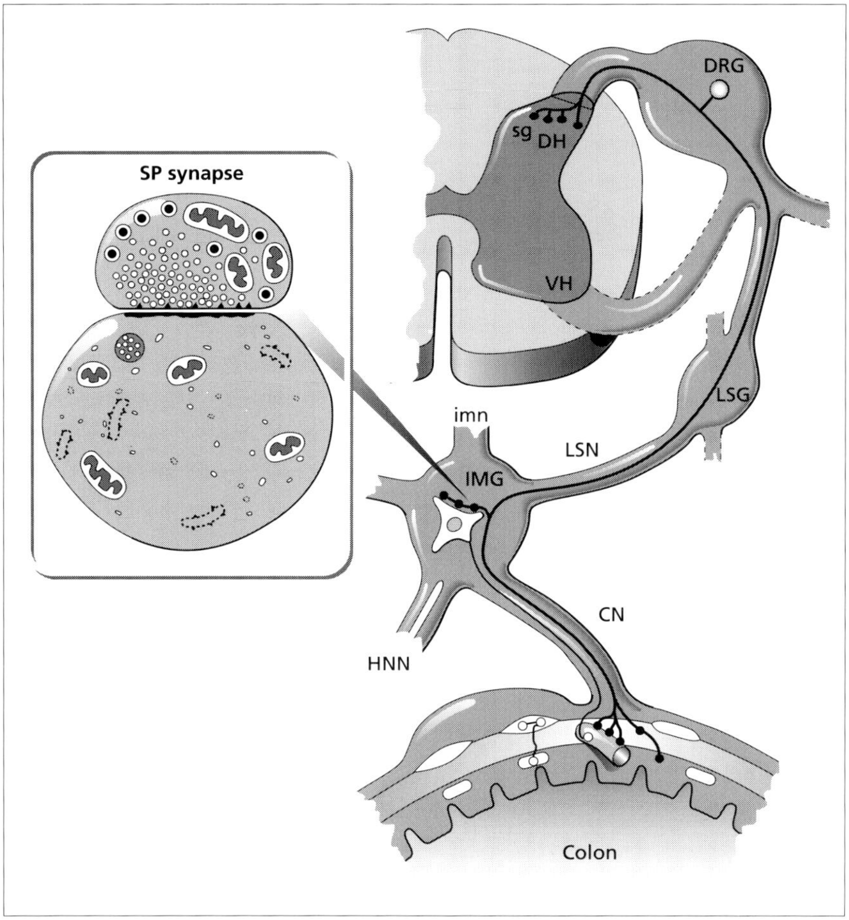

Fig. 2.21 Organisation of substance P (SP) containing visceral afferent from the colon. The afferent fibre is a bipolar neurone with its cell body in the dorsal root ganglion (DRG). The sensory nerve terminals are in the wall of the colon, and before leaving the gut wall, send collaterals to blood vessels. The axon leaves the gut and enters the inferior mesenteric ganglion (IMG) via a colonic nerve fascicle (CN). Again it gives off collaterals which innervate cells in the IMG. The main axon then runs in the lumbar splanchnic nerve (LSN) to the lumbar sympathetic ganglion (LSG) of the paravertebral chain and so to the dorsal root ganglion. The central branch enters the dorsal horn of the spinal cord (DH) and synapses with cells in the substantia gelatinosa (sg). (imn) intermesenteric nerve. (HNN) hypogastric nerves. (VH) ventral horn. Adapted from Matthews & Cuello (1982).

Fig. 2.20 *Continued*
This has properties intermediate between the other two types, and releases transmitter both to the blood stream and through efferent synapses (e) with local neurones. (C) Principal sympathetic neurone. This cell has afferent synapses on dendrites (d) and dendritic spines, and releases transmitter from varicose nerve endings (y). From Matthews & Raisman (1969).

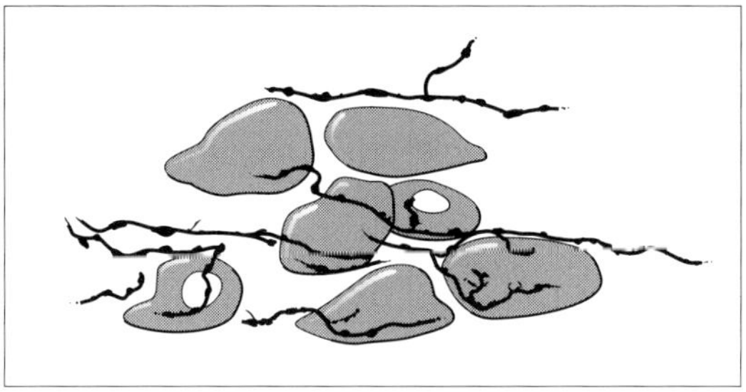

Fig. 2.22 Drawing of substance P containing varicose nerve terminals innervating ganglion cells in the inferior mesenteric ganglion of the rat. Adapted from Matthews & Cuello (1982).

the viscera and can trigger both somatic and visceral reflexes. The sensory fibres are normally small myelinated fibres (classed as Aδ fibres), or are unmyelinated (C fibres).

A subpopulation of the C fibres containing peptides, such as substance P and calcitonin gene-related peptide (CGRP), are now thought to have a dual sensory and motor function. Activation of these nerves results not only in propagation of action potentials to the central nervous system and nociceptive responses, but also action potential invasion of collaterals, which may release peptides that have a motor or secretory function in the viscera. Branches of these fibres may also have actions on neurones in the prevertebral and paravertebral ganglia (see Figs. 2.21 & 2.22). Capsaicin, the 'hot' component of peppers in the capsicum family, can interact with nerve terminals in this group, and activate them. The burning sensation that results from eating peppers is due to non-selective activation of these nociceptive fibres. At high doses the drug can kill the nerve cells, and if capsaicin is applied systemically (under anaesthesia) to neonatal rats, they grow up into adults that do not respond to painful stimuli. Capsaicin application has been used to study the role of these sensorimotor fibres in autonomic reflexes.

2.8 Concept of autonomic reflexes and interactions with the somatic system

Autonomic reflexes can be defined as reflexes in which the autonomic nervous system supplies the output or motor arm of the reflex. An obvious example is the reflex control of blood pressure. This involves baroreceptors in the arterial system responding to changes in blood pressure, sensory nerves running to the brainstem, an integrating centre in the medulla and the sympathetic and parasympathetic nerves adjusting the cardiac output and the peripheral resistance (Fig. 2.23; see also Section 8.1.6).

The baroreceptor reflex is an example of a reflex that operates without any perceptual input, and without any involvement of the somatic motor system. It could thus be regarded as an example of a purely autonomic reflex. However, the situation is not always as straightforward as this, and many autonomic reflexes involve the somatic motor system to a greater or

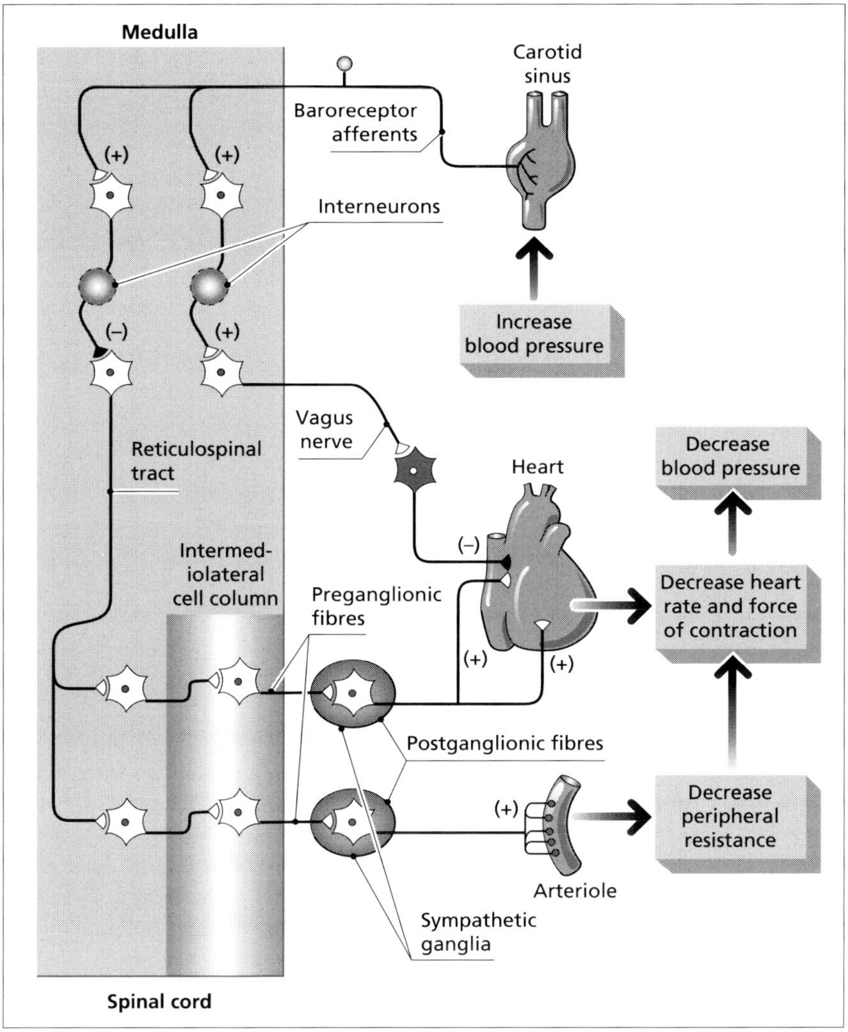

Fig. 2.23 Diagram to illustrate the reflex control of the blood pressure. An increase in peripheral blood pressure is perceived by the baroreceptors in the carotid and aortic arch sinuses. Afferent impulses ascend to the brainstem, and trigger reflex slowing of the heart through activation of the vagus. The afferent impulses also inhibit neurones in the medulla that normally provide excitatory drive to the sympathetic preganglionic neurones in the intermediolateral cell column of the spinal cord, resulting in a reduced sympathetic drive to the heart, and dilation of blood vessels. The overall effect is a reduction in blood pressure.

lesser extent. Often the sensory trigger for the reflex enters our conscious awareness and an element of voluntary control is involved. For example, in temperature regulation, cooling will trigger both autonomic adjustments of the vasculature through the sympathetic nervous system, and shivering, which is produced by contractions of the skeletal muscle and initiated through the somatic motor nerves. Perception of the skin temperature also occurs, and will lead to appropriate behavioural responses.

Another example is the micturition reflex responsible for emptying the urinary bladder. In this case, stimulation of sensory nerves in the bladder wall during filling leads to a perception of bladder fullness and initiates a desire to void. Urination is achieved under voluntary control, through not only the co-ordinated activation of the sympathetic and parasympathetic nervous systems, but also the somatic nervous system, which is involved in the control of striated muscles in the external urethral sphincter and the pelvic floor muscles.

The local integration centres for various autonomic reflexes may also differ. The peristaltic reflex in the gut, for example, is integrated within the gut wall, and there is a reflex contraction to stretch in the colon that appears to be integrated at the level of the inferior mesenteric ganglion. In neither case does the sensory information reach the central nervous system. Integrating centres for autonomic reflexes also exist in the spinal cord – for instance, in the control of blood pressure through the sympathetic nerves, and for the reflex contraction of the bladder by the parasympathetic pelvic nerves. These are normally controlled and co-ordinated by descending impulses from higher brain centres, but their presence is revealed in patients suffering from spinal cord lesions that cut off the higher control.

Autonomic reflexes are of great importance in the maintenance of homeostasis – a term introduced in 1929 by the American physiologist Walter B. Cannon to designate the constancy of the internal environment. Homeostasis requires complex integration of many reflex and hormonal

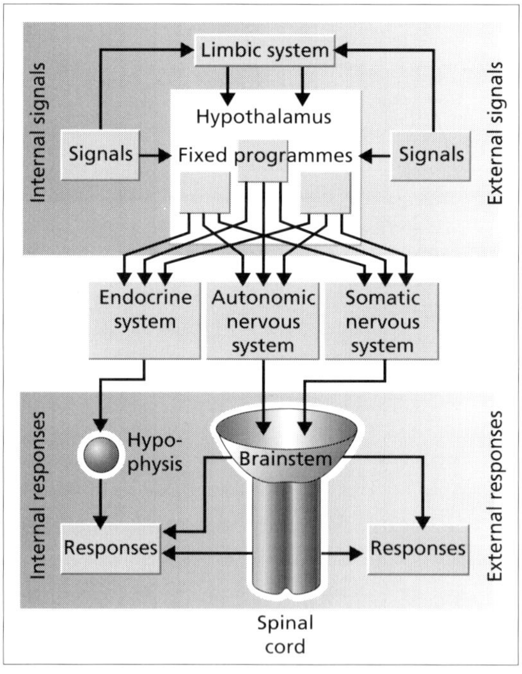

Fig. 2.24 Diagram of the functional organisation of the hypothalamus in relation to its role in homeostasis.

mechanisms. Most of this integration takes place in the hypothalamus, which receives input from many of the afferent systems and has reciprocal innervation with the thalamus and cortex, and the limbic system. The hypothalamus exerts a major control over the brainstem and its autonomic centres, and also the pituitary gland (Fig. 2.24).

Further reading

Furness, J.B. & Costa, M. (1987) *The Enteric Nervous System.* Churchill Livingstone, Edinburgh.

Gabella, G. (1976) *Structure of the Autonomic Nervous System.* Chapman and Hall, London.

Hamilton, W.J. (1976) *Textbook of Human Anatomy.* Macmillan, London.

References

Dogiel, A.S. (1899) Ueber den bau der Ganglien in den Geflechten des Darmes und der Gallenblase des Manschen und der Säugetiere. *Arch Anat Physiol Leipzig, Anat Abt* (Jg 1899): 130–58.

Dowling, J.E. (1992) *Neurons and Networks.* Harvard University Press, Cambridge, Massachusetts.

Furness, J.B. & Costa, M. (1987) *The Enteric Nervous System.* Churchill Livingstone, Edinburgh.

Haines, D.E. (1985) *Correlative Neuroanatomy.* Urban & Schwarzenberg, Baltimore.

Hamilton, W.J. (1976) *Textbook of Human Anatomy*, 2nd edn, Macmillan.

Kandel, E.R., Schwartz J.H. & Jessel, T.M. (1991). *Principles of Neuroscience*, 3rd edn, Elsevier, London.

Matthews M.R. (1989) Small, intensely fluorescent cells and the paraneuron concept. *J. Electron Microscopy Technique* **12**, 408–16.

Matthews, M.R. & Cuello, A.C. (1982) Substance P-immunoreactive peripheral branches of sensory neurons innervate guinea-pig sympathetic neurons. *Proc. Natl. Acad. Sci. USA* **79**, 1668–72.

Matthews M.R. & Raisman G.J. (1969) The ultrastructure and somatic efferent synapses of small granule-containing cells in the superior cervical ganglion. *Anat. Lond.* **105**, 255–82.

Matthews, M., Connaughton M. & Cuello, A.C. (1987) Ultrastructure and distribution of substance P-immunoreactive sensory collaterals in the guinea-pig prevertebral sympathetic ganglia. *J. Comp. Neurol.* **258**, 28–51.

Olson, L. & Malmfors, T. (1970) Growth characteristics of adrenergic nerves in the adult rat. *Acta Physiol. Scand.* (Suppl 348), 1–142.

3 : Electrical Properties of Neurones

3.1 Introduction

The purpose of this chapter is to introduce the neurones in the autonomic nervous system and the mechanisms that enable them to carry messages throughout the body. It will concentrate on the peripheral neurones, since these are easier to study, although it must be remembered that neurones in the central nervous system play a major role in the integration of sensory signals and the activation of the motor neurones in the autonomic nervous system. We will look at the passive and active properties of neurones.

3.2 Passive electrical properties of neurones

3.2.1 Biophysical properties of the neurone

At the surface of the neurone, the cell membrane acts as a barrier and prevents ions present in the external fluid from mixing rapidly with those in the internal solution. The membrane has a high electrical resistance, about 1000 Ω cm^2 in a resting axon, and an electrical capacitance of 1 microfarad cm^{-2}. These are the values that might be expected for a bimolecular layer of lipid with a thickness of 5 nm, a dielectric constant of 5 and an electrical resistivity of 2×10^9 Ω cm. The high resistivity of the membrane is in striking contrast to that of the axoplasm and external fluid, these being about 30 and 20 Ω cm, respectively. During the nerve impulse, the conductivity of the membrane increases about one hundredfold, and sodium and potassium move down their concentration gradients. As we will see later, these ionic movements provide the immediate source of energy for the conduction of the nerve impulse.

3.2.2 Ionic composition

One of the most important functions of the plasma membrane is to maintain a specific ionic composition of the cytosol, which is different from the composition of the extracellular fluid, and this ensures that ionic gradients exist across the membrane. These gradients are responsible for the transmembrane potential difference that occurs in all living cells, and they can be utilised in the production of action potentials and synaptic potentials. Early estimates of the intracellular ionic concentration were fairly inaccurate, since they relied on chemical estimates of the total tissue ions and a value for the extracellular volume, the latter being very difficult to assess accurately. In early years, the only certainty was that the cytoplasm contained high levels of potassium, and relatively low levels of Na^+ and Cl^-. The recent techniques of ion-sensitive microelectrodes and the development of ion-sensitive fluorescent or luminescent probes have allowed more accurate estimates of the intracellular ionic concentrations. Some representative examples of intracellular and extracellular ionic concentrations in mammalian cells are given in Table 3.1, which also includes the calculated Nernst potential for each ion (see Section 3.2.4).

Experiments with radioactive tracers show that all the ions can cross the cell membrane. Two important questions arise from inspection of the data in Table 3.1: what is the effect of the ionic gradients on the membrane potential and how are these ionic gradients established and maintained?

Table 3.1 Typical ion concentrations and Nernst potentials in mammalian cells.

Ion	Intracellular concentration (mmol/l)	Extracellular concentration (mmol/l)	Nernst potential at 38°C
K^+	150	4.5	−92.9
Na^+	9	140	+72.7
Cl^-	(3–50) 30	100	−31.9
HCO_3^-	12	24	−18.4
Ca^{2+}	0.0003	2.4	+119
Mg^{2+}	0.4	1.5	+17.3
X^-	118	28	RP −50 to −70 mV

RP: resting potential.
The Cl^- concentration inside cells may vary over the range shown in parentheses. The Nernst potential is calculated using the value outside the parentheses.
X represents the net negative charge of macromolecules.

3.2.3 Ions and charge distribution

Considering any single ion species in solution, if it is distributed at different concentrations on each side of a membrane that it can permeate, then ions will tend to move across the membrane by diffusion in both directions. However, since one side has a higher concentration, the ions from this side will initially tend to cross the membrane more frequently because there are more of them. As soon as more ions move in one direction than in the other, there will be a difference in charge on each side of the membrane.

Now, although in free solution the effect of the charge is rapidly dissipated, the membrane has capacitative properties. This allows a charge difference to be 'felt' across it. The lipids in the membrane can be thought of as having attached dipoles along their length. Dipoles are small flexible parts of a molecule with positive and negative charge that can change orientation in response to an electric field. Thus, net charge near the outside of the mem-

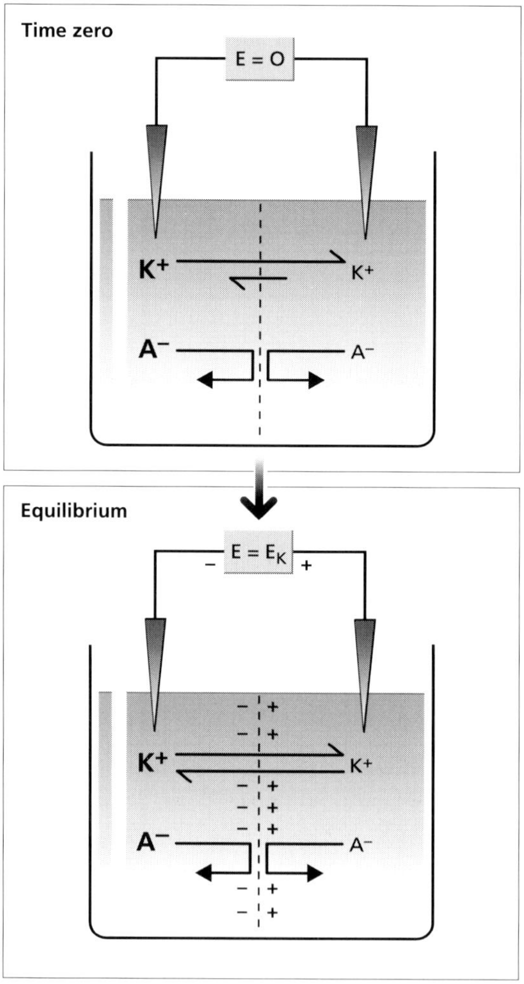

Fig. 3.1 How a membrane potential is set up across a membrane that is only permeable to K^+. Initially, two solutions of KA (a salt that fully dissociates into K^+ and A^-) at different concentrations are added each side of the membrane. The anions cannot cross the membrane, but the K^+ ions immediately begin to diffuse across. More K^+ ions penetrate from left to right because of their higher concentration, and they thus begin to build up a charge separation, with the right-hand chamber becoming positive to the left-hand chamber. The potential gradient increases the energy required for K^+ to cross the membrane from left to right, and finally a steady state is reached when K^+ flows equally in both directions. The potential is then equal to the Nernst potential for K^+.

brane will flip the nearest dipole, which will flip its neighbour, and so on across the membrane, so that the charge nearest the intracellular fluid will be the opposite of that on the outside. In reality, this means that, at any instant of time, there will be rather more positive ions adjacent to one side of the membrane than there would be in free solution, and rather more negative ions adjacent to the other side. The membrane is allowing the ions to feel the attraction of the opposite charge across them. This build-up of charge on the cell surface can affect the probability of ions moving across the membrane.

3.2.4 The Nernst potential

Consider K^+ ions (Fig. 3.1). If the normal concentration gradient were suddenly established across the membrane, then initially more K^+ ions would move out from the cell than back into the cell. However, their actual movement would set up a charge difference across the membrane, which would then reduce the number leaving, because an ion would now require more energy to penetrate into the positive extracellular environment. Eventually, the charge build-up on the membrane would be sufficient to slow down the rate of K^+ ions leaving the cell until it equalled the rate of K^+ ions entering. Once this happened, a steady state would result, and no net K^+ movement would now occur. This state of events actually happens faster than can be measured. It is obvious that the larger the concentration gradient of the ion, the greater the amount of charge build-up necessary to reach the steady state. This relationship is formalised by the Nernst potential:

$$E_K = \frac{RT}{zF} \ln \frac{[K]_o}{[K]_i}$$

where E_K is known as the equilibrium potential or Nernst potential of the potassium ion (defined as the internal potential minus the external potential); $[K]_o$ and $[K]_i$ are the potassium concentrations (or strictly potassium activities; Box 3.1) outside and inside the fibre; R is the gas constant (8.314 J $deg^{-1}mole^{-1}$); T is the absolute temperature; z is the valency of the ion; and F is the Faraday (96500 coulombs $mole^{-1}$). If the ionic gradients are known, it is possible to calculate the Nernst potential for any ion. This has been done in Table 3.1.

3.2.5 Resting potential and constant field equation

Although it is easy to see how the membrane potential arises if the membrane is only permeable to a single ion, the situation is obviously much more complicated in real cells, which have membranes permeable to many different ions, each with a different ionic gradient. Every ion that diffuses through the membrane will contribute to the resultant membrane potential. The more net ions that can cross, the greater the contribution of each particular ionic species. This means that three things will be important:

1 the permeability of the membrane to the ion in question;
2 the driving force operating on the ion;
3 the actual concentration of the ion on the two sides of the membrane.

If the ion cannot diffuse through the membrane, then it will not contribute to the membrane potential. The larger the driving force, the greater the tendency for net movement of an ion, and thus movement of charge. If there were identical driving forces and identical permeabilities, the actual number of ions moving would depend on the absolute concentrations present. All these factors are taken account of in the Goldman constant field equation:

$$E = \frac{RT}{zF} \ln \sqrt{\frac{P_{Na}[Na]_o + P_K[K]_o + P_{Cl}[Cl]_i +}{P_{Na}[Na]_i + P_K[K]_i + P_{Cl}[Cl]_o +}}$$

The terminal plus signs allow for the inclusion of other permeant ions. Usually their concentration or permeability is so small that they can be ignored.

This equation is theoretically derived on the assumption that the difference in charge across the membrane is uniformly distributed within the membrane – hence the term 'constant field' – but the relationship between membrane potential, concentrations and permeabilities can actually be derived for any pattern of charge in the membrane, and the equation is a good predictor of the membrane potential (although it does not include any contribution of electrogenic processes).

Box 3.1 Properties of ions in solution

In solution, each ion carries a charge. The charge density at the surface of the ion will depend on its size. With monovalent ions, for instance, the charge density of K^+ will be less than that of Na^+, since K^+ is a larger ion, and the single charge is therefore spread over a larger area of space. The effect of this charge drops off very quickly with distance from the ion. However, the water molecules, although carrying no net charge, are weakly polarized, being negative at one end and positive at the other, and the charge on the ions is sufficient to attract water molecules to them, and develop hydration shells around the ions (Fig. B3.1.1). The size of the hydration shell will depend on the charge density on the ion. This means, for instance, that although Na^+ is a smaller ion than K^+, in solution it carries a larger water shell, and behaves as if it were bigger. This water shell and the rapid drop of electrical potential with distance mean that, in weak solutions, the ions stay separate, and there is little tendency for interaction between negative and positive ones – they do not 'see' each other. However, in stronger solutions, there is a small interaction between them, which reduces their speed of movement in solution, a phenomenon that is reflected in the specific activity of the

Continued

Box 3.1 *Continued*

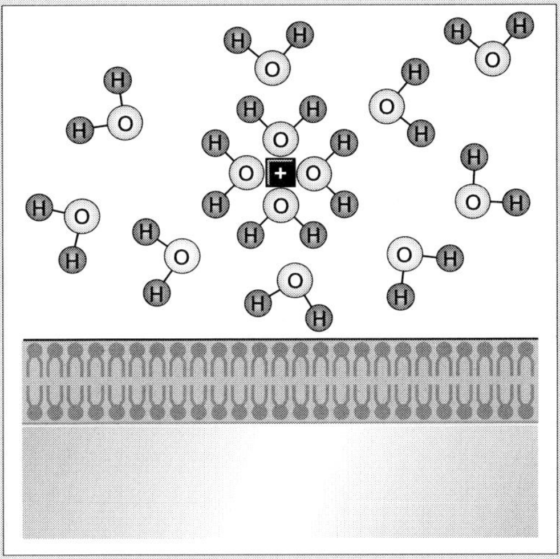

Fig. B3.1.1 Ions in solution attract water molecules and become surrounded by a hydration shell, because the distribution of electrons in water molecules results in the molecules being weakly polarized. The size of the water shell depends on the charge density at the surface of the ion. For ions of the same valency, the larger ions have a smaller water shell than the smaller ions. The water shell slows the diffusion of the ion, and makes it more difficult for the ion to penetrate the non-polar environment of the lipid bilayer, since much energy is necessary for the ion to leave its polar water shell.

ions – this would be 1 in an infinitely dilute solution, when concentration and activity are the same, but is less than 1 in solutions of physiological strength. In theory, when calculating Nernst or Goldman potentials, activity should be used rather than concentration.

From an energetic point of view, if the existing membrane potential is the same as the equilibrium potential for a particular ion, then no energy needs to be expended in keeping the ionic gradient for that ion constant, and the ion can be considered to be passively distributed. If the two values differ, then there will be an electrochemical driving force equivalent to the difference between the two values, resulting in the net passive movement of that ion across the membrane. However, if the ions are in a steady state, the cell must be expending energy to move equal numbers of the ion in question in the opposite direction. In practice, it is rare to find any ions passively distributed – although this appears to be approximately the case for Cl^- ions in the frog skeletal muscle, which has an unusually large Cl^- permeability (it is not true in mammalian skeletal muscle or nerves).

3.2.6 Origin of the uneven distribution of ions across the cell membrane

The ions are unequally distributed because of the presence inside the cell of charged macromolecules (Box 3.2) and the presence in the membrane of mechanisms to transport ions across it actively.

Ion pumps, or primary active transport systems, are proteins that translocate ions against their electrochemical gradients using the energy derived from adenosine triphosphate (ATP) breakdown. The most important mechanism is the Na^+ pump, or the Na^+,K^+-ATPase molecule, which translocates three Na^+ ions out of the cell in exchange for two K^+ ions into the cell for each molecule of ATP hydrolysed (Fig. 3.2). This mechanism is responsible for preventing net ion flow into the cells and osmotic lysis – in many cells blocking this pump with the alkaloid ouabain results in cell swelling. It is also responsible for the low intracellular Na^+ and high intracellular K^+ in all cells. Other primary active transport systems that are present in cell membranes are the H^+ pump and the Ca^{2+} pump, which are responsible in part for removing these reactive ions from the cells against their electrochemical gradients. Apart from the pumps, there are secondary active transport proteins that can move an ion up its electrochemical gradient by coupling it with the downhill movement of another ion. A list of some of the various pumps and co-transport and counter-transport mechanisms that have been identified is given in Table 3.2. Many of these mechanisms couple the movement of other ions and molecules to Na^+ movement. Because the inside of the membrane is negatively charged, the inward

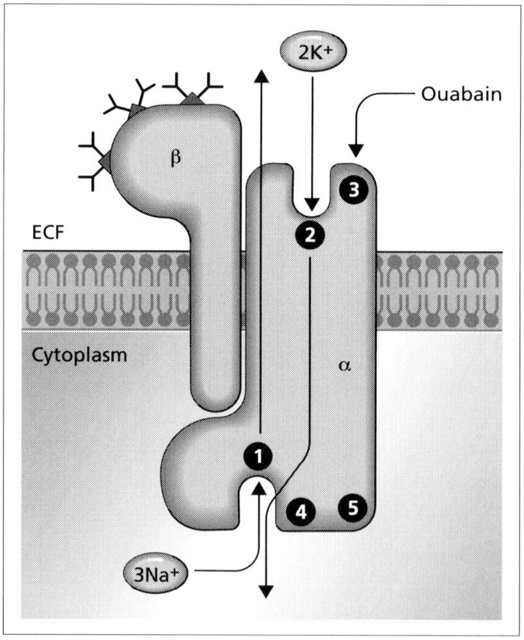

Fig. 3.2 Diagrammatic structure of the Na^+ pump (Na^+,K^+-ATPase). The pump is a heterodimer, with a large α subunit (molecular weight about 100K) and a smaller β subunit (55K). Both subunits extend through the membrane. The β subunit is a glycoprotein, and the α subunit is the ion transporter. (1) The intracellular binding site for Na^+. (2) The extracellular binding site for K^+. (3) The extracellular cardiac glycoside binding site. (4) A phosphorylation site. (5) An ATP binding site. From Horisberger *et al.* (1991).

Box 3.2 Macromolecules and ionic distribution

One important factor resulting in the unequal distribution of ions across the cell membrane is the fact that the cell contains macromolecules that are charged. In fact, there is a net negative charge on intracellular macromolecules that are either part of the cell structure or are non-permeant macromolecules. Now, since there must always be equal numbers of positive and negative charges, if a significant number of non-permeant (or 'fixed') negative charges are present on the inside, it follows that the number of permeant negatively charged ions must be less intracellularly than the cations. In the extracellular medium, there will be roughly equal numbers of permeant anions and cations. There is therefore of necessity an uneven distribution of permeant anions – in practice intracellular [Cl^-] will be less than extracellular [Cl^-]. However, this situation generates an interesting problem. If we consider a purely passive situation, we know that permeant ions can only be passively distributed if their Nernst potentials are the same as the membrane potential, and since there can only be one membrane potential, this means that the gradient for permeant cations must be equal and opposite to the gradient for permeant anions:

$$E_{Cat} = \frac{RT}{zF} \ln \frac{[Cat]_i}{[Cat]_o} = E_{An} = \frac{RT}{zF} \ln \frac{[An]_o}{[An]_i}$$

$$\frac{[Cat]_i}{[Cat]_o} = \frac{[An]_o}{[An]_i}$$

$$[Cat]_i \times [An]_i = [Cat]_o \times [An]_o$$

This is known as the Gibbs–Donnan equilibrium, which states that ions can only be passively distributed across a membrane if the product of the permeant anions and cations on one side is equal to the product of the permeant anions and cations on the other side (Fig. B3.2.1).

We also know that:

$$[Cat]_o = [An]_o \text{ and } [Cat]_i > [An]_i$$

To use an example, if the concentrations of extracellular permeant cations and anions were both 150 mmol/l and that of intracellular cations 300 mmol/l and intracellular anions 75 mmol/l, this would fulfil the requirements for passive distribution:

$$[Cat]_o \times [An]_o = 150 \times 150 = 22\,500$$
$$[Cat]_i \times [An]_i = 300 \times 75 = 22\,500$$

However, the osmolarity of the two solutions depends on the sum of the particles. In this case:

$$[Cat]_o + [An]_o = 150 + 150 = 300$$
$$[Cat]_i + [An]_i = 300 + 75 = 375$$

Continued on p. 54

Box 3.2 *Continued*

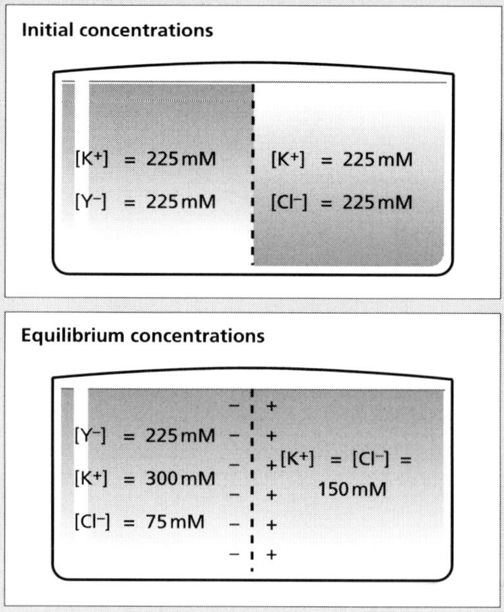

Fig. B3.2.1 Setting a Gibbs–Donnan equilibrium. The two chambers cannot change volume, and the membrane between them is permeable to K^+ and Cl^- but not Y^-. Initially, equal concentrations of KCl and KY are added each side of the membrane. The salts are fully dissociated, and there is no concentration gradient across the membrane for K^+, but an infinite right to left concentration gradient for the permeable Cl^-. Movement of Cl^- down its concentration gradient will generate a transmembrane potential which will affect the movement of K^+, and result in a net movement of K^+ also from right to left. Equilibrium is reached when the concentration gradients for K^+ and Cl^- are equal and opposite (i.e. E_K and E_{Cl} are equal and the same as the membrane potential). However, under these conditions, the osmolarity of the left compartment will be greater than the right, resulting in a hydrostatic pressure gradient.

and the osmolarity of the inside medium would be 75 mosmol greater than the outside, in addition to which there would be the osmotic contribution of the non-permeant ions. This would result in a totally unstable situation – water would enter down the osmotic gradient, this would disrupt the Gibbs–Donnan equilibrium, ions would enter down their new driving forces, the intracellular osmolarity would tend to rise, and water would enter again. This cycle would continue until the cells burst. The only way around this is if ions are transported out of the cell by pumps. Presumably, cell membranes could only have evolved to surround replicating charged macromolecules if active ion pumps evolved at the same time.

Table 3.2 Pumps and ion transport processes.

Ion pumps	
	Na^+,K^+-ATPase
	H^+,K^+-ATPase
	Ca^{2+}-ATPase
Co-transporters	
	Na^+-glucose
	Na^+-amino acid
	Na^+-HCO_3^-
	Na^+-Cl^-
	K^+-Cl^-
	Na^+-K^+-$2Cl^-$
Counter-transporters	
	Na^+/H^+
	$3Na^+/1Ca^{2+}$
	Na^+/Mg^{2+}
	Cl^-/HCO_3^-

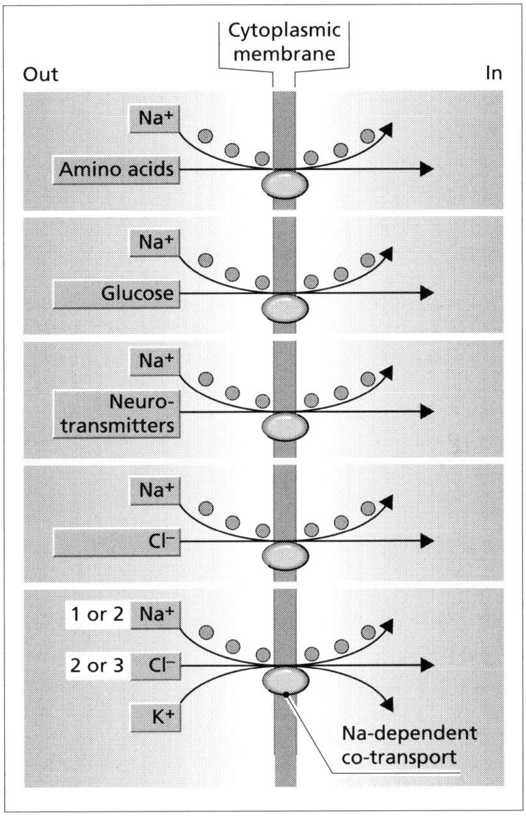

Fig. 3.3 Sodium-dependent co-transport. Several mechanisms exist in the plasma membrane which use the potential energy of the Na gradient to transport other ions or molecules against their chemical or electrochemical gradients.

driving force for Na^+ ions is very large, since both the chemical and electrical gradients operate in the same direction. This then provides a large potential energy source that can be tapped to provide uphill movement of other ions and molecules (Fig. 3.3). Na^+ ions entering the cell on these carriers are then pumped back out. The steady state concentrations of all the permeant ions will depend on the balance of their pumped and leaked movements, and the types and amounts of the various channels and translocators present.

3.2.7 Electrogenic vs. non-electrogenic ion movements

Net passive ion movement through channels is in fact current, and generates changes in membrane potential. Ions moved in combination with translocators may be electrically silent or generate current (i.e. be electrogenic), depending on the coupling ratio. Thus, if the translocator exchanges one hydrogen ion, for example, leaving the cell with one Na^+ ion entering, the exchange is neutral and thus electrically silent. In the case of the Na^+ pump, however, three Na^+ ions are pumped out for only two K^+ ions in, resulting in a net outward current that will contribute to the membrane potential. In this instance, the current is moving cations to the outside, and so will tend to hyperpolarize the membrane. The Goldman constant field equation takes no account of any electrogenic contribution of ion translocators, and for correct prediction of the membrane potential, any electrogenic contribution must be added:

$$E = \frac{RT}{zF} \ln \sqrt{\frac{P_{Na}[Na]_o + P_K[K]_o + P_{Cl}[Cl]_i +}{P_{Na}[Na]_i + P_K[K]_i + P_{Cl}[Cl]_o +}} + r$$

where r = electrogenic contribution.

The potential generated by electrogenic currents is normally only significant for the Na^+ pump, and then rarely contributes more than a few mV in the steady state. The rate of turnover of the Na^+ pump will depend on the rate of entry of Na^+ into the cell down its electrochemical gradient, both through leak pathways and during secondary active transfer. Examples of other electrogenic translocators are Na^+-glucose co-transport and Na^+/Ca^{2+} exchange (three Na^+ ions transported in exchange for one Ca^{2+}). These probably contribute little to the membrane potential in the steady state.

3.3 Active properties of neurones

3.3.1 Action potentials

Action potentials are transient changes in membrane potential that are regenerative in nature and triggered by a smaller change that takes the membrane potential beyond a certain threshold. Under identical conditions, action potentials are all-or-none events – either the stimulus is large enough to cross the threshold, in which case the membrane generates a full-sized action potential, or it is not. Because of their nature, action potentials spread from their site of initiation at a speed dependent on the physical properties of the cells. They presumably evolved to enable signals to be

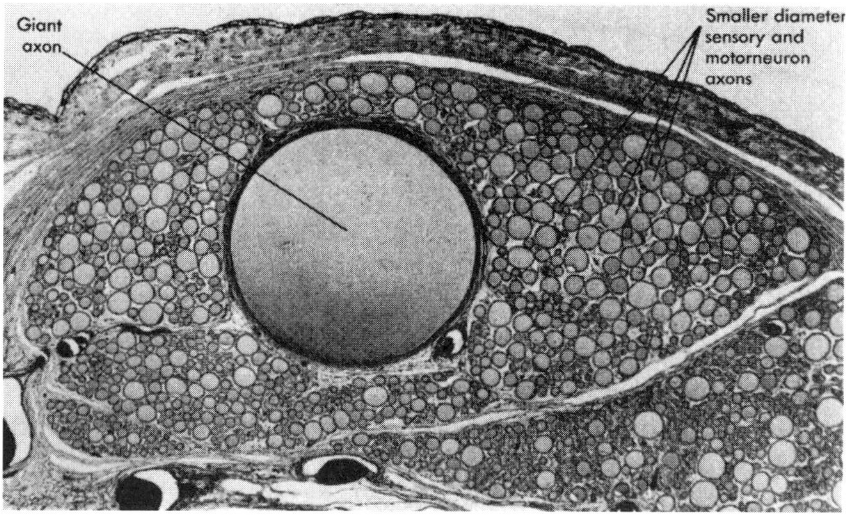

Fig. 3.4 Cross-section of the mantle of the squid, showing a nerve containing many normal nerve fibres and one giant axon. Reproduced from Moffet *et al.* (1993) with permission of The McGraw-Hill Companies.

passed rapidly from one part of a cell to another. In an electric wire, current can flow over very large distances as long as the wire is insulated, because current does not leak out. Unfortunately, cell membranes are by their very nature leaky to the ions that carry the current, and currents injected into cells would dissipate rapidly if a mechanism had not evolved to boost the current constantly. The action potential is such a mechanism. Cells that can generate action potentials are said to be excitable. In excitable cells in animals, an action potential is almost invariably a transient depolarization. Action potentials arriving at their destination are used to trigger secondary events. They have been best studied in nerves such as the squid giant axon (Fig. 3.4) and frog myelinated nerve fibres, cells specialised for rapid transmission of information over long distances. In axons, the action potential finally triggers the release of chemical transmitter from the nerve ending. In other excitable cells such as muscle, the action potential will trigger contraction, and in endocrine and exocrine glands will trigger exocytosis.

The upstroke of the action potential depolarisation is caused by inward current flowing through ion channels down electrochemical gradients. In cells specialised for rapid conduction, the ion carrying the inward current is Na^+, but in cells where rapid conduction is not as important, the ion is usually Ca^{2+}. Both of these ions have a large inwardly directed driving force operating on them, but the far greater number of Na^+ ions allows larger currents to be generated, and as we will see below, the size of the current is important in determining the speed with which the action potential can spread. Ca^{2+} entering the cells in the Ca^{2+}-based action potentials is very reactive and can directly trigger cellular events. This type of action potential probably evolved first. In Na^+-based action potentials, the Na^+ entering has little effect on its own, and the action potential has to activate voltage-sensitive Ca^{2+} channels and let Ca^{2+} in to trigger cell processes. Na^+-based action potentials probably evolved later specifically for rapid conduction.

3.3.2 Requirements for action potential production

In order for a membrane to be able to generate an action potential, a small triggering stimulus in the form of a depolarization (caused by an approaching action potential, by neurotransmitters, by generator potentials in sensory neurones, or by electrical stimuli applied by physiologists) must result in opening of enough voltage-sensitive channels to allow a net inward current flow. This will generate more depolarization, and further opening of the channels, setting up a positive feedback situation resulting in the rapid depolarisation of the membrane towards the equilibrium potential of the ion in question. If these inward current channels remained open, a new depolarized steady membrane potential would be set up, in accordance with the constant field equation. Repolarization requires closure of these channels, and this is achieved by their inactivation, which is usually also triggered by depolarization, but occurs more slowly than channel opening. More rapid repolarization can be achieved by simultaneous opening of K^+ channels, which brings the membrane potential closer to the K^+ equilibrium potential (Fig. 3.5).

The studies by Hodgkin and Huxley and their colleagues of action potentials in the squid giant axon provided the classical model of the action potential generation in nerve, and more details are given in Box 3.3.

3.3.3 Threshold potential

The threshold is a precisely defined point. Like the resting potential, the threshold potential is one at which there is no net current flowing through the membrane, and, in theory, if the membrane properties remained absolutely constant, so would the membrane potential (normally, spontaneous fluctuations in channel opening cause small changes in potential that will eventually exceed the threshold and trigger the action potential). The local circuit current flowing during the stimulating depolarization is outward, and carried largely by K^+ ions (since the passive membrane is most permeable to them). The depolarization will, however, cause opening of the voltage-sensitive inward current channels (Na^+ or Ca^{2+}), and inward current through these will reduce the net outward current, and at one particular potential, the threshold, the inward and outward currents will be equal. With no net current flowing, there is obviously then no tendency for the membrane potential to change. If the threshold is exceeded, the net inward current will depolarize further and a positive feedback situation will occur,

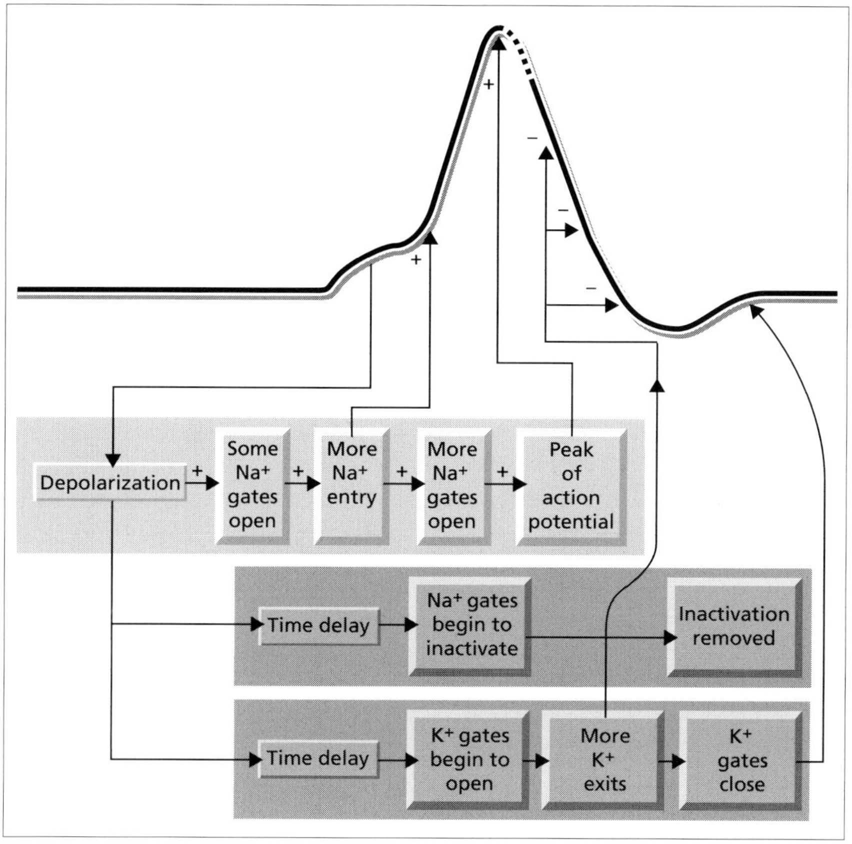

Fig. 3.5 Mechanisms underlying the nerve action potential. An initial depolarization opens sufficient Na channels to allow the generation of a net inward Na current. A positive feedback reaction is initiated, since the net inward current further depolarizes the membrane, thus opening more Na channels, resulting in the rapid upstroke of the action potential to a value approaching the Na equilibrium potential. The depolarization also activates K channels, and inactivates the Na channels, but with a delay. These two delayed events result in the repolarization of the membrane. The deactivation of the K channels and the removal of the Na channel inactivation are also slow processes. Thus, as the membrane approaches the resting potential during repolarization, the Na channels are still inactivated and the K channels still open, the P_K/P_{Na} ratio is larger than in the resting state, and the membrane potential hyperpolarizes towards the K equilibrium potential until the K channels close, and the resting permeability ratio is restored.

Box 3.3 Action potentials in nerves

Measurement of the permeability changes during the nerve action potential. Detailed estimation of the permeability changes and currents flowing through the membrane in an action potential would be extremely difficult in the normal axon, because everything is changing both spatially along the axon and in time. The transient changes in the permeability of the cell membrane were first measured when a method

Continued on p. 60

Box 3.3 *Continued*

(voltage clamp) was devised in which it was possible to use a feedback circuit to step the membrane potential to a desired value, and hold it there while measuring the resulting time-dependent changes in the current that were initiated by the potential change (Fig. B3.3.1). It should be appreciated that, in order to depolarize a membrane experimentally, the depolarizing electrode (cathode) causes outward flow of current across the membrane, as predicted by Ohm's law. This is simply a current flowing in response to an imposed voltage, and is sometimes called passive current. However, if the depolarisation opens channels that allow ions to flow through them, the resulting currents will be determined by the electrochemical gradients operating on the ions, and the selectivity of the channels. Under these circumstances, inward current flow (cations entering or anions leaving the cell) will depolarize the cell, and outward current flow (anions entering the cell or cations leaving it) will hyperpolarize it. These are not currents flowing directly in response to a potential change, but result from the potential change allowing the tapping of the energy stored in the ionic gradients across the cell membrane, and are sometimes called active currents. Under voltage clamp conditions, the membrane potential change that is caused by these passive and active currents is detected as soon as it begins, and

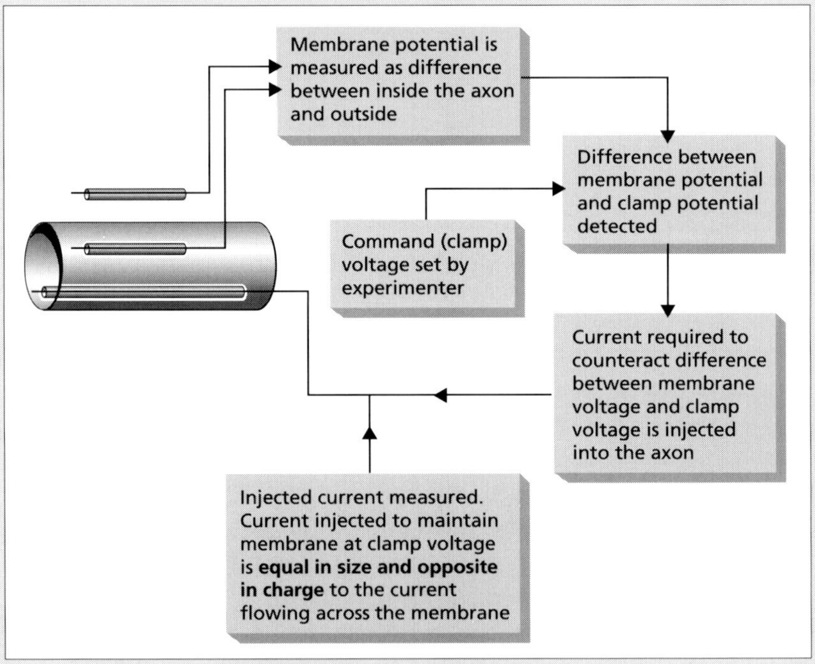

Fig. B3.3.1 Diagram of the voltage clamp apparatus for the squid giant axon.

Continued

Box 3.3 *Continued*

is compensated for by delivering equal and opposite current through current electrodes on each side of the membrane, thus clamping the voltage at the desired value. Measurement of the applied current thus reflects the current flowing through the membrane at that potential. It should be pointed out that, in these studies, it is essential for accurate interpretation that the whole area of membrane through which the currents pass should be clamped uniformly at the same voltage – any spatial non-uniformities will result in lateral current flow through differently polarized areas of membrane, which could not be distinguished from the transmembrane flow. The squid giant axon is an ideal preparation, since it is large enough to allow electrodes to be inserted along the length of the axon to be clamped, and allows great uniformity of voltage (Fig. 3.4).

Voltage clamp studies. In 1952, Hodgkin & Huxley, using experimental data obtained from voltage clamp studies in the squid giant axon, were the first to provide a detailed description of the ionic mechanisms underlying action potential generation in nerves (see Hodgkin, 1957). They analysed records of the active currents generated during depolarizing pulses of various amplitudes and time courses, and devised methods for separating them into Na^+ and K^+ currents (Fig. B3.3.2). They showed that the current amplitudes were linearly related to the voltage, allowing them to estimate membrane conductance using Ohm's law (V = I/G, where V is the voltage, I is the current, and G is the

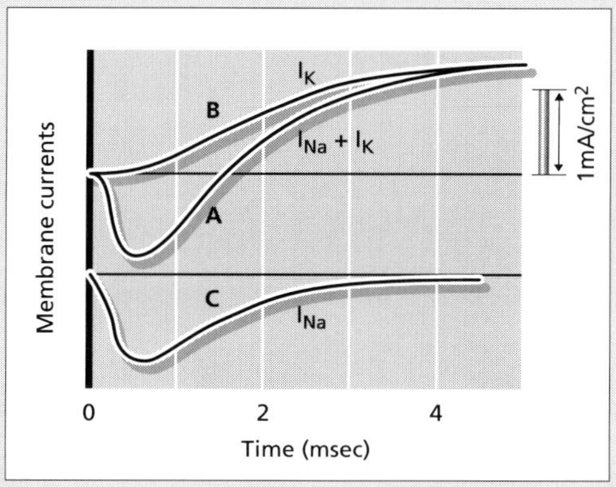

Fig. B3.3.2 Separation of the net ionic current in response to a depolarizing pulse into sodium and potassium currents. The net current in A shows that, on depolarization to 0 mV, there is an initial inward current which reverses to become a constant outward current. Curve B shows the currents flowing when there is no driving force on the Na ions. This is achieved by replacing most of the external Na by the non-permeant monovalent ion choline, so that the intracellular and extracellular Na concentrations are the same. This curve is the K current I_K. The sodium current I_{Na} can then be obtained by subtracting I_K from the net current. This is shown in curve C.

Continued on p. 62

Box 3.3 *Continued*

conductance, the reciprocal of resistance). Hodgkin and Huxley then derived a series of empirical equations accurately describing the conductances through Na^+ and K^+ channels as a function of membrane potential and time. They were then able to calculate the expected shape and conduction velocity of the propagated action potential (Fig. B3.3.3).

Model of an action potential. According to the Hodgkin–Huxley model, the membrane potential can effect the opening and closing of a series of gates that determine whether or not ions can flow through the channels. The nerve membrane has two types of voltage-sensitive channel, Na^+ channels and K^+ channels, both of which have four 'gates'. The Na^+ channel has two kinds of gate: three are activation gates, which are closed at the resting potential, and one is an inactivation gate, which is open at the resting potential. The K^+ channel has four activation gates. The rate constants of the gate opening and closing are instantaneous and continuous functions of voltage. During the action potential, the following sequence occurs (Fig. B3.3.4). Depolarization of the membrane causes first a rapid opening of the 'activation gates' of the Na^+ channels, resulting in an inward Na^+ current. This Na^+ current causes further depolarization, which results in the opening of more gates and further inward current. This regenerative process leads to the upstroke of the action potential, and since the membrane is now more permeable to Na^+ ions than to any other ion, the membrane potential rapidly approaches the equilibrium potential for Na^+ ions (within 0.5 ms). The depolarization then triggers two further changes, which have slower kinetics: inactivation of the Na^+ channels (closing the inactivation gates), and simultaneous opening of the 'activation gates' of the K^+ channels. These processes reduce the inward Na^+ current and approaches its resting value, the activation gates for both the Na^+ and the K^+ channels begin to close, those for the Na^+ channels closing more

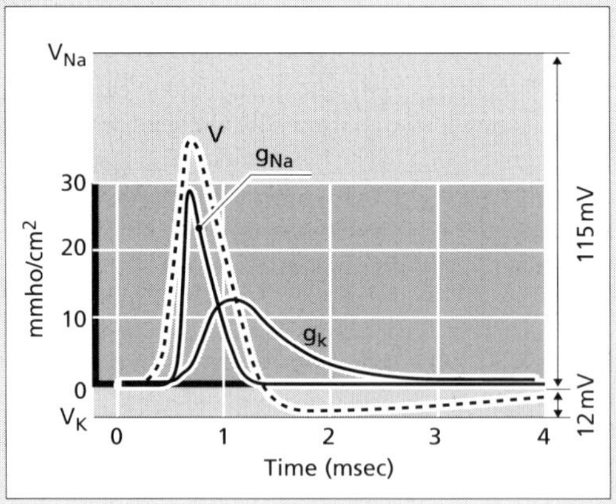

Fig. B3.3.3 The dotted outline (and right ordinate) shows the theoretical action potential obtained by Hodgkin and Huxley from their equations. The time course of the sodium conductance change (g_{Na}) and the potassium conductance change (g_K) is drawn with solid lines (left ordinate). V_{Na} and V_K are the equilibrium potentials for Na and K.

Continued

Box 3.3 *Continued*

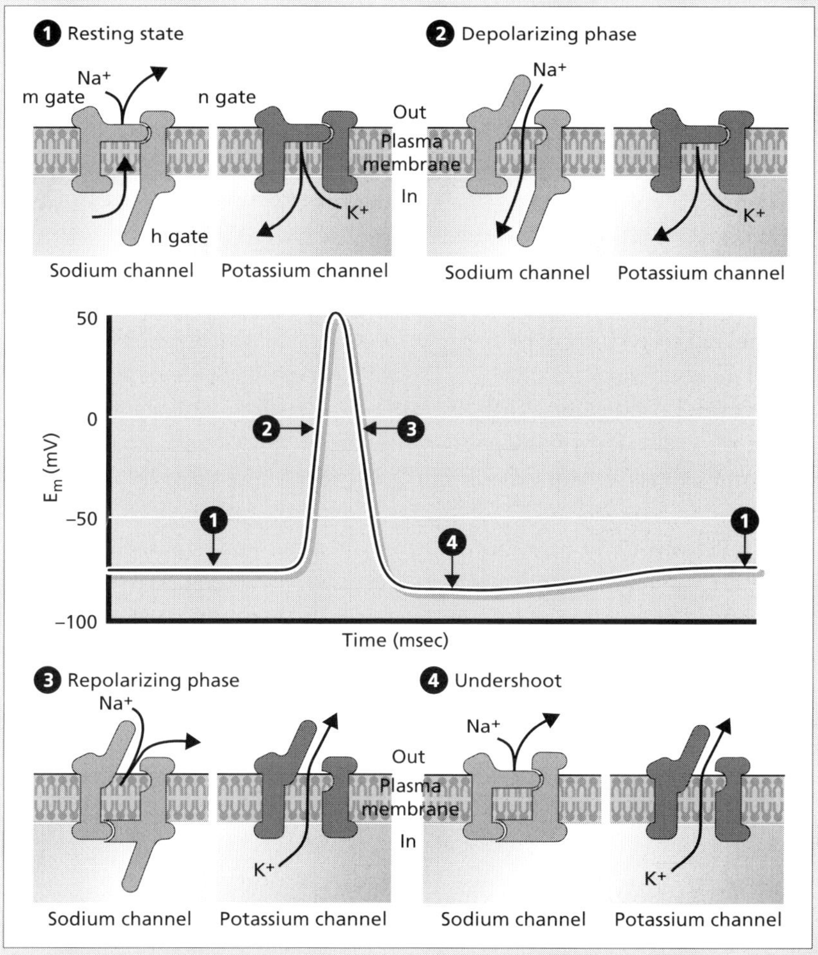

Fig. B3.3.4 Interpretation of the Hodgkin–Huxley model in terms of the gating of the sodium and potassium channels. In this figure, only one of each type of gate is shown for convenience. In the model, there are three independently acting Na activation gates (m gates), and four K activation gates (n gates). Any single gate can close the channel. In the resting state (1), at any instant of time, the majority of the m gates are closed, and the h (inactivation) gates open in the Na channel. The majority of the n gates of the K channel are closed. (2) Depolarization opens the m gates rapidly, accounting for the rising phase of the action potential. (3) After a delay, the K channel n gates begin to open and the Na channel inactivation gates to close, allowing repolarization to occur. (4) For a period after repolarization, the h gates are beginning to open and the n gates close, but until the gates return to normal, the increased K conductance is associated with an after-hyperpolarization, and the threshold for initiation of a new action potential is increased, accounting for the absolute and relative refractory periods.

Continued on p. 64

Box 3.3 *Continued*

rapidly than for the K^+ channels. At this stage, the membrane has a higher permeability to K^+ than in its resting state, and both activation and inactivation gates of the Na^+ channels are closed, so that the membrane potential approaches the potassium equilibrium potential. This is the negative after-potential, or after-hyperpolarisation. It is a transient event, as the activation gates of the K^+ channels finally close, and the inactivation gates of the Na^+ channels also reset themselves (Fig. B3.3.4).

Soon after the action potential, whilst the Na^+ channels are inactivated and the K^+ channels still open, the membrane is initially unable to respond to a further depolarisation, and is thus refractory. This is because further depolarization simply keeps the Na^+ channels shut and K^+ channels open. Later, as the Na^+ channel inactivation decays progressively and some of the K^+ channels shut, the membrane enters a relatively refractory state in which another action potential can be triggered, but only with a much larger depolarization (Fig. B3.3.5). Several milliseconds are required for resetting the gates before the normal sensitivity to depolarization returns. The small gain of Na^+ and loss of K^+ ions that have occurred are restored in due course by the Na^+ pump. (It is interesting to note that in the squid giant axon, the amounts gained or lost are so small that even if the Na^+ pump has been poisoned, so little change in ionic concentration occurs that the axon can still fire several thousand action potentials. This will not be the case in very small axons, in which the large surface area to volume relationship will result in more rapid changes in ionic concentration.)

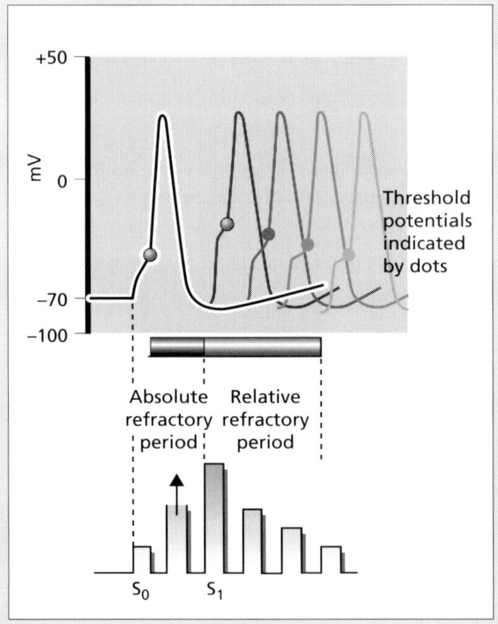

Fig. B3.3.5 Diagram showing the recovery of the nerve after an action potential. The lower part shows the relative size of the depolarizing pulses needed to trigger a second action potential. In the absolute refractory period no action potential can be triggered.

with further depolarization opening more channels and generating more depolarization (Fig. 3.6).

The threshold potential may vary under different circumstances, as in the relatively refractory period. It is very dependent on the state of the voltage-sensitive channels. If some of the inward current channels are inactivated, then a larger depolarization will be required to open enough of the available channels. Also, if some of the outward current channels are still activated, then more inward current channels will need to be opened to balance the outward current. Inactivation of the inward current channels, although it is a slower process than activation, is often more voltage-sensitive, and if the rate of the stimulating depolarization is slow enough, inactivation may cause the threshold to rise faster than the depolarization, in which case an action potential will not be produced.

The types of voltage-sensitive channel and the rates of activation and inactivation vary widely between and within tissues. In most conducting axons, Na^+ channel inactivation is so sensitive to depolarization that if a long depolarizing stimulus is applied, only a single action potential is generated, because the Na^+ channels remain inactivated until the stimulus is switched off. However, where the action potential is initiated (in sensory nerve terminals or at the axon hillock), differences in the channels mean that a constant stimulating current can produce repetitive firing, although commonly the frequency declines with time (adaptation). The lack of repetitive

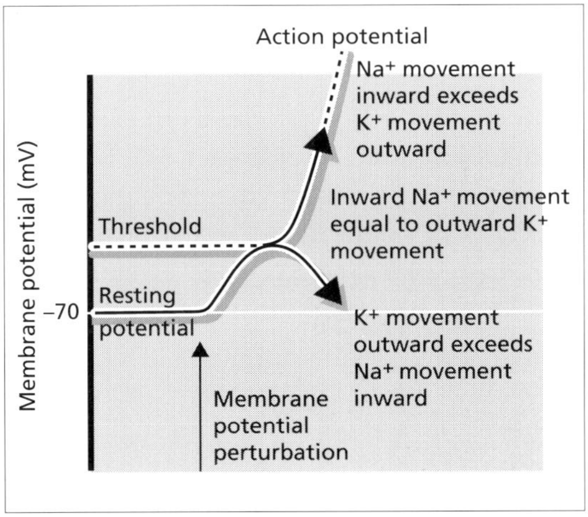

Fig. 3.6 Negative and positive feedback processes and membrane activation. A depolarizing stimulus will be associated with an outward K current (increased driving force for K ions). The depolarization will, however, open Na channels with a resultant inward Na current. At threshold these two currents are equal. If the depolarization does not reach threshold, the outward K current will repolarize the membrane (a negative feedback process). If the depolarization exceeds threshold, a net inward Na current will flow, resulting in further depolarization and opening of more Na channels (positive feedback process).

firing to sustained depolarization in conducting axons prevents spurious initiation of trains of action potentials when their blood supply is accidentally cut off, for instance by applied pressure, leading to depolarization.

3.3.4 Initiation of action potentials *in vivo*

In neurones, the action potentials arise either close to the sensory nerve terminal in sensory neurones, or at the axon hillock in motor or interneurones. In sensory neurones, the first part of the nerve terminal is normally specialised for generating inward current in response to a sensory stimulus. This part has different properties from the conducting axons, and is frequently electrically inexcitable. Local circuit current spreads and depolarizes the adjacent spike initiation site, which is excitable, but again contains different channels from those in the conducting axon. This region, unlike the main axon, can generate repetitive firing in response to a sustained depolarization, and normally the frequency is related to the degree of depolarization. In motor neurones, the axon hillock region again has the property of generating repetitive action potentials in response to sustained depolarization. In this case, however, the cell body and dendritic tree of the neurone, through their synaptic input, generate inward or outward currents, depending on whether the incoming synapse is excitatory or inhibitory. The axon hillock then acts as an integrating membrane, summing outward (depolarizing) or inward (hyperpolarizing) local circuit currents to generate a final response (Fig. 3.7).

3.3.5 Electrical behaviour of autonomic ganglion cells

Although the production of action potentials in motor neurones is quite well understood, microelectrode recordings made from the soma of ganglion cells have shown that the cells can display a range of action potential shapes and electrical behaviours. As expected, action potentials can be evoked by depolarizing current injection, and by stimulating the postganglionic nerves. This latter procedure evokes antidromic action potentials that travel backwards along the axons to invade the soma. In most, but not all neurones, action potentials can be elicited orthodromically through synaptic activation by stimulation of the preganglionic fibres. Neurones that appear to have no synaptic input are present in many ganglia, particularly in the enteric nervous system, and are probably sensory neurones. Several ganglia contain neurones that fire spontaneous action potentials with pacemaker depolarizations, and some neurones fire spontaneously with synaptic input – presumably from pacemaker neurones within the ganglion. The shapes of the action potential vary markedly, and are characteristic of the neurone, as are the presence or extent of any after-hyperpolarization. Several classifications of the ganglion cells in specific

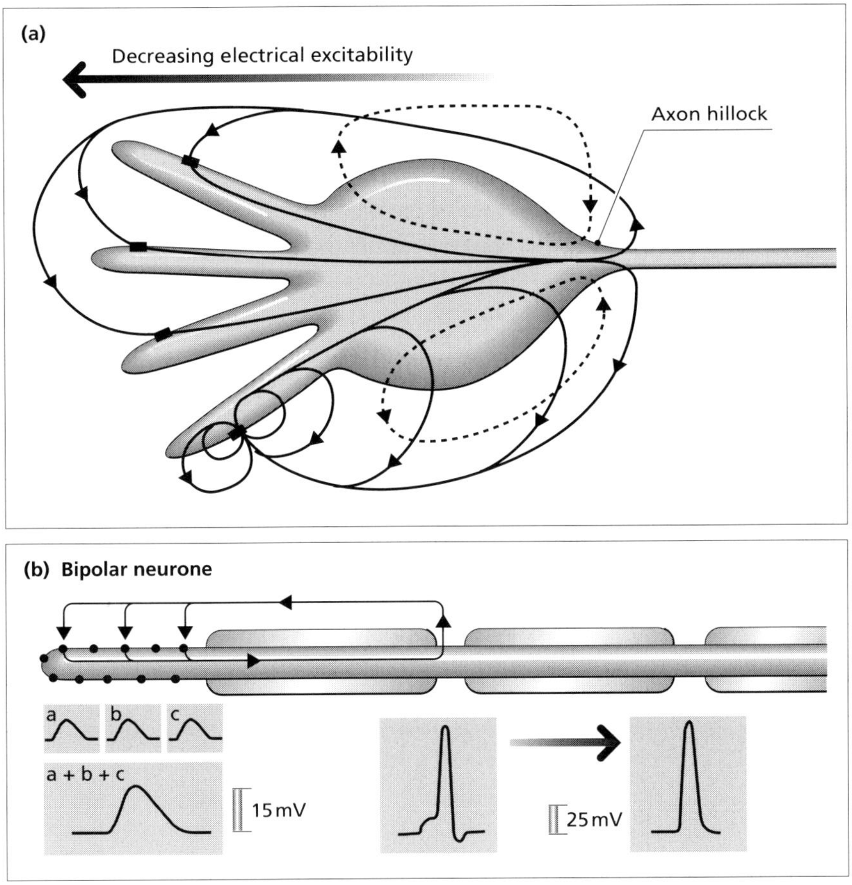

Fig. 3.7 Initiation of action potentials. (a) In motor and interneurones, the action potentials arise in the axon hillock or proximal axon, where the threshold is lowest. Activation of ion channels at synapses on the dendrites and soma results in transmembrane current; inward synaptic current (solid lines) is excitatory and outward synaptic current (dotted lines) is inhibitory. The local circuit currents sum at the axon hillock. Net outward current is associated with depolarization of the membrane and repetitive triggering of action potentials. (b) In sensory nerves, inward current is generated in the nerve terminal by activation of sensory receptors. The terminal normally has a high threshold, but this declines along the axon. Local circuit currents spread along the axon, and action potentials arise at the point where the threshold is low enough for the local circuit current to depolarize above threshold. In myelinated axons, this is often at the first node of Ranvier.

ganglia have been made using the individual electrical characteristics of the cell. The types and properties of the channels responsible for the characteristic features of ganglion cell action potentials are being studied in many laboratories. The presence of these different types of neurone highlight the fact that ganglia are not just simple relays in the autonomic pathways, but are complex structures in which information may be modified as well as transmitted.

3.4 Conduction of action potentials

3.4.1 Frequency coding

Since the information transmitted along individual axons is in identical bits, information about the degree of activation of the neurone can only be carried as a frequency code, reflecting the time intervals between successive nerve action potentials. The relationship between stimulus intensity and frequency of action potentials will depend on the channel properties at the spike initiation site, but the maximum frequency that an axon can conduct will depend on how soon the membrane can generate another action potential after a previous one, i.e. on the refractory period of the axon. Action potentials in nerves usually last on the order of 1–2 ms, and the axons are relatively refractory for a period slightly outlasting this. Thus, the maximum frequency is usually less than 500 impulses per second (500 Hz). However, there can be quite large differences in the speed at which action potentials are propagated (see 3.4.3).

3.4.2 Factors involved in action potential propagation

The regenerative all-or-none property of the nerve action potential is the necessary mechanism for long-distance signal transmission. If an action potential is experimentally induced in the centre of an axon, the inward current flowing through the segment of membrane undergoing an action potential discharges the membrane capacitance on both sides of it, resulting in depolarization and local circuit currents that flow out of the axon and complete the circuit. This depolarization then triggers action potentials in both adjacent membrane segments, and these initiate exactly the same cycle in the membrane ahead, and so on, resulting in an action potential propagating away from the initiation site in both directions. Normally, however, the action potential is initiated at one end of the axon, either near the axon hillock of the cell body or near the sensory nerve terminal, in response to local currents initiated by neurotransmitters or sensory transduction mechanisms (Fig. 3.8). Retrograde local circuit current will not activate the membrane behind an advancing action potential, because it leaves the membrane it has passed through refractory.

3.4.3 Factors affecting conduction velocity

Action potentials travel faster in large nerves than in small ones, and myelinated nerves conduct action potentials faster than unmyelinated ones of the same overall diameter (Fig. 3.9).

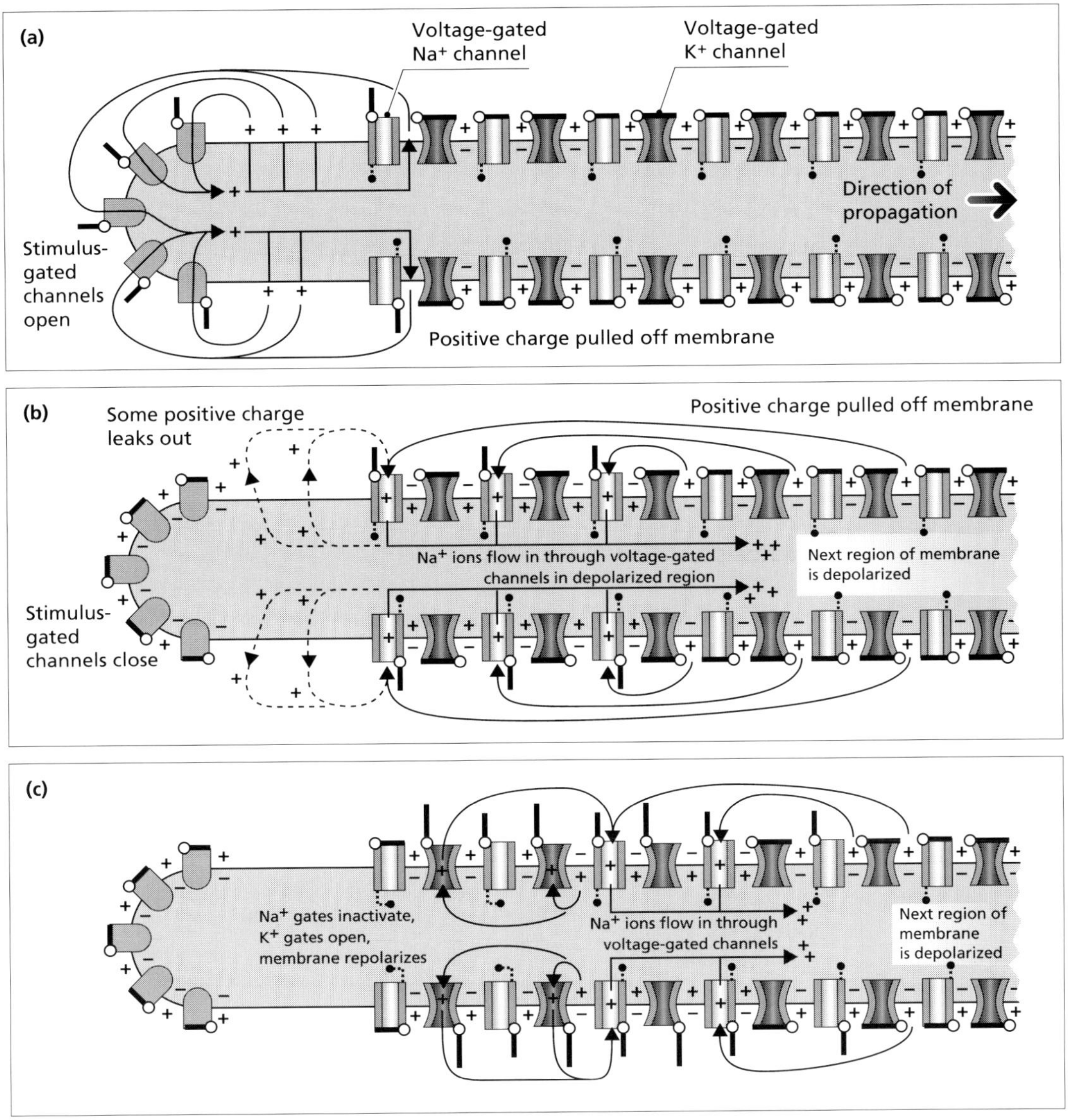

Fig. 3.8 Initiation and propagation of an action potential. (a) Inward current flowing through channels activated by sensory mechanisms pulls positive charge from the membrane of the axon and the depolarization begins to open voltage-sensitive Na channels. (b) Inward current entering through the Na channels depolarizes adjacent regions, and triggers further opening of Na channels away from the terminal. (c) Local depolarization causes delayed inactivation of Na channels and activation of potassium channels, repolarizing the membrane behind, and preventing retrograde propagation.

Passive properties

Conduction velocity is determined by the spread of current ahead of an action potential, and how fast this can depolarize the membrane to threshold. This is dependent on the passive electrical properties of the nerve fibre.

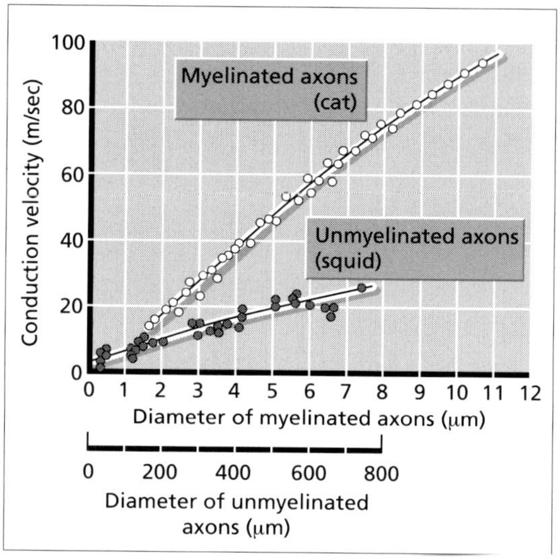

Fig. 3.9 Conduction velocities in myelinated and unmyelinated axons as a function of diameter. Note the different scales for the diameter. The myelinated axons are from a cat nerve, and the unmyelinated ones from the squid. In both types, the conduction velocity increases with diameter, but squid unmyelinated axons need to be about 100 times the diameter of the myelinated fibres to achieve the same velocity. Some of the difference arises from the temperature difference (mammalian body temperature 38 °C and squid axons at room temperature).

The important physical characteristics are the time constant τ, which describes the time taken for the membrane potential to change in response to a current flow (Fig. 3.10), and the length (or space) constant λ, which describes the spread of current down the nerve (Fig. 3.11). These *constants* are determined by the membrane resistance and capacitance, the longitudinal resistance of the axon and the resistance of the extracellular space (Box 3.4). The amount of inward current available from the invading action potential is also an important factor in determining the conduction velocity.

There is a tendency for students to think of the action potential as a Morse code blip running down the nerve. However, if one considers for a moment the shape the nerve action potential would have if it were frozen for an instant in time, the total length occupied instantaneously by an action potential would depend on the duration of the action potential and the conduction velocity. For example, if the duration of the action potential was 2 ms and it was conducted at 10 m/s, then the action potential would be spread over a 2-cm length of the axon.

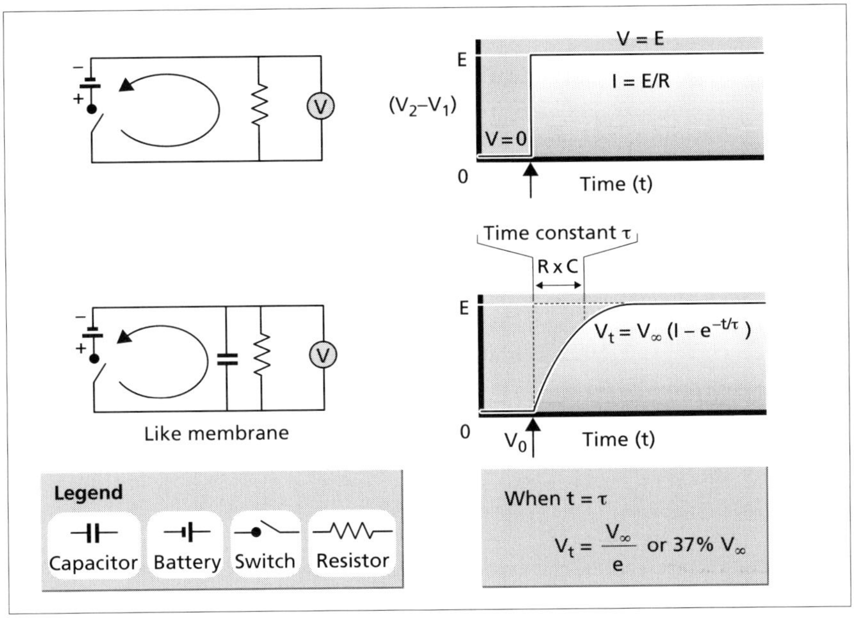

Fig. 3.10 Shape of voltage response to an applied current in a circuit with and without a capacitor. In the right panels, the switch is closed at the arrow. In the top panels, a step change in voltage is recorded across a resistor when the current flows, with an amplitude determined by the resistance, according to Ohm's law. In the lower panels, the effect of adding a capacitor in parallel with the resistor is seen. The voltage now rises exponentially to the steady state value, with a time constant equal to the product of the resistance and capacitance.

Box 3.4 Time and space constants

We need first to consider the response of a passive membrane to current injection. Because the membrane can be thought of as a resistance and capacitance in series, it does not respond instantly to a step change in current in the way that a pure resistance would, but has a delayed response (see Fig. 3.10). The majority of the current initially flows into the membrane capacitance, charging or discharging it, and it is only as the membrane charge is built up that the current flows across the resistance. When the capacitance is fully charged, all the current flows across the resistance, and voltage can now be predicted by Ohm's law. In a simple resistance–capacitance circuit, or with uniform current flow across a passive membrane, the time course of the change is exponential, and the time constant τ, i.e. the time taken for the voltage to change by 63% of its final value, is the product of the resistance and the capacitance:

$$\tau = RC$$

Continued on p. 72

Box 3.4 *Continued*

This means that, in the axon, the voltage response to any current flow will be delayed. From Fig. B3.4.1 it can be seen that, if depolarization to a particular value is needed to trigger an action potential, the larger the current flow, the faster this value is reached. This is why fast conductance velocities need large currents, and probably why the Na^+ channel evolved, since with its properties and the larger Na^+ concentrations, much larger inward currents can be generated than with Ca^{2+} channels.

The current flow is, however, never uniform across the membrane in life. The geometry of current flow from a source can be predicted from a knowledge of the relative resistances that it will meet – more current will flow through lower resistance pathways. The resistances encountered by a local circuit current in an axon will be the internal axonal resistance, the membrane resistance, and the resistance of the extracellular fluid. The first two will be greater than the extracellular fluid resistance, which is often ignored (Fig. B3.4.2).

As the axon diameter increases, although both the longitudinal resistance and the membrane resistance will drop, the longitudinal resistance drops more, because the longitudinal resistance in a unit length of axon (r_i) is related to the resistivity of the axoplasm (R_i) by

$$r_i = R_i/\pi a^2$$

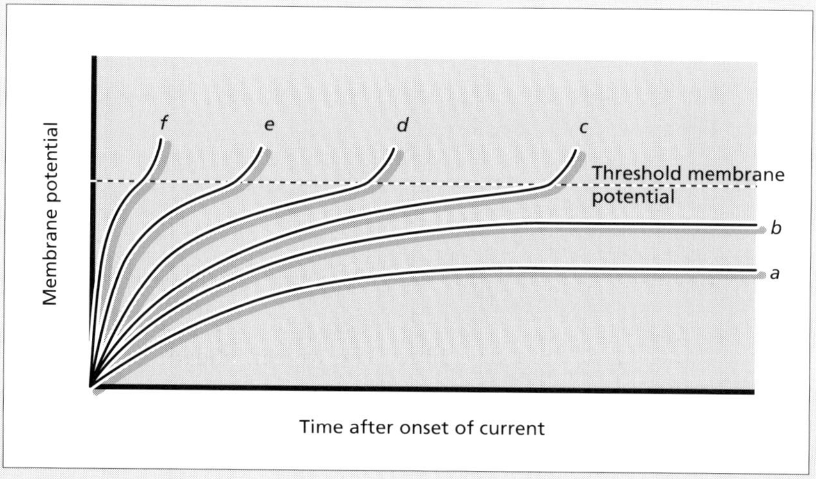

Fig. B3.4.1 Schematic diagram to show the effect on a nerve membrane potential of increasing the strength of a depolarizing current. The current strength increases from a to f. Currents from c to f lead to action potential generation. As can be seen, the rate at which the membrane potential changes increases as the current strength increases; this is because larger currents can discharge the membrane capacitance more quickly. In this diagram it is assumed that the threshold will remain constant during the current pulse. In reality the threshold may increase with time.

Continued

Box 3.4 *Continued*

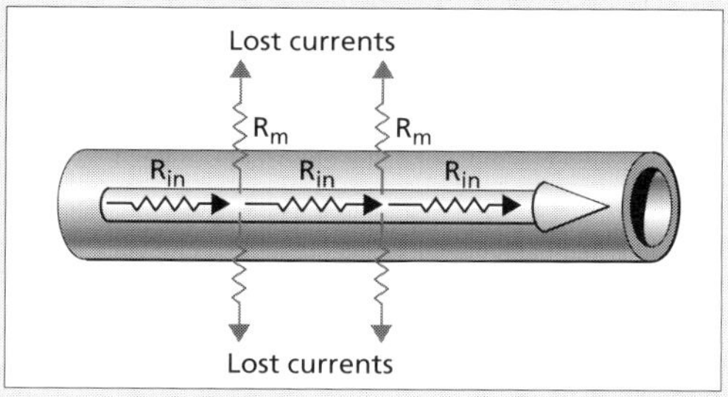

Fig. B.3.4.2 Current flow in an axon.

whereas the membrane resistance of a unit length of axon (r_m) is related to the resistance of a unit area of membrane (R_m) by

$$r_m = R_m / 2\pi a$$

This means that the larger the axon, the further the current will flow, and the longer the length constant will be. If current enters the axon uniformly around it at one position, the spread of current will decay exponentially along it, with a length (or space) constant λ where

$$\lambda = \sqrt{\frac{r_m}{r_i + r_o}}$$

and r_m is the membrane resistance and r_i and r_o the axonal and extracellular resistances.

Myelination

In myelinated fibres, the Schwann cells wrap around the axon to produce the myelin sheath, as described earlier (Figs 2.8 & B2.1.1, pp. 23 & 24). The sheath is interrupted at intervals by the nodes of Ranvier. In this type of nerve, conduction does not proceed continuously, but jumps from node to node (Fig. 3.12). This is termed *saltatory conduction,* and greatly increases the conduction velocity of the nerve fibre. The myelin sheath adds parallel layers of membrane, and thus from an electrical point of view increases the resistance and decreases the capacitance of the internodal current pathway out of the nerve (in a parallel circuit, resistance adds normally, but the total capacitance is the sum of the reciprocals of the individual capacitances). The decrease in capacitance reduces the amount of charge on the membrane associated with the membrane potential, and the increased resistance greatly reduces current loss from this region, so that local circuit current leaves the nerves predominantly at the nodes of Ranvier, where the action potential generating machinery resides, and little current is lost charging up the internodal capacitance. In theory, the length of the nodes that would allow propagation would be determined by the length constant, and

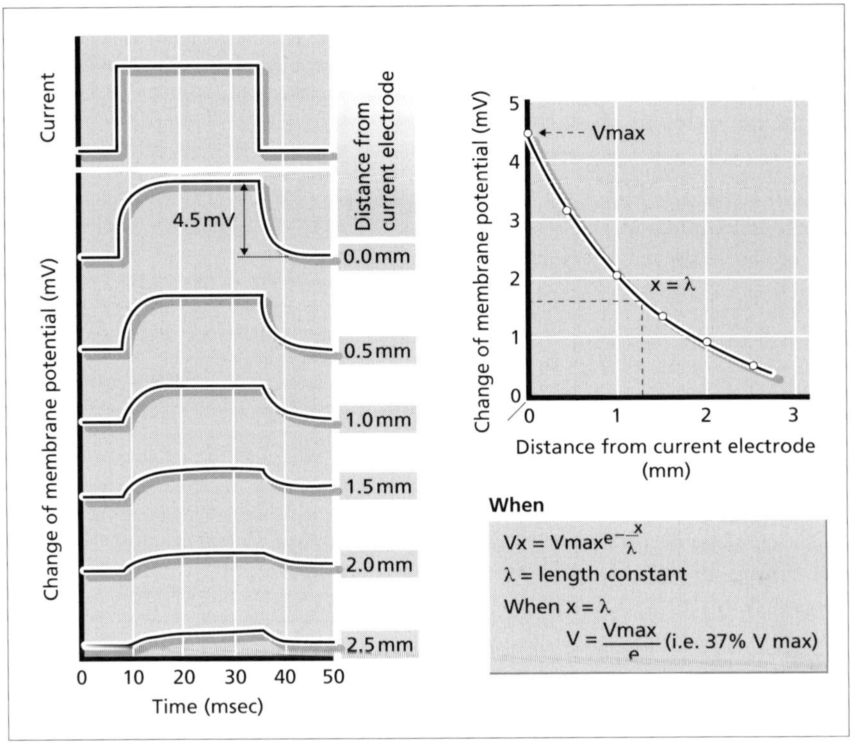

Fig. 3.11 Theoretical voltage changes recorded at increasing distances along a cylindrical unmyelinated axon in response to a square current pulse applied at one point. The maximum voltage declines exponentially with distance, in this example with a length constant of 1.3 mm.

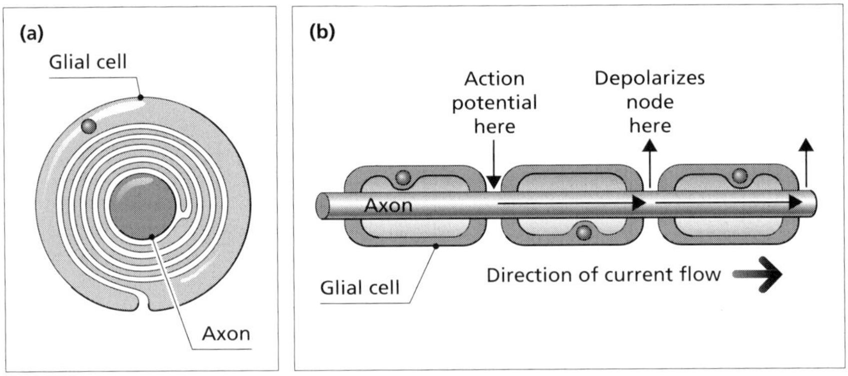

Fig. 3.12 Propagation of an action potential along a myelinated fibre. (a) Cross-section of an internodal region showing how a glial cell wraps around the axon to form the myelin sheath. (b) An action potential, occurring at one node of Ranvier, generates local circuit current which depolarizes the nodes ahead of it.

propagation would occur as long as the current was large enough to activate the next node. In practice, the internodal distance is considerably shorter than this, because as we have seen earlier, even though current flow is instantaneous in all parts of a circuit, the time taken for the voltage to reach threshold is long for a small current, and this would counteract the gain in distance. The internodal distance is nicely calculated in nature to give the optimum increase in velocity; this also has the advantage that there is a considerable safety factor built in, preventing failure of propagation. The safety factor for transmission can, however, become an important variable affecting information transfer under some conditions – for example, after anaesthesia and at branch points (where the invading local circuit current has to depolarize a larger area of membrane). Failure can also occur at high frequencies.

In the nodes of Ranvier, the Na channels are much more densely packed than in unmyelinated nerves, which may be one reason why myelinated nerves need higher concentrations of local anaesthetics to block them. It is interesting that, in mammalian nodes, the voltage-sensitive K channels are absent. At the temperature of warm-blooded animals, Na channel inactivation proceeds rapidly enough to repolarize the nodes without necessitating an increase in K permeability. The action potentials thus do not have an after-hyperpolarization. This is probably an economical measure, since without the contaminating outward current, less Na ions are involved in the action potential, and therefore less energy is needed pumping them out.

Further reading

Aidley, D.J. (1989) *The Physiology of Excitable Cells*, 3rd edn. Cambridge University Press, Cambridge.

Bennett, M.R. (1972) *Autonomic Neuromuscular Transmission.* Cambridge University Press, Cambridge.

Hammond, C. (1997) *Cellular and Molecular Neurobiology*. Academic Press, London.

Hille, B. (1991) *Ionic Channels of Excitable Membranes*, 2nd edn. Sinauer Associates Inc., Sunderland, Massachusetts.

Hodgkin, A.L. (1957). Ionic movements and electrical activity in giant nerve fibres. *Proc. Roy. Soc. B.* **148**, 1–37.

References

Hodgkin & Huxley (1952). *See Hodgkin, A.L. (1957).*

Horisberger, J.D., Lemas, V., Kraehenbuhl, J.P. & Rossier, B.C. (1991) Structure function relationship of Na-K-ATPase. *Ann. Rev. Physiol.* **53**, 565.

Moffet, D.F., Moffet, S.B. & Schauf, C.L. (1993) *Human Physiology: Foundations and Frontiers.* Mosby, St Louis.

4: Neuromuscular and Synaptic Transmission

4.1 Introduction

The terminal branches of a nerve form connections with an effector cell, which are called synapses (particularly when the connection is with another neurone) or junctions (for instance, neuromuscular junctions). At these sites, action potentials travelling down the nerves release chemicals (transmitters) from the presynaptic element, which interact with the postsynaptic cell. Commonly, the interaction involves the transmitter binding to and activating a specific postjunctional receptor. The transmitters may be excitatory (leading to activation of the postjunctional cell) or inhibitory (leading to suppression of activity in the postjunctional cell). Excitatory transmitters normally depolarize the postjunctional cell, and the transient depolarization caused by a single action potential is known variously as an end-plate potential (EPP, on striated muscle), an excitatory postsynaptic potential (EPSP, on neurones) or an excitatory junction potential (EJP, on autonomic effectors such as smooth and cardiac muscles). Inhibitory transmitters also often cause changes in the membrane potential of the postjunctional cell, usually hyperpolarising. These are called inhibitory postsynaptic potentials (IPSPs) or inhibitory junction potentials (IJPs). These potential changes are particularly important when the postsynaptic cell is excitable. It should be pointed out, however, that many transmitters can produce their effects through mechanisms that bypass the membrane potential changes. This is particularly true for autonomic effectors.

In this chapter, all the processes involved in the chemical transmission of the signal between a nerve and the cell that it innervates will be discussed. This will include the anatomy of the junctions, the identity of the transmitters, their synthesis, storage and release, prejunctional and postjunctional consequences of their release and processes involved in the termination of their action. Some of these processes are covered in more detail in Chapters 5 and 6. First, the well-studied events that are known to occur at the neuromuscular junction (NMJ) will be used to highlight the similarities and very significant differences between neuromuscular transmission in the somatic and autonomic nervous systems, and, finally, ganglionic synaptic transmission will be considered.

4.1.1 Changing perspective

Transmission in the autonomic nervous system clearly involves transmission at both ganglionic and postganglionic synapses. Many textbooks imply that the ganglia in the autonomic nervous system act as simple relays between preganglionic and postganglionic neurones. They also suggest that, in contrast to the discrete neuromuscular junctions in the somatic nervous system, the postganglionic neurones of the autonomic system release transmitter diffusely from their nerve terminals, which then diffuses through the extracellular fluid and bathes the entire surface of the effector cell. Both of these are misconceptions. Ganglia turn out to be important integrating centres, and more detailed electron microscopy and electrophysiological studies have demonstrated a very much more precise innervation of the final effectors than was originally believed. The idea of a diffuse innervation was based largely on the fact that, in contrast to skeletal muscle in which bath-applied acetylcholine is pretty ineffective, natural agonists can easily activate or inhibit smooth and cardiac muscles when applied exogenously, implying that the bath-applied agonist has easy access to the receptors. Also, nerve varicosities in random cross-sections of autonomic effectors are often some distance from the nearest effector cell, and little evidence of any junctional specialisation is seen. Careful studies of serial sections with the electron microscope have revealed a different picture.

4.2 Organisation of neuro-effector junctions

4.2.1 Skeletal muscle

Nerves innervating fast skeletal muscles contact the muscle at well-defined specialised regions of the muscle fibres called end plates. The nerves are myelinated nerves of the α class, they divide as they enter the muscle, and a single neurone will innervate a group of muscle fibres, normally with a branch ending on each muscle fibre at the motor end plate. This group of muscle fibres, which is scattered through the muscle, constitutes a single motor unit. The number of muscle fibres in a motor unit depends on several factors, such as the sensitivity of control needed by the muscle, and the diameter of the nerve fibre. There may be less than ten or up to several hundred, depending on the muscle. As each axonal branch reaches the fibre it innervates, myelination stops, and the unmyelinated fibre, which is about 1 μm in diameter, divides into smaller branches which extend for about 100 μm before terminating (Fig. 4.1). The length of contact with the muscle fibre at the end plate varies between species.

Each of the muscle fibres in a skeletal muscle is electrically isolated from its neighbours, but all muscle fibres in a motor unit are synchronously activated by the innervating neurone, an action potential invading the nerve terminal and releasing enough transmitter to depolarize each muscle fibre beyond the threshold for initiation of an action potential in the muscle fibre. The transmission is thus all-or-none: if the stimulus applied to the nerve is large enough to fire it, the end-plate potential will be large enough to activate its muscle fibre, and an all-or-none twitch will result. The response of a single muscle fibre is not graded with stimulus strength. Thus, the minimum contractile force that a skeletal muscle can produce will be caused by a single action potential in a neurone innervating the smallest motor unit of the muscle, all fibres of which will generate a synchronous twitch. Increases in force can be achieved both by increasing the number of nerve fibres activated, and by repetitive firing in them, which produces a tetanic response of the muscle fibres (Fig. 4.2). The transmitter in vertebrate NMJs is acetylcholine, acting through nicotinic receptors.

4.2.2 Postganglionic autonomic junctions

In contrast, in the postjunctional autonomic nerves, all the innervating nerves are unmyelinated. The nerves branch extensively on entering the tissue, and the terminal branches alternately increase and decrease in

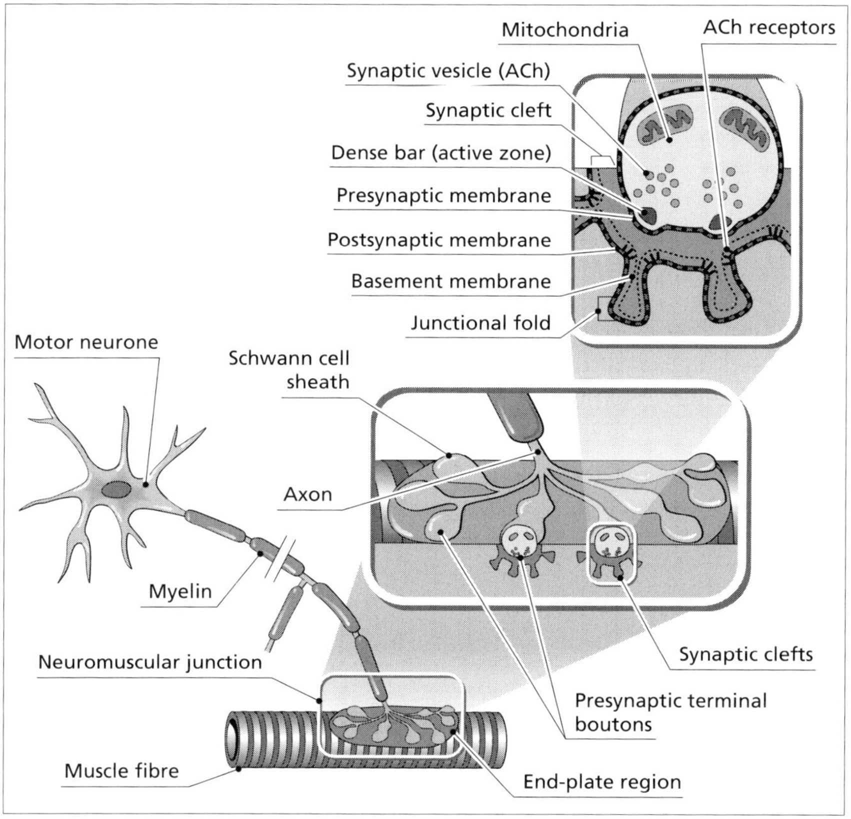

Fig. 4.1 A skeletal muscle neuromuscular junction. The motor neurone branches to supply several muscle fibres. At each muscle fibre, the nerve terminal loses its myelin sheath and forms an end plate which innervates the muscle via several branches. The enlarged views of the end plate show the branches lying in shallow grooves on the muscle. The grooves have junctional folds, and in the axon terminals, there are distinct active zones aligned above the junctional folds.

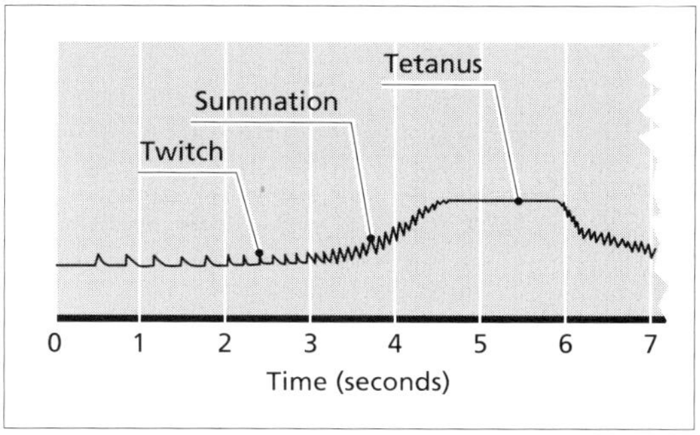

Fig. 4.2 Diagram to show the force developed by a skeletal muscle fibre in response to repetitive stimulation with increasing and then decreasing frequency. Initially, there are individual twitch responses, but as the frequency increases they begin to fuse, and the force increases until finally it reaches a maximum tetanic force, which may be several times the twitch force.

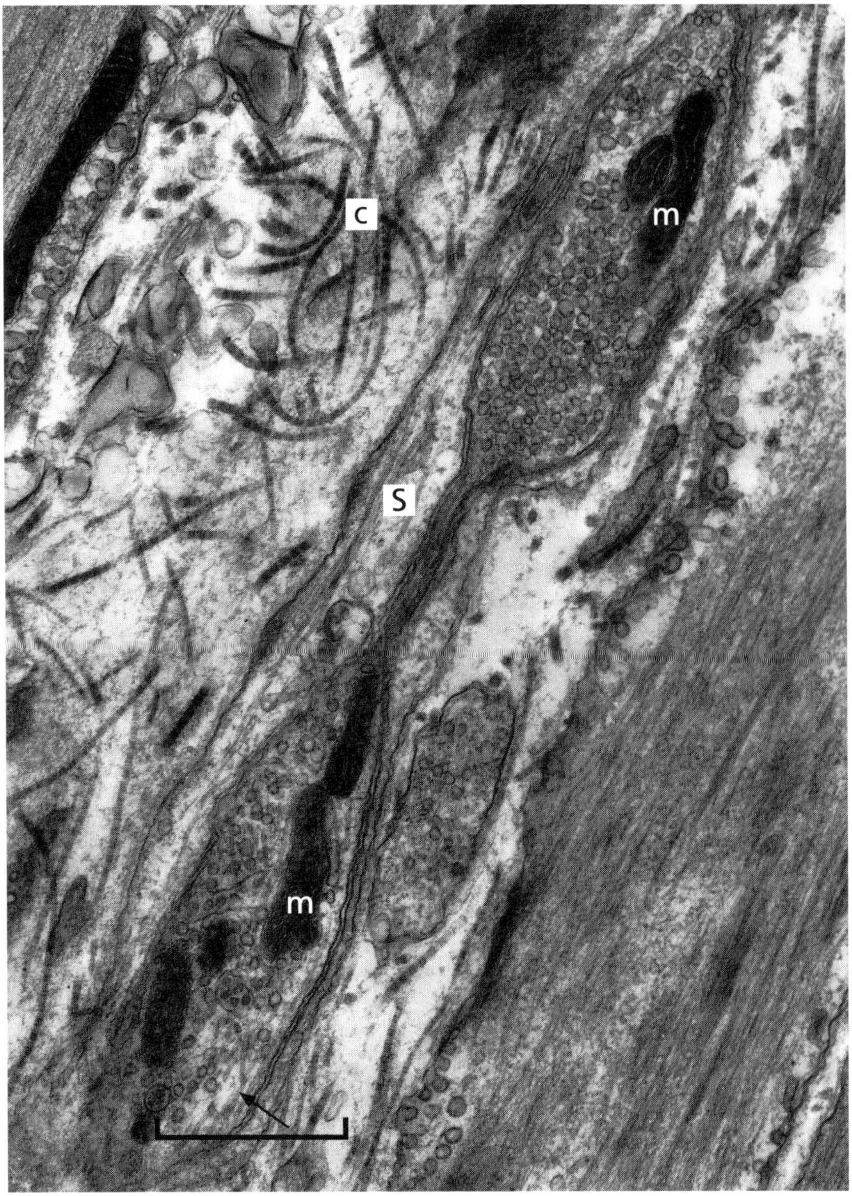

Fig. 4.3 Electron micrograph of autonomic neuromuscular junctions in the rat urinary bladder. Longitudinal section of axon. In this electron micrograph of the bladder muscle coat, a terminal axon, extending from the bottom left corner to the top right corner, is made up of two expansions or varicosities and a narrow intervaricose segment. The entire profile of the axon is sheathed by a Schwann cell (S). The varicosities are packed with vesicles and mitochondria (m) and a few microtubules (arrow); the intervaricose segment is occupied by microtubules. At the bottom right and top left corner are muscle cells, sectioned longitudinally. In the spaces between cells are collagen fibrils in various orientations (c). Scale bar: 1 μm. Micrograph kindly supplied by G. Gabella.

diameter every few microns, giving them a characteristic beaded or varicose appearance (Figs. 4.3 & 4.4). These varicosities contain the synaptic vesicles, and are specialised for the release of transmitters from the prejunctional axons. Terminal branches of each individual fibre may have several hundred varicosities, and a single neurone may have 20000 or more. The number of varicosities close to each effector cell varies depending on the tissue. In densely innervated smooth muscles, such as vas deferens or in arterioles, there may be more than one varicosity per single smooth muscle, but in less densely innervated tissue, many cells may have no varicosity near to them. The other difference between striated muscle and smooth or cardiac muscle is that, in the majority of cases, muscle cells within the latter

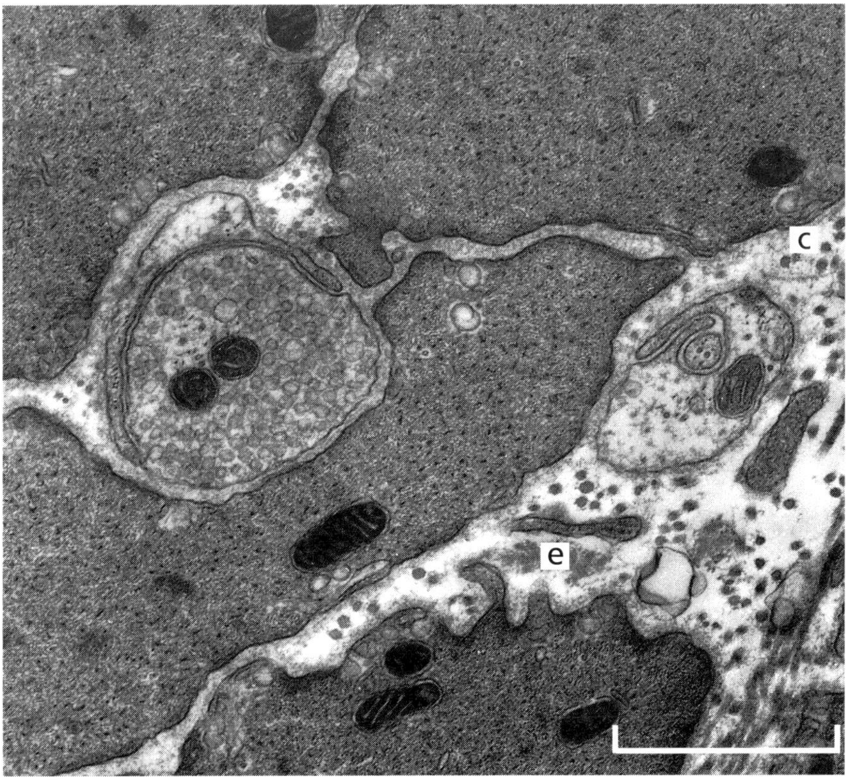

Fig. 4.4 Electron micrograph of autonomic neuromuscular junctions in the rat urinary bladder. Cross-section of axon. This section through the muscle coat of the urinary bladder, shows part of the profile of four smooth muscle cells, of irregular shape and close to each other. Between the muscle cells are two axons, one sectioned through an expansion or varicosity, the other sectioned through an intervaricose portion. The varicosity is packed with vesicles, two mitochondria and a few microtubules, and it is only partially wrapped by a Schwann cell process; the uncovered portion of the varicosity lies very close to the surface of a muscle cell and is a site of neuromuscular transmission. In contrast, the intervaricose axonal profile is fully sheathed by a Schwann cell process and contains only two microtubules and a few neurofilaments. In the intercellular space there are collagen fibrils (c) and some small elastic fibres (e). Scale bar: 1 μm. Micrograph kindly provided by G. Gabella.

two are electrically coupled, and do not behave as separate units. Thus, a single effector cell in the autonomic nervous system may be affected by transmitter released from several different nerves – either directly, or indirectly through local current flow from neighbouring cells. In contrast to the skeletal NMJ, junction potentials recorded from single smooth and cardiac muscles are graded in size with the strength of stimulus applied to the nerve (Fig. 4.5). This is because larger stimulus strengths will activate more nerve fibres, and increase the amount of transmitter affecting a single cell.

Another major difference is that many different transmitters can be released from postganglionic autonomic nerves. The main ones are acetylcholine from parasympathetic and some sympathetic neurones, and noradrenaline from most sympathetic neurones. These 'classical' neurones will also often release more than one active compound, and these may be co-transmitters, or modulators of transmission. Apart from this there are a number of non-adrenergic, non-cholinergic nerves containing a variety of excitatory or inhibitory transmitters.

4.3 Fine structure of neuro-effector junctions

The chemicals released from nerve terminals are packaged into synaptic vesicles, which vary depending on the transmitter involved, but are characteristic features of all secretory nerve terminals. The presynaptic and postsynaptic elements are separated by a synaptic cleft, which may vary in width depending on the tissue, but is normally small, 20–100 nm. Postsynaptic specialisations are present at some, but not all, junctions.

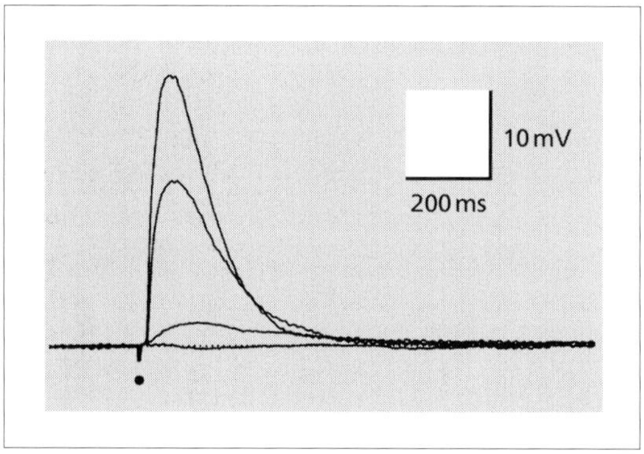

Fig. 4.5 Excitatory junction potentials recorded with intracellular microelectrodes from a smooth muscle cell in a strip of guinea-pig urinary bladder, in which the postjunctional parasympathetic nerves were stimulated with single voltage pulses (0.5 ms) of increasing stimulus strength. Action potentials in the smooth muscle were blocked by including 10 μM nifedipine in the bathing solution. The junction potential increases in size with increased stimulus strength. The resting potential of the cell was –52 mV. From Bramich & Brading (1996).

4.3.1 The skeletal neuromuscular junction

This has been examined in great detail. In different species, the nerve terminals end either with several naked branches lying in gutters on the muscle surface, as seen in the frog (Fig. 4.6), or in ovoid clusters of swollen nerve endings that indent the surface of the muscle fibre, as seen in mammals (see Fig. 4.1). In either case, the synaptic clefts are narrow, only about 50–100 nm in diameter, and the nerve terminals contain small clear synaptic vesicles of about 50 nm in diameter. In the frog, the end-plate region extends for as much as 0.5 mm along the fibre, and this has allowed detailed analysis of the junctional structure. Each branch runs in a gutter, and the gutter contains periodic deep transverse folds or clefts that occur at intervals of about a micron, and penetrate for a similar distance (Fig. 4.7). In mammals, and particularly humans, these clefts are deeper. The surface of the nerve terminal

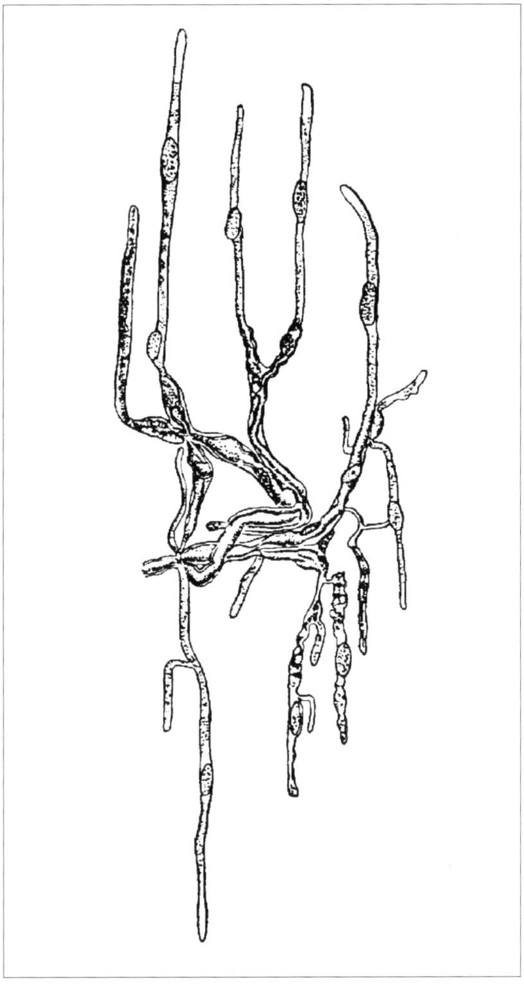

Fig. 4.6 Drawing showing the terminal arborization of an axon innervating a single frog skeletal muscle fibre. From Kuhne (1887). The terminal branches are sheathed in Schwann cells; their nuclei are visible along the branches.

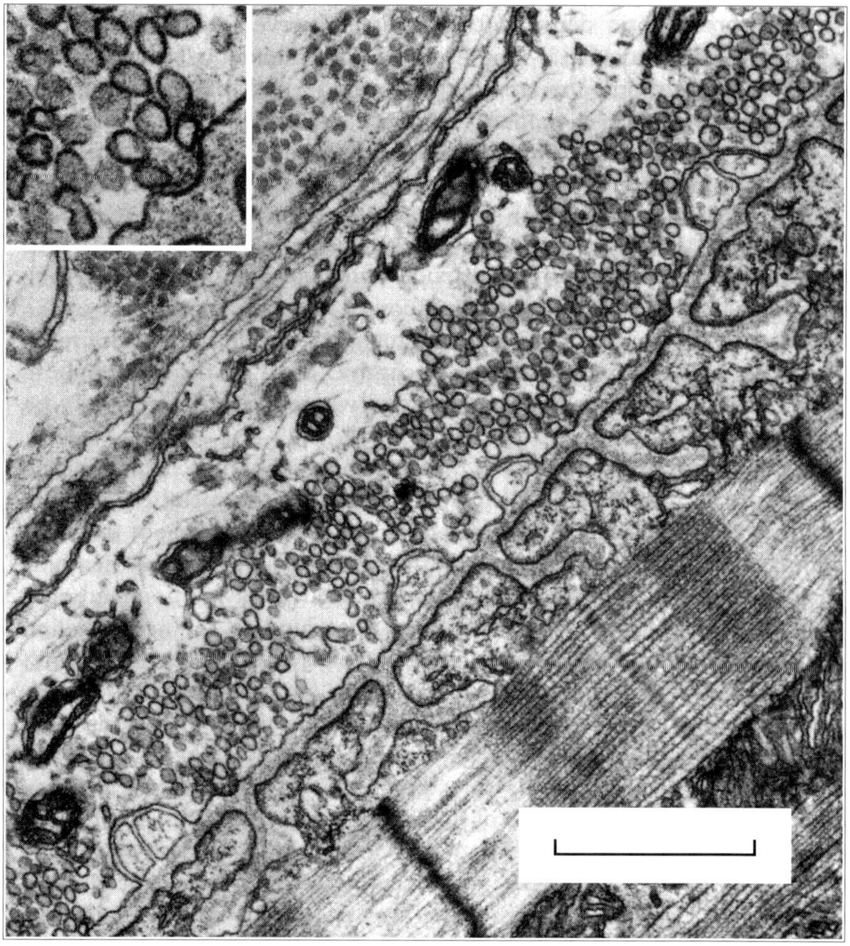

a

Fig. 4.7 Detailed structure of a frog neuromuscular junction. (a) Electron micrograph of a longitudinal section of a frog neuromuscular junction. Note the postjunctional folds lying above the sarcomere, and the clusters of vesicles around electron-dense tufts in the presynaptic nerve membrane that overlie the folds (inset shows one at higher magnification). Finger-like processes of a Schwann cell penetrate between the pre- and postsynaptic membranes at intervals along the axon. Scale bar: 1 μm. Reprinted from Heuser (1976) by permission of the publisher, Academic Press Limited, London. (b) Three- dimensional view of pre- and postsynaptic membranes showing active zones with adjacent rows of synaptic vesicles as well as places where the vesicles are undergoing exocytosis. The split membranes show predicted images of the structures in freeze fracture. The membrane leaflet nearest the cytoplasm is the P (protoplasmic) face, and the one nearest the outside is the E (external) face. Adapted from Kuffler *et al.* (1984).

that lies above these folds contains a ring of specialised transmitter release sites, which can be seen with electron microscopy in freeze-fractured preparation as a double row of intramembrane particles, and in cross-sections as electron-dense tufts associated with clusters of clear synaptic vesicles, about 50 nm in diameter (Fig. 4.8). The particles mark the position of

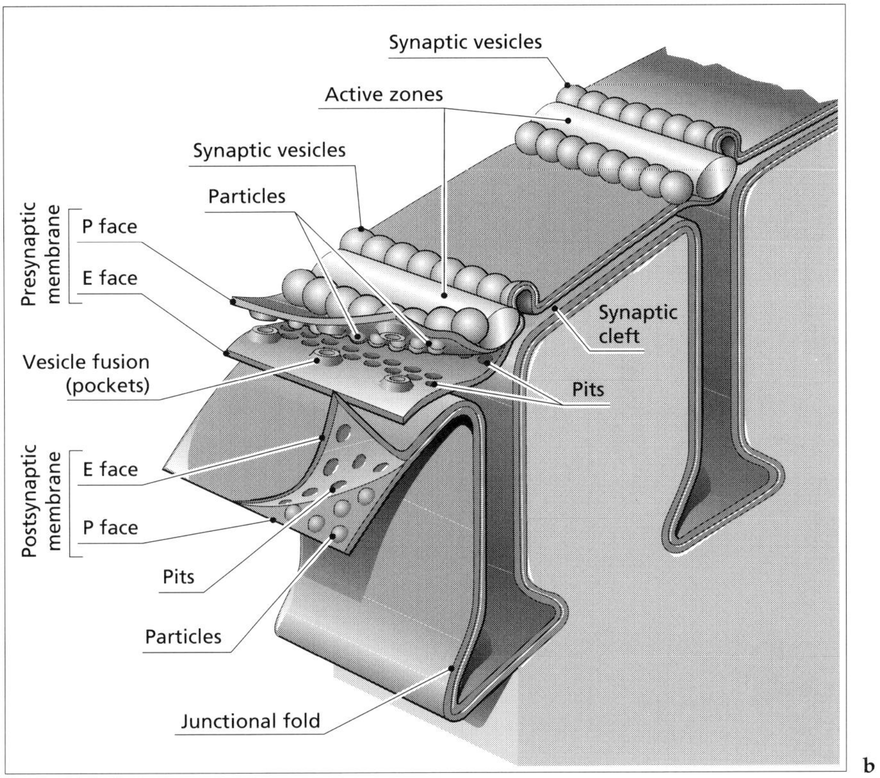

Fig. 4.7 *Continued.*

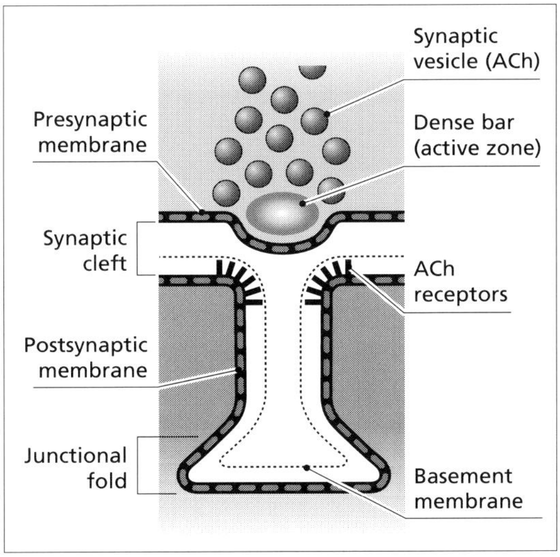

Fig. 4.8 Diagram of detailed arrangement of release site and postjunctional fold of a skeletal neuromuscular junction.

voltage-sensitive Ca channels. There may be about 500 of these rows (or release zones) in each frog neuromuscular junction, and each row has release sites for about 40 vesicles, suggesting that a single NMJ has about 20 000 release sites. For a single motor nerve, this number has to be multiplied by the number of muscle fibres in a motor unit. The acetylcholine receptors are localised in the membranes at the top and the sides of the clefts immediately under the release zones, and acetylcholinesterase molecules are associated with the basal lamina in the synaptic cleft. The whole nerve terminal is covered by a Schwann cell, which sends out periodic finger-like processes that run embracing the terminal between the active zones (Fig. 4.7).

4.3.2 The autonomic neuro-effector junction

In contrast to these massive structures, the varicosities that are the equivalent structures in the autonomic nerves are very small, with dimensions of one to a few microns, each probably only having a very few release sites. Again in contrast with the skeletal NMJ, there is rarely any morphological evidence of postsynaptic specialisations. Although random cross-sections do not often show close contacts between nerves and muscle, careful reconstructions using serial sections and electron microscopy show that, in the majority of tissues, at least part of every varicosity is bare of Schwann cell and forms a close contact (35–75 nm) with an effector cell (Fig. 4.9). The varicosities may contain predominantly small clear vesicles (presumably cholinergic) or predominantly small dense-cored vesicles (presumably adrenergic), or mainly large dense-cored vesicles, although these are also often present in small numbers in the other varicosities (Fig. 4.10). Acetylcholinesterase is present in the membrane of many nerve terminals, particularly those containing small clear vesicles.

4.3.3 Release sites

A combination of light microscopy, looking at the histological reconstruction of neurones from serial sections, and electron microscopy, providing more detailed studies of junctional structure, allows rough estimations of the numbers of release sites in various neurones. It is instructive for students to remember that whether we are talking about somatic or autonomic motor neurones, or sensory neurones, the numbers of release sites are likely to be considerable – although the exact number that can be supported by a neurone will depend on the supply of material from the nucleus, and will decline with the diameter of the axon (since access will depend on the cross-sectional area, which in turn depends on the square of the radius). However, even in the smallest unmyelinated postsynaptic nerves, there are probably tens of thousands of potential release sites, and with the exception of some powerful and specialised inputs, such as the skeletal neuromuscular junc-

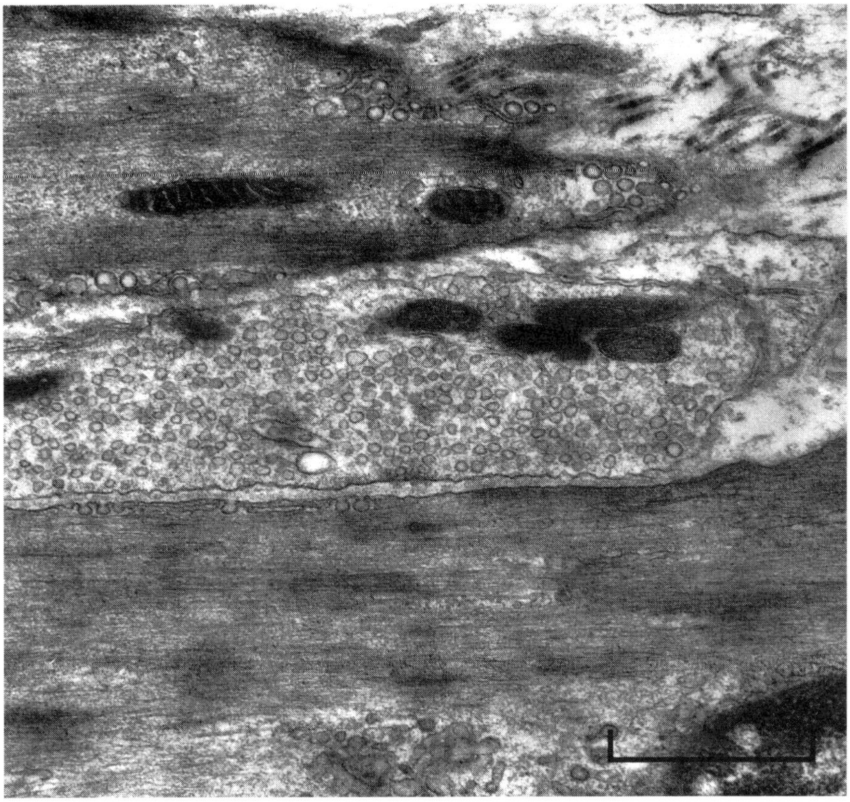

Fig. 4.9 Autonomic neuro-effector junction. This electron micrograph shows a longitudinal section of a muscle bundle in the rat urinary bladder. Two muscle cells are cut longitudinally, and show filaments and organelles; at the bottom right corner part of the nucleus is visible. Between the muscle cells is an expanded axon, or varicosity, which is packed with vesicles and mitochondria; this axon is unsheathed and its membrane lies very close to the surface of the muscle cells. In the top right corner are collagen fibrils. Scale bar: 1 μm. Micrograph kindly supplied by G. Gabella.

tion, the release sites are likely to be affecting a large population of postsynaptic cells. Certainly, on a structural basis, simple one-to-one coupling does not occur, and the nervous system innervates diffusely, and with enormous convergence and divergence of inputs.

4.4 Synthesis, storage and metabolism of transmitters

In this section, we will outline what is currently known of the synthesis, storage and metabolism of the two most important transmitters in the autonomic nervous system, acetylcholine and noradrenaline; we will then look in more detail at the experimental approaches that have allowed us to understand the mechanisms of transmission.

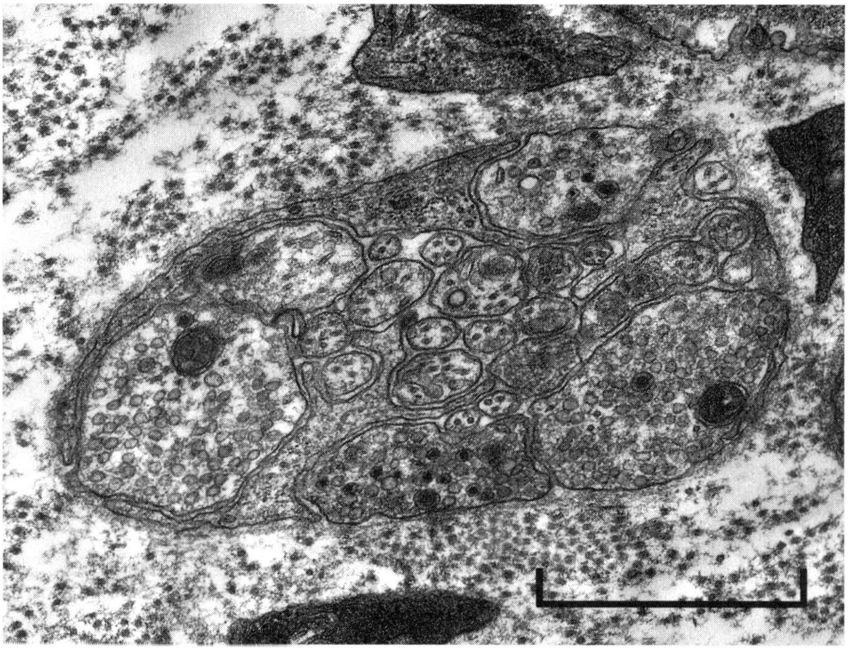

Fig. 4.10 Section of a small intramuscular nerve bundle in a guinea-pig large intestine. The bundle, which is surrounded by collagen fibrils and, at a distance, by processes of fibroblasts, consists of approximately two dozen axons, partly separated from each other by laminar and convoluted processes of Schwann cell. The axons display mainly microtubules, except for a few which are packed by small agranular vesicles or by a mixture of small granular and agranular vesicles. Some large granular vesicles can also be seen. Scale bar: 1 μm. Micrograph kindly supplied by G. Gabella.

4.4.1 Acetylcholine

Acetylcholine is synthesised in the cytoplasm of the nerve terminal by acetylation of choline using the enzyme choline acetyltransferase, an enzyme found only where acetylcholine synthesis occurs, and thus used as a marker for cholinergic nerves (Fig. 4.11). Choline comes largely from the extracellular space, and is taken up into the nerve terminals by a special choline transport mechanism, using the energy of the Na gradient (Na choline co-transport). The choline concentration in the extracellular space is determined by the concentration in the blood (normally about 10 μmol/l), and the breakdown of secreted acetylcholine by extracellular acetylcholinesterases. Normally, about 50% of the choline released by the breakdown of acetylcholine is taken up again. The acetyl groups come from the acetylated form of coenzyme A (acetyl-CoA). The rate-limiting step for acetylcholine synthesis is the availability of choline.

The uptake of choline can be prevented experimentally by the application of hemicholinium, a molecule related to choline that competes with it for occupancy of the carrier, but is not itself transported. The cytoplasm of

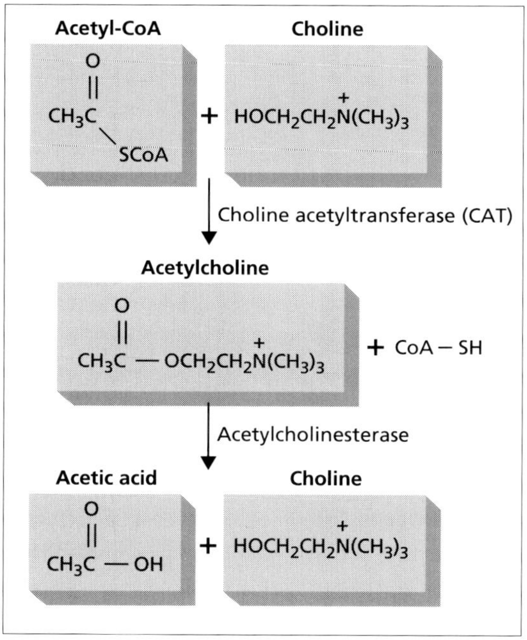

Fig. 4.11 Synthesis and metabolism of acetylcholine.

the nerve terminal also contains acetylcholinesterase, and breakdown and resynthesis of acetylcholine are constantly occurring in the cytoplasm. Blocking the cytoplasmic acetylcholinesterase by membrane-permeable blockers, such as physostigmine (eserine), increases the free acetylcholine in the nerve terminal, but this is not released. Once synthesised, acetylcholine is taken up into vesicles (see Fig. 4.12). The cholinergic nerve terminal thus contains vesicular and cytoplasmic acetylcholine, but the majority is vesicular. Evidence suggests that recently synthesised acetylcholine is preferentially released in neurotransmission. More recently filled vesicles appear to exchange acetylcholine with the cytoplasmic pool, but the probability of a vesicle being released and its ability to exchange acetylcholine seem to diminish with time. The arrangement of the junction and the drugs affecting transmission are shown in Fig. 4.12.

4.4.2 Noradrenaline

In adrenergic neurones, the precursor for noradrenaline is the aromatic amino acid L-tyrosine. This is taken up by adrenergic neurones from the extracellular space. In the cytosol, L-tyrosine is converted by hydroxylation to L-dihydroxyphenylalanine (L-DOPA) by the enzyme tyrosine hydroxylase, a reaction that needs molecular oxygen and a co-factor. This is a specific and rate-limiting step in the synthesis of catecholamines, and the reaction can be regulated by feedback inhibition, tyrosine hydroxylase being inhibited by the end-product, noradrenaline. Tyrosine hydroxylase

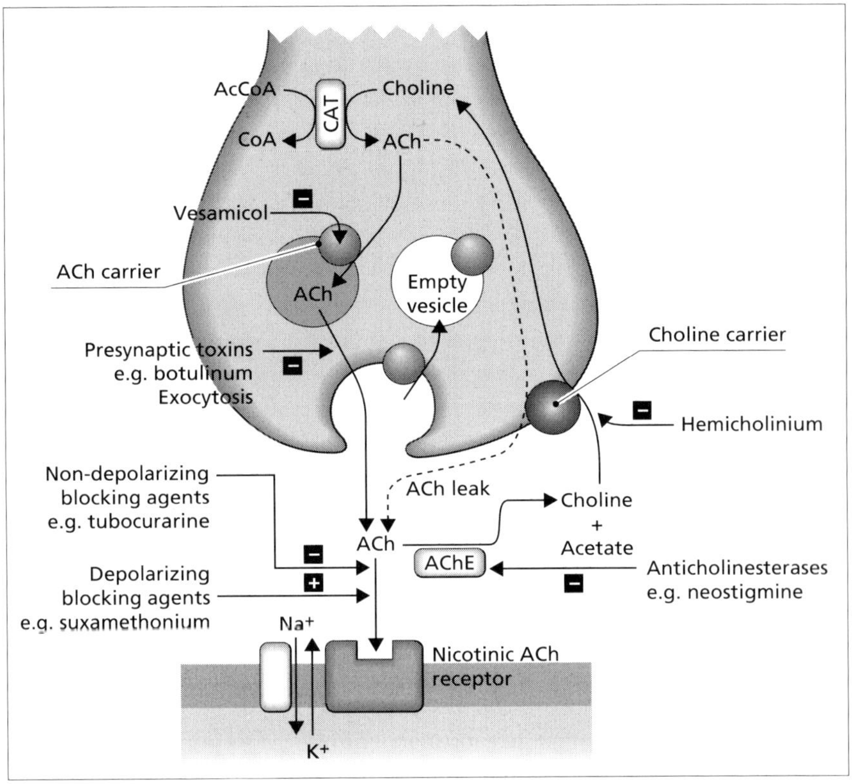

Fig. 4.12 Events and sites of drug action at a cholinergic synapse. Acetylcholine (ACh) is synthesized in the cytoplasm, and availability of choline is the rate-limiting step. Choline uptake can be blocked with hemicholinium. Uptake of ACh into the vesicles can be blocked by vesamicol. Exocytosis of the vesicles can be prevented by certain toxins, such as botulinum toxin. ACh acts on nicotinic receptors in this example, and its action can be prevented by competitive antagonists, such as tubocurarine. ACh is normally broken down by junctional acetylcholinesterase (AChE). Anticholinesterases prolong its action. Continuous activation of the nicotinic receptors by depolarizing neuromuscular blockers, such as suxamethonium, can cause inactivation of the surrounding voltage-sensitive Na channels and thus block transmission. Adapted from Rang *et al.* (1995).

activity can also be regulated by phosphorylation, through a Ca calmodulin-dependent kinase, which increases its activity and allows long-term regulation so that catecholamine synthesis can keep up with secretion. L-DOPA is then converted into the first catecholamine of the series, dopamine, by the enzyme DOPA decarboxylase, a cytoplasmic enzyme that is fairly non-specific in its requirements, and is also involved in the synthesis of 5-hydroxytryptamine (5-HT) and histamine. Dopamine is then taken up into vesicles (see below). In some neurones, dopamine is the final transmitter, but in adrenergic nerves it is converted within the vesicle to noradrenaline by the enzyme dopamine-β-hydroxylase, which is present in the vesicle (mostly bound to the wall, although there is a small amount of

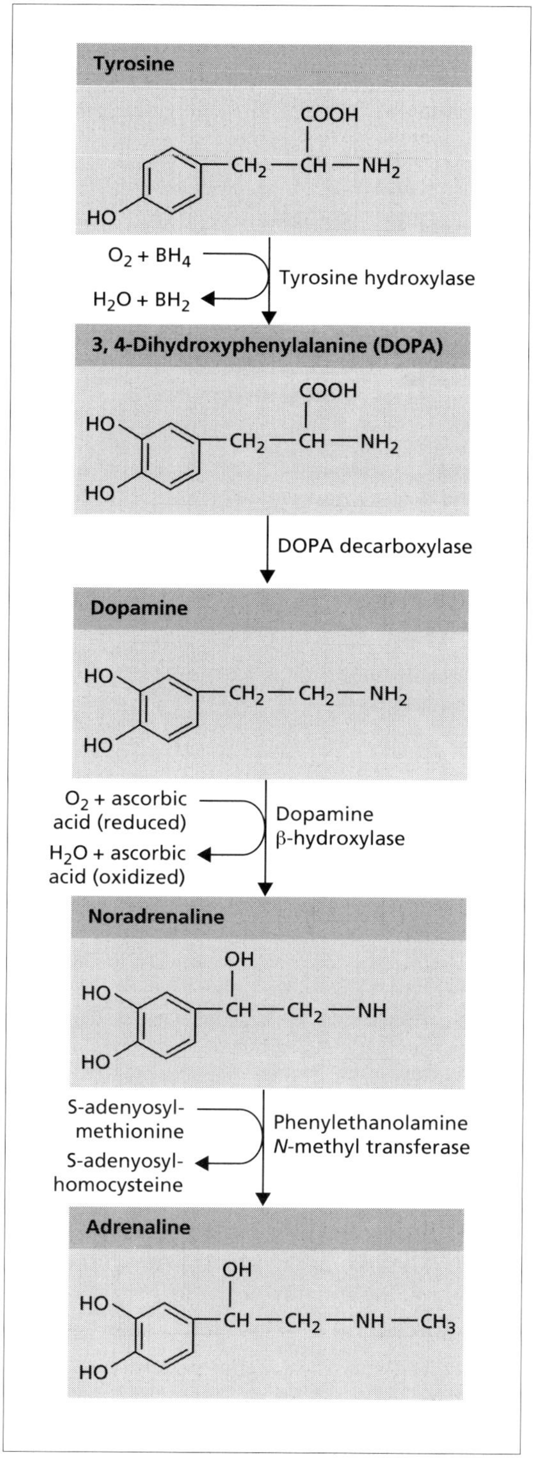

Fig. 4.13 Biosynthesis of catecholamines. The first two steps occur in the cytoplasm, but dopamine-β-hydroxylase is only present in the vesicles, and so dopamine is taken up into the vesicles for synthesis to noradrenaline. In tissues that synthesise adrenaline, the enzyme phenylethanolamine *N*-methyltransferase is a cytoplasmic enzyme, and so noradrenaline has to leave the vesicles to be methylated, and then retaken up for exocytosis.

enzyme that is released during exocytosis) (Fig. 4.13). In cells that secrete adrenaline, noradrenaline has to return to the cytoplasm for the addition of a methyl group by the enzyme phenylethanolamine *N*-methyltransferase (PNMT), before re-uptake into vesicles.

After release, noradrenaline is taken up into the nerve terminal unchanged through a specific Na-dependent carrier (uptake 1), which can also transport adrenaline. This is a powerful uptake mechanism, and it is also responsible for lowering the concentration of adrenaline in the blood stream after its release from the adrenal medulla. The catecholamines can then either be taken up into the vesicles, or metabolised in the cytoplasm. There are no extracellular enzymes in the synaptic cleft, so removal of catecholamines relies on diffusion and cellular uptake. Some uptake is through a different carrier (uptake 2) into non-neural cells such as smooth muscle. Neurones contain monoamine oxidase (MAO), which is bound to the surface of mitochondria, and which converts catecholamines to their corresponding aldehydes, a first step in their further degradation. Smooth muscle and non-neural cells also contain catechol-*O*-methyltransferase (COMT), which produces a methoxy derivative that can then be oxidised by MAO. MAO can be inhibited, causing an increase in cytoplasmic catecholamines and also an increase in the vesicular pool, resulting in an enhanced adrenergic transmission (Fig. 4.14).

4.5 Filling, release and re-formation of synaptic vesicles

Filling of synaptic vesicles is achieved again through a carrier-mediated transport using the energy of a proton gradient, generated by a proton pump. This is a membrane adenosine triphosphatase (ATPase) that transports hydrogen ions electrogenically into the vesicle, thus generating an inside positive potential across the vesicle wall and a proton gradient. How this is used in filling the vesicle depends on the transmitter involved (Fig. 4.15).

In cholinergic nerves, the vesicle membrane is probably permeable to chloride, and the potential generated by electrogenic H^+ movement allows passive Cl^- uptake. A specific carrier couples proton diffusion down its gradient with acetylcholine uptake, allowing concentration of acetylcholine chloride, the final concentration being limited by the osmolarity of the vesicle contents. The vesicles also contain some adenosine triphosphate (ATP). In vesicles from electric organs the actylcholine : ATP ratio is 3–7 : 1.

In adrenergic nerves, the carrier allowing uptake of dopamine into the vesicles can also transport noradrenaline and adrenaline. The catecholamine is thought to be transported across the vesicle membrane in its uncharged form, and is then protonated once inside the vesicle, rendering it impermeable. The vesicles also contain a protein, chromogranin A, which can bind catecholamines, and ATP (about four molecules for each catecholamine molecule). The final concentration of noradrenaline is

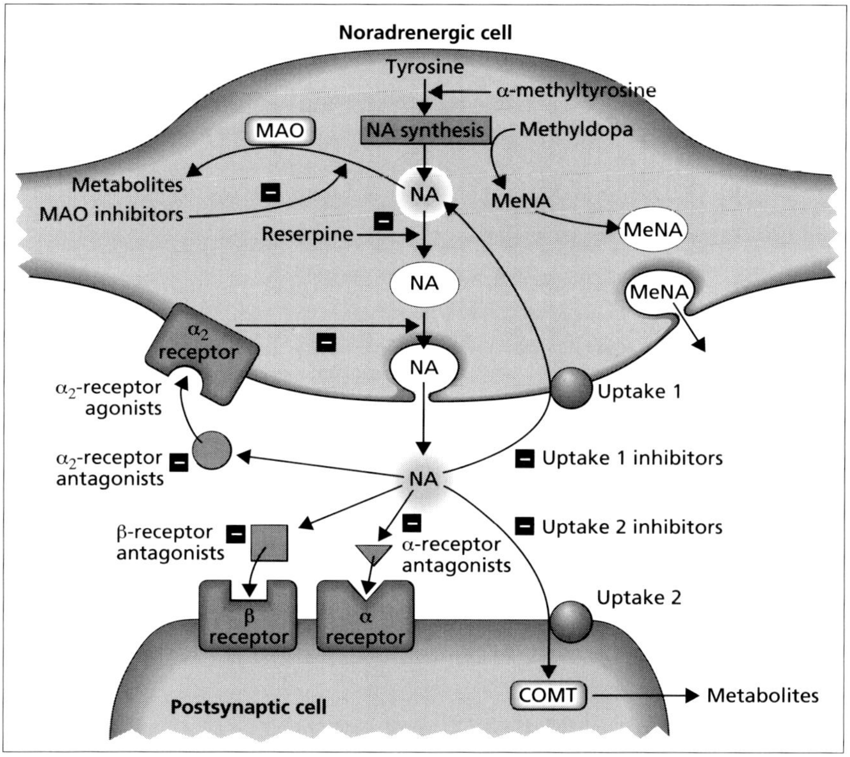

Fig. 4.14 Events and sites of action of drugs at a noradrenergic nerve terminal. Synthesis of noradrenaline (NA) can be competitively inhibited by α-methyltyrosine. Supplying the cell with methyldopa can lead to the synthesis and release of the false transmitter methylnoradrenaline (MeNA). NA in the cytoplasm is metabolized by monoamine oxidase (MAO), and the NA content of the varicosity can be increased by MAO inhibitors. Reserpine selectively blocks the uptake of catecholamines into the synaptic vesicles. After release, NA can act postsynaptically on various classes of catecholamine receptor, and can also act presynaptically to reduce its own release through α_2 adrenoceptors. Various antagonists can block its actions. NA is removed from the cleft by uptake mechanisms into the pre- or postsynaptic cell, which can be blocked by uptake inhibitors. Postsynaptically, it is metabolized by catechol-*O*-methyltransferase (COMT). Adapted from Rang *et al*. (1995).

considerably greater than occurs with acetylcholine, concentrations reaching between 0.3 and 1 mol/l, presumably because the catecholamine is largely bound, and thus osmotically inactive. The uptake of catecholamine into the vesicle can be blocked specifically by reserpine, which does not, however, appear to block the accumulation of ATP.

Release of vesicles is triggered by the entry of calcium into nerve terminals, which occurs through voltage-activated calcium channels, opened by the depolarization produced by the invasion of the nerve action potential (Box 4.1).

It now seems clear that quantal release does not involve anything as simple as vesicles undergoing Brownian motion, randomly striking the

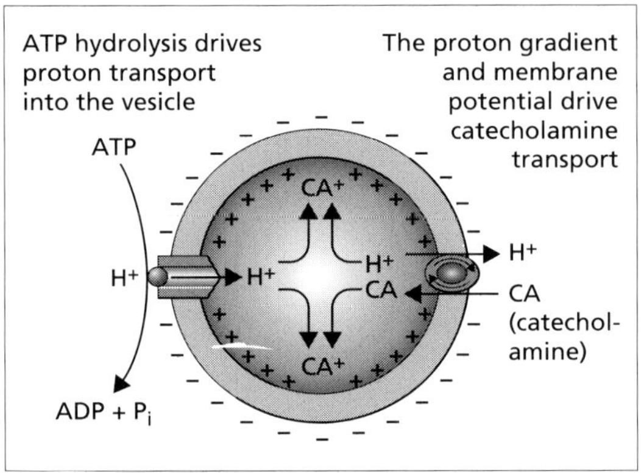

Fig. 4.15 Schematic diagram of postulated mechanism of catecholamine uptake into synaptic vesicles. A proton pump is used to accumulate H^+ in the vesicle utilizing ATP as a substrate. The H^+ gradient is then used to take up catecholamines into the vesicle through a neutral counter-transport mechanism. Once inside the vesicle the catecholamine is protonated. Adapted from Hall (1992).

Box 4.1 Factors regulating nerve terminal Ca concentration and exocytosis

There appear to be at least two types of voltage-sensitive calcium channel involved in neurotransmitter release. Analysis of the two types of channel is based on the effect of two toxins – *w-conotoxin*, which blocks calcium influx through channels that are termed *N-type* channels, and *funnel-web spider toxin*, which blocks calcium influx through channels termed *P-type* channels. Experiments with these toxins indicate that nerve-evoked transmission at the frog skeletal neuromuscular junction involves N-type channels, whereas that at the mammalian skeletal neuromuscular junction involves P-type channels. However, the calcium channels involved in transmitter release from neurones in the mammalian autonomic nervous system seem to vary unpredictably. Other types of calcium channel may also be involved.

If Ca entry triggers vesicle release, then it is important functionally that the free $[Ca]_i$ should decline rapidly. This occurs both by intracellular buffering (binding to proteins and uptake into vesicular elements similar to muscle sarcoplasmic reticulum) and by removing Ca from the nerve terminal. There is evidence that both Ca ATPase and Na/Ca exchange may be involved here (Fig. B4.1.1).

Just how Ca triggers exocytosis is not known, but evidence strongly suggests that it acts co-operatively and that the binding of several Ca ions (up to four) is needed for each vesicle fusion, giving a steep relationship between release probability and free $[Ca]_i$ (Fig. B4.1.2). This latter feature, combined with Ca removal, probably accounts for

Continued

Box 4.1 *Continued*

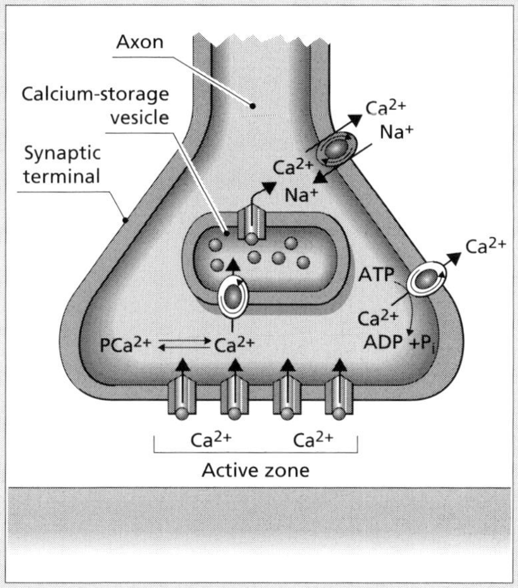

Fig. B4.1.1 Calcium influx and removal from a presynaptic nerve terminal. The invading action potential depolarizes the nerve terminal and activates voltage-sensitive calcium channels. Calcium entering can trigger exocytosis, but is then buffered by intracellular proteins (P), or taken up into calcium storage vesicles before being extruded from the nerve terminal either by Na/Ca exchange, or by a Ca ATPase. Adapted from Hall (1992).

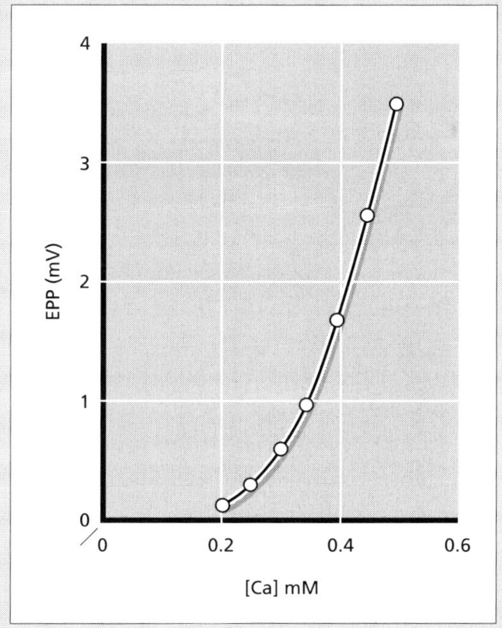

Fig. B4.1.2 Relationship between end-plate potential (EPP) size and extracellular calcium concentration in a frog neuromuscular junction. From Dodge & Rahamimoff (1967).

Continued on p. 96

Box 4.1 *Continued*

the phenomenon of facilitation. Ca entry resulting from the invading action potential will saturate a proportion of the binding sites involved in triggering release. However, since the co-operative effect of several bound Ca ions is required, as Ca buffering and extrusion begin to lower $[Ca]_i$, Ca dissociation from the binding sites will rapidly reduce the release probability, which will decline to baseline values while the free $[Ca]_i$ is still elevated above normal. A second action potential arriving during this time will thus elevate $[Ca]_i$ to a higher level, increasing the release probability and the size of the junction potential (Fig. B4.1.3).

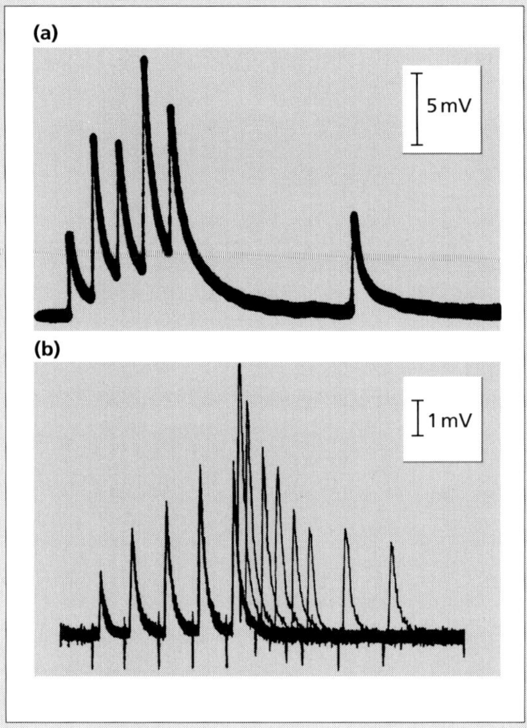

Fig. B4.1.3 End-plate potentials recorded with an intracellular microelectrode in a bathing solution containing 12 mM $MgCl_2$ to reduce the release of quanta. (a) Recording during a train of five shocks (stimulus interval 20 msec) followed by a single test shock 140 msec later. Note summation and facilitation of end-plate potentials. (b) Averaged responses showing the effect of leaving different time intervals before the test shock. The release probability is increased after the train, and declines with time, presumably as intracellular free calcium concentrations fall back to normal. From Mallert & Martin (1967).

plasma membrane and releasing their contents, as was initially proposed. Complex events occur to fill vesicles, move them towards the release sites, dock them with the membrane, initiate membrane fusion and transmitter release and bring about membrane retrieval. The process of exocytosis of

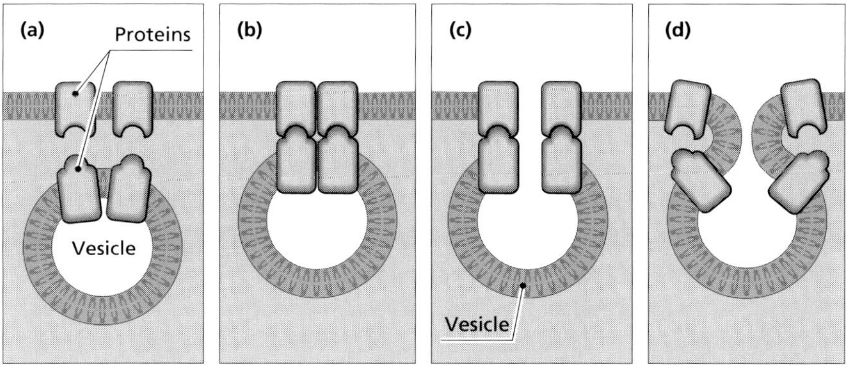

Fig. 4.16 Possible mechanism for exocytosis. Interaction between specific proteins in the vesicle and on the membrane of the synaptic terminal may occur, resulting in pore formation. Phospholipids from the membrane may then insert themselves between the subunits of the pore to enlarge it and allow the two membranes to fuse. Adapted from Almers (1990).

vesicles from glands and other non-neuronal secreting cells, such as mast cells, is undergoing extensive study, both electrophysiological (following increases in membrane capacitance as vesicles fuse with the plasma membrane) and biochemical. Some of the processes involved are described in Chapter 6. Synapses are too small for these detailed studies, but several specific proteins have been found associated with vesicles: one of these is synapsin, which can bind with cytoskeletal proteins, such as actin, and to vesicles, and is thought to play a role in vesicle transport; another is synaptophysin, which resembles gap junction protein and may be involved with the initial pore formation between the vesicle and plasma membrane, which is then followed by pore widening and vesicle fusion (Fig. 4.16).

After exocytosis, the membrane is retrieved through coated pits, which become incorporated into cisternae, from which vesicles are re-formed (Fig. 4.17).

4.5.1 Presynaptic receptors

It is perhaps not surprising, considering the complex nature of the release process, that release can be enhanced or inhibited by transmitters and neuromodulators acting on presynaptic receptors. Some examples of presynaptic receptors and their effects are shown in Table 4.1. The mechanisms that are involved have only been elucidated in a few cases, but are likely to include second-messenger-mediated phosphorylation of proteins. In most instances, the primary transmitter has an inhibitory presynaptic effect on its own input – auto-inhibition. This seems to be important in preventing unnecessary amounts of transmitter release. The presynaptic nerve terminal normally also has several other receptors that can be affected by circulating or

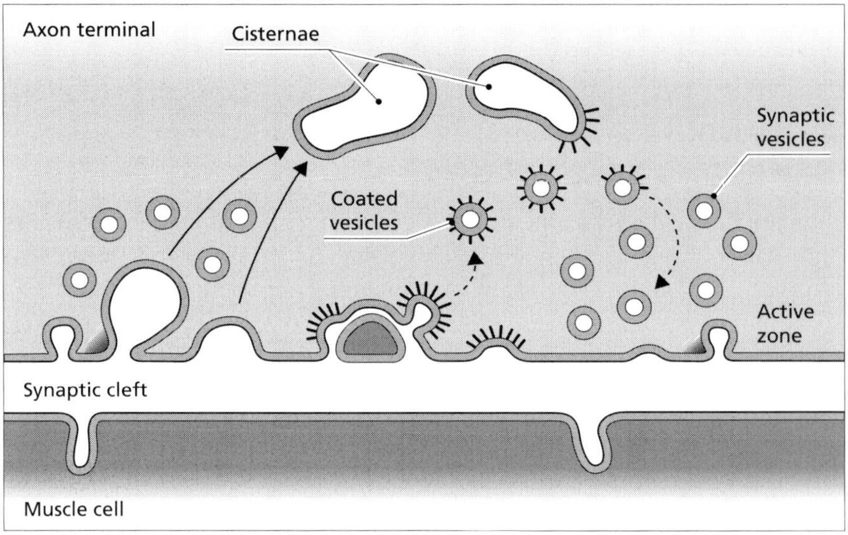

Fig. 4.17 Recycling of the vesicle membrane. Exocytosis occurs at the active zones, and the vesicle membrane is incorporated into the presynaptic membrane. Membrane, including intramembrane particles, is retrieved via coated pits, which form coated vesicles. These may fuse with the cisternae from which synaptic vesicles are re-formed (dotted arrows). After intensive stimulation uncoated pits may form to retrieve excess membrane (but not specifically retrieving membrane particles). Adapted from Miller & Heuser (1994).

Table 4.1 Some examples of presynaptic receptors.

Mediator	Receptor type	Neurone	Effect
Acetylcholine	M_2	Parasympathetic*	Inhibitory
		Sympathetic	Inhibitory
	Nicotinic	Somatic motor	Excitatory
		Parasympathetic	Excitatory
		Sympathetic postganglionic	Excitatory
Noradrenaline	α_2	Sympathetic*	Inhibitory
		Somatic motor	Excitatory
Adrenaline	β_2	Sympathetic	Excitatory
Dopamine	D_2	Sympathetic	Inhibitory
Serotonin	5-HT_1	Sympathetic	Inhibitory
ATP	P_2	Sympathetic*	Excitatory
		Parasympathetic*	Excitatory
Adenosine	P_1	Sympathetic	Inhibitory
Histamine	H_2	Sympathetic	Inhibitory
Angiotensin II	AT_1	Sympathetic	Excitatory
Enkephalin	δ	Sympathetic	Inhibitory

These receptors are on the nerve terminals releasing transmitters to the effector cells.
* Autoreceptors, i.e. presynaptic receptors mediating the effects of the released transmitters.

locally produced agonists, co-transmitters and neuromodulatory peptides, and can enhance or suppress the probability of vesicular release.

4.6 Detailed studies of junctional transmission at the vertebrate neuromuscular junction

Our present understanding of the mechanisms underlying neurotransmission started with the elegant electrophysiological studies of Katz and colleagues in the early 1950s (see Katz, 1962). Fatt and Katz carried out their experiments on amphibian nerve-muscle preparations using intracellular and extracellular recording techniques to measure the postjunctional response to acetylcholine released from the somatic motor nerves. Since in the normal preparation activation of the nerves produces all-or-none action potentials in the muscle, which obscure the details of the junctional process, they frequently used preparations in which neuromuscular transmission had been blocked either by the nicotinic receptor antagonist *d*-tubocurarine, or by reducing transmitter output through elevation of extracellular Mg or reduction in extracellular Ca concentrations. Under these conditions, the stimulation is subthreshold, and no action potentials or contraction are elicited.

4.6.1 End-plate potentials

When the skeletal muscle fibre is impaled with a microelectrode near the end-plate region, stimulation of the motor nerve innervating the muscle elicits a depolarizing EPP. Subthreshold EPPs have a rapid rise time of about 1 ms, and decay roughly exponentially in about 20 ms (Fig. 4.18). They are caused by activation of nicotinic receptors, resulting in the opening of non-selective cation channels and a net inward current, which depolarizes the membrane towards the equilibrium potential of the channels (about –10 mV). The local current flow spreads along the muscle fibre for a few mm, so that the size of the EPP declines with distance from the end plate, its size and time course being determined by the passive electrical characteristics of the muscle. In normal muscle, the EPPs are always suprathreshold, i.e. they are always large enough for triggering a muscle action potential by activating the adjacent voltage-sensitive Na channels. It has recently been shown that voltage-sensitive Na channels cluster in the postsynaptic folds, so that they are optimally placed to respond to the local circuit current.

4.6.2 Miniature end-plate potentials

If the microelectrode impalement is close enough to the end plate, small random spontaneous depolarizations are recorded – miniature end-plate potentials (MEPPs). These arise from the random impact of multimolecular

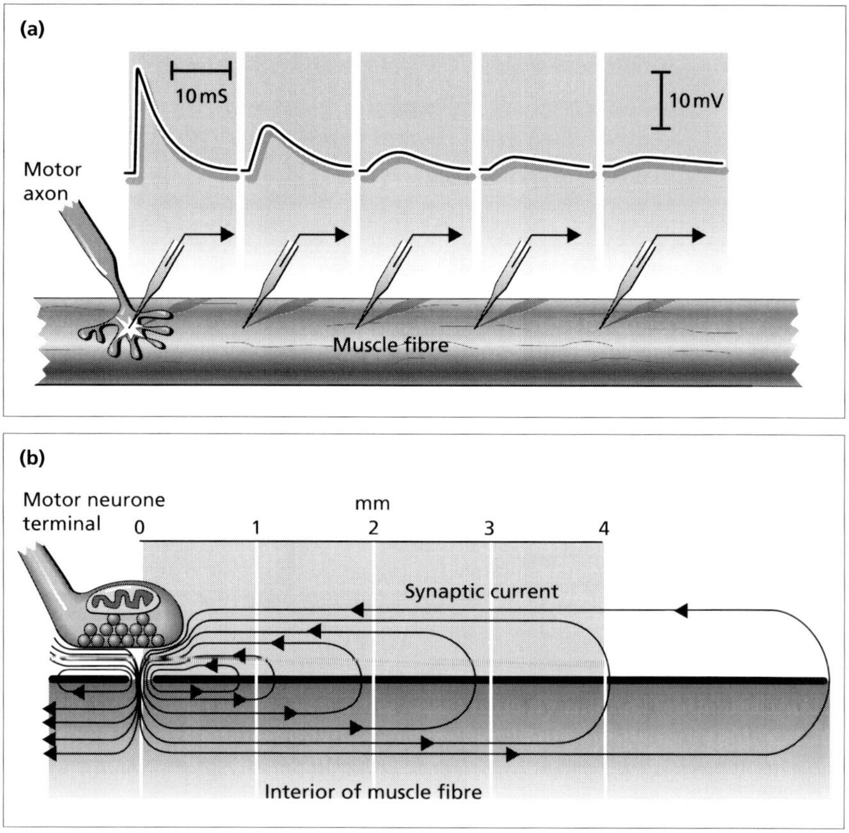

Fig. 4.18 Generation and spread of a subthreshold end-plate potential. (a) End-plate potentials recorded at increasing distances from the neuromuscular junction. (b) Current flow following transmitter release. The size and time course of the end-plate potential are determined mainly by the electrical properties of the muscle fibre (length and time constant).

packets of acetylcholine upon the nicotinic receptors on the surface of the muscle fibre at the end-plate region. They have a similar time course and similar pharmacological characteristics to the evoked EPPs, being potentiated by anticholinesterases and reduced by nicotinic receptor blockers. Their size depends on the diameter of the muscle fibre, being larger in small muscle fibres (these have higher longitudinal resistance, so that more current leaves the muscle near the end plate, giving rise to a larger potential), but on average they vary between about 0.2 and 2 mV, and their size is normally distributed (Fig. 4.19).

4.6.3 The quantal nature of transmission

The exact relationship between the spontaneous MEPP and the nerve-evoked EPP was elucidated by del Castillo and Katz in 1954 (see Katz, 1962). It was found that the amplitude of the EPP could be reduced progressively

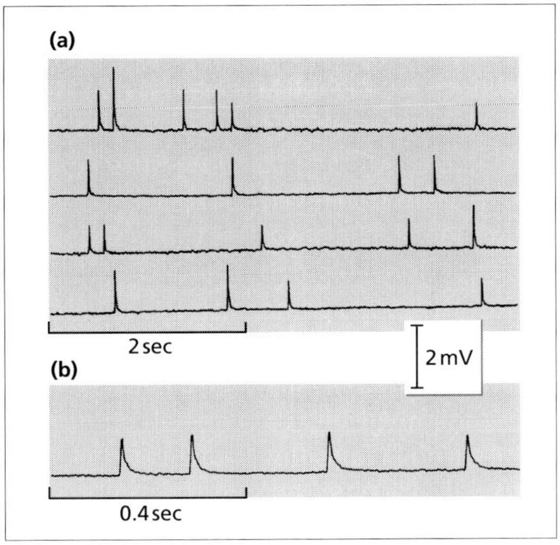

Fig. 4.19 Spontaneous miniature end-plate potentials recorded with an intracellular microelectrode at the end plate. (a) Note the randomly varying size and frequency of the events. (b) Potentials recorded with an expanded time base, showing abrupt rising phase and roughly exponential falling phase.

by increasing the Mg^{2+} and reducing the Ca^{2+} concentration. As their size approached that of the MEPP, many nerve stimuli failed to evoke an EPP, and the size of the evoked EPPs when they occurred fluctuated in amplitude in a random but stepwise manner, the step unit having a similar amplitude to the MEPP. In other words, the smallest evoked EPPs had the same amplitude distribution as the MEPPs, but there were also EPPs with amplitudes of about twice or three times the MEPP amplitude. Based on these observations, it was suggested that the EPP was composed of an integral number of all-or-none units (quanta), identical in size to the MEPP, the release of each unit following the arrival of a nerve action potential being determined in a probabilistic manner. This constituted the 'quantal hypothesis' (Box 4.2), which proposed that evoked neurotransmitter release occurred in standard multimolecular 'packets' (identical with the spontaneously released units), the size of which was independent of the event that caused the release. Students should note that, at the time when this hypothesis was formulated, there was in fact no evidence about what the quanta were in reality.

4.6.4 The vesicle hypothesis

The quantal hypothesis of chemical transmission was thus widely accepted in the early 1950s, without a morphological correlate of the quantum. However, the refinement of the technique of electron microscopy, which had recently been invented, soon allowed the identification of vesicles in the presynaptic terminals of neurones. The question naturally arose as to whether a single quantum could be equated with the amount of acetylcholine sequestered within a single vesicle. Elegant work by Kuffler and colleagues on the snake NMJ (Kuffler & Yoshikama, 1975) provided a good

Box 4.2 Tests of the quantal hypothesis

This hypothesis – that evoked neurotransmitter release occurred in standard multimolecular packets (or quanta) identical with the spontaneously released units, the size of which was independent of the event that caused the release – was tested statistically. When transmitter release was greatly suppressed, the observed fluctuations in EPP amplitude could be fitted by a 'Poisson series', whose 'unit class' was identical to the mean amplitude of spontaneously occurring MEPPs (Fig. B4.2.1). In this analysis, the mean quantal content (number of quanta in an EPP) was determined either by dividing the mean amplitude of the EPP by the mean MEPP amplitude, or from the prediction of the Poisson distribution using the number of failures (Katz 1966). Both methods produced closely similar results, providing strong

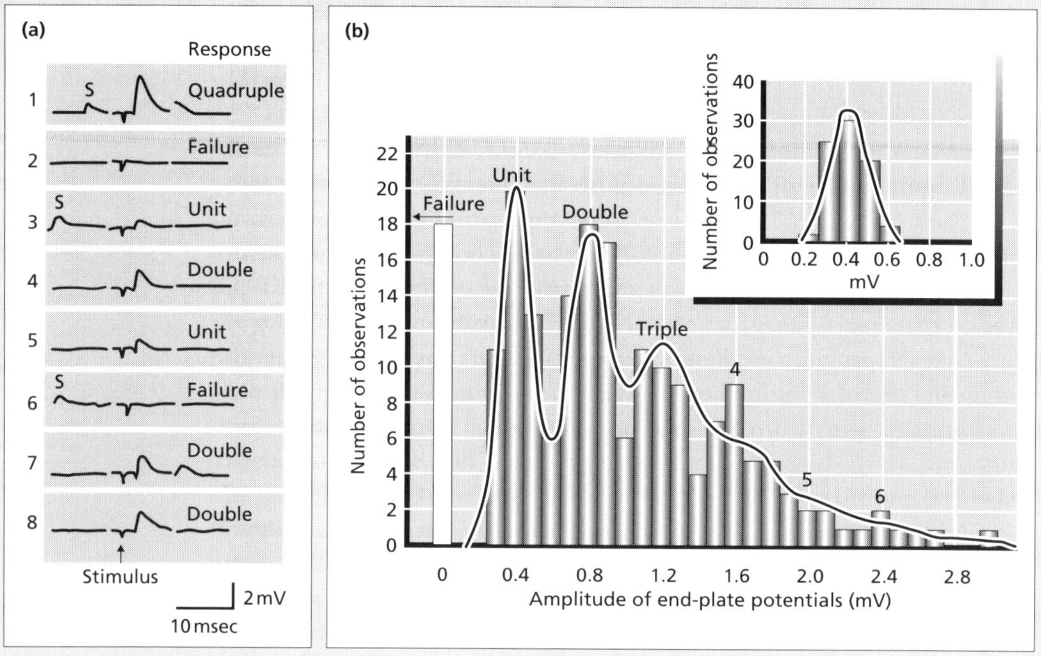

Fig. B4.2.1 Quantal release of transmitter at the neuromuscular junction. (a) End-plate potentials (EPPs) evoked by nerve stimulation in a preparation in which quantal release has been suppressed by bathing in a low calcium–high magnesium solution. Of the eight records shown, two stimuli failed to release any transmitter, in two the stimulus released a single quantum (roughly the same size as the spontaneous EPPs – S), in three it released two quanta, and in one it released four quanta. (b) Response size histograms. After a long train of stimuli, the size of each response was measured, and plotted as a histogram. The inset shows the normal distribution of the spontaneous EPPs. The solid line for the evoked EPPs shows the theoretical distribution predicted for quantal release. (a) Adapted from Liley (1956). (b) Adapted from Boyd & Martin (1956).

Continued

Box 4.2 *Continued*

support for the quantal hypothesis. Studies at other neuromuscular junctions and at chemical synapses have confirmed the quantal nature of the neurotransmitter release process.

The distribution of amplitudes of the evoked postjunctional or evoked postsynaptic potentials under normal conditions can actually rarely be fitted by Poisson statistics. The release process envisaged by Katz is inherently binomial. There is a population of n quanta and a uniform probability of releasing a single quantum p ($0 < P < 1$). The probability that a site will not release a quantum is q ($q = (1 - p)$) and the mean quantal content (m) = $n \cdot p$. Using the binomial equation requires separate estimations of n and p, which cannot be achieved unambiguously. However, if the number of quanta released is very small in comparison with the total number, as occurred in the experiments of Katz and colleagues, the binomial process simplifies to a Poisson distribution, which is easier to apply.

In a re-analysis of neurotransmitter release at the frog neuromuscular junction, Wernig (1975) suggests that, under normal conditions, p approaches 1, n being ≈ 100–200. The actual value of n would be expected to depend on the size of the nerve terminal investigated. This estimate of n is of the same order of magnitude as the number of 'active zones' described morphologically at these junctions, which are thought to be the regions of the nerve terminal specialised for neurotransmitter release. On the basis of these observations, it has been suggested, that under normal conditions, each active zone has only one active release site.

estimate of the number of acetylcholine molecules present in a quantum (less than 10 000), and calculations show that this number could sensibly be concentrated into the volume of a vesicle. The idea of transmitters being packaged in vesicles and released in an all-or-none manner became known as the vesicle hypothesis – a hypothesis that has subsequently been considered to hold true for chemical transmission in a wide variety of species and tissues.

However, although quantal release is widely accepted, the vesicle hypothesis has not been accepted by all scientists for cholinergic nerves, although it is well established for adrenergic ones. Acetylcholine is synthesised in the cytoplasm, and biochemical analysis shows that newly synthesised acetylcholine is preferentially released. After labelling with radioactive choline, the decline in radioactivity in the perfusate of stimulated synapses occur in parallel to the decline in cytoplasmic rather than vesicular acetylcholine. It has therefore been suggested that the cytoplasmic acetylcholine rather than the vesicular is the source of the quanta. The main technical problems for acetylcholine are that there are no markers that allow it to be visualised microscopically, and acetylcholine in vesicles may exchange with free acetylcholine in the cytoplasm, making it difficult to follow the source of the quanta using radiotracer experiments. There is also good evidence that acetylcholine can indeed leak out of the cytoplasm, although in a non-quantal fashion. When acetylcholine release is measured biochemically at the skeletal neuromuscular junction, it can be detected from unstimulated preparations. The MEPPs can account for only about 1% of the acetylcholine detected. It therefore seems that, apart from spontaneous and evoked quantal acetylcholine release, there is a substantial 'leakage' of acetylcholine from nerve terminals and Schwann cells.

Establishing vesicular release for sympathetic nerves has been easier. Adrenergic vesicles contain binding proteins for the catecholamines and enzymes that can be made electron-dense, or labelled by immunostaining. Thus, the vesicles can be visualised in the nerve terminals, extracted from tissues with their contents intact, and analysed, and their release can be followed both microscopically and by monitoring tissue perfusates.

4.6.5 The calcium hypothesis

The demonstration by Katz and colleagues (Katz, 1962) that the number of quanta released in response to nerve stimulation is dependent on the extracellular Ca^{2+} concentration indicated the importance of Ca^{2+} in neuromuscular transmission. In addition, they found that acetylcholine release could still be evoked by focal depolarization of the nerve terminal in preparations in which propagation of the nerve impulse had been blocked by tetrodotoxin (TTX). However, this release only occurred in the presence of Ca^{2+}. These early studies led to the idea that the release of neurotransmitter is dependent on the entry of Ca^{2+} into the nerve terminal. The calcium hypothesis is now widely believed to hold true for all nerves.

These detailed studies on the NMJ have given it the status of a model synapse. It has certainly proved true that there are many similarities between the processes involved here and other synapses, but it should be remembered that the NMJ is unique in being an all-or-none synapse, in which physiological modulation of the transmission does not occur. This is far from the case with the junctions in the autonomic nervous system, and we will now consider what is known about them.

4.7 Transmission to autonomic effectors

Until recently, little was known about the characteristic features of neurotransmitter release from postganglionic autonomic nerve terminals on an impulse-to-impulse basis. Much of our knowledge initially came from biochemical measurements of the release of tritium-labelled catecholamines from electrically stimulated preparations, and these led to some interesting conclusions.

Folkow and colleagues measured the release of noradrenaline from the vasoconstrictor nerves of cat calf muscle. They found that the fraction of the total noradrenaline released by a nerve action potential was about 1/50000 of the total noradrenaline content of the vasoconstrictor nerve endings. They made two assumptions: first, that most of the noradrenaline in the tissue is contained in vesicles in the varicosities; second, that the majority of the varicosities release neurotransmitter when excited by a nerve action potential. Estimates were made of the number of vesicles in a varicosity and the number of molecules of noradrenaline contained in a vesicle, and the fractional release of the noradrenaline store per nerve impulse was determined. The results suggested that only 1–3% of the neurotransmitter content of a vesicle is released per nerve impulse. An alternative explanation proposed by the same research group was that not all varicosities are capable of discharging neurotransmitter when depolarized by an action potential. This hypothesis requires that a noradrenergic varicosity discharges neurotransmitter only once in response to every 30–100 nerve impulses, i.e. release is intermittent.

Recording the membrane potential responses of autonomic effectors, such as cardiac and smooth muscles, to excitation of the nerves innervating them is more difficult than for the skeletal muscle, because of the smaller cells and the frequent presence of spontaneous myogenic activity, and it gives little information about release from individual varicosities. The problems arise from the far greater complexity of the innervation. As explained earlier, single effector cells may be innervated by several different nerves, which may be excitatory or inhibitory, and electrical coupling between effector cells means that the postsynaptic responses seen reflect the responses of a large number of cells and synapses. Problems about selectively activating nerves are discussed in Box 4.3.

4.7.1 Transmission in the guinea-pig vas deferens

The most detailed studies of any autonomic neuro-effector junction have been carried out on the guinea-pig vas deferens. This has the advantage of showing no spontaneous activity, and thus being mechanically quiescent unless action potentials are initiated in it in response to nerve stimulation. It is also very densely innervated by the sympathetic nervous system, and the hypogastric nerve to it can be easily isolated and stimulated. Figure 4.20a shows a fluorescent histochemical image of the dense innervation of the guinea-pig vas deferens. Figure 4.20b shows the innervation of the vas deferens as revealed by confocal microscopy; the dense innervation and characteristic 'string-of-beads' appearance of the varicose terminals are clearly evident.

Microelectrode recording

When a smooth muscle cell in the wall of the vas deferens is penetrated with a microelectrode and a single stimulus is applied to the hypogastric nerve,

Box 4.3 Selective activation of postganglionic autonomic nerves

Although it is possible in some cases to stimulate the nerve trunk innervating an autonomic effector, in most situations – and particularly in many smooth muscles – the only method of activating the nerves is by field or transmural stimulation of intrinsic nerve fibres. When this is done, it is not only the nerve fibres that are subjected to the applied voltage, but also the muscle fibres and other cells within the preparation. It is therefore important to establish whether or not the recorded electrical activity results solely from nerve excitation. Normally, pulses of more than 1 ms duration are needed before smooth muscle cells are directly excited, because of the very large area of membrane that has to be discharged. Activation of nerves can usually be achieved with pulses of less than 0.1 ms, which allows them to be selectively activated. In order to confirm that the activity recorded is in fact nerve-evoked, it is essential to demonstrate that it is abolished by agents that block nerve impulse propagation. Since the action potential in smooth muscle is generated by the activation of voltage-gated Ca^{2+} channels, whereas the action potential in neurones involves voltage-gated sodium channels, it is possible to use Na^{+} channel blockers, such as TTX to block nerve-mediated responses selectively.

When a tissue is innervated by many different types of nerve fibre, a degree of selective activation may be achieved by judicious variation of the pulse width and intensity of the applied stimulus, but this is only effective if the nerve populations are of distinctly different sizes. If the transmitters involved are known, it may be possible to achieve some selectivity by the use of selective nerve-blocking drugs. Activation of adrenergic nerves can be prevented by the adrenergic neurone-blocking agents guanethidine or bretylium. Similarly, botulinum toxin can be used to block neurotransmitter release from cholinergic fibres.

an EJP is evoked lasting some 300–2000 ms. In the absence of nerve stimulation, spontaneous excitatory junction potentials (SEJPs) occur every few seconds. Figure 4.21 shows EJPs in response to a train of stimuli, and SEJPs in an unstimulated preparation. During the train of stimuli the EJPs show marked facilitation, and a single SEJP can be seen following the fifth EJP. Examples of EJPs and SEJPs are shown in Fig. 4.21. The time courses of EJPs are some two to three times slower than those of the SEJPs, and this differs from the corresponding EPPs and MEPPs recorded at the skeletal neuromuscular junction, which have similar but much shorter time courses. In the skeletal neuromuscular junction, where muscle fibres are electrically isolated and usually innervated by a single nerve terminal, it is possible to analyse statistically the quantal content of EPPs using the amplitude distri-

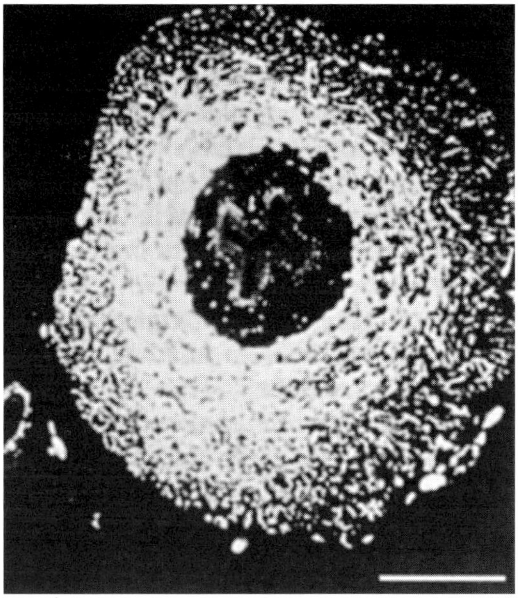
(a)

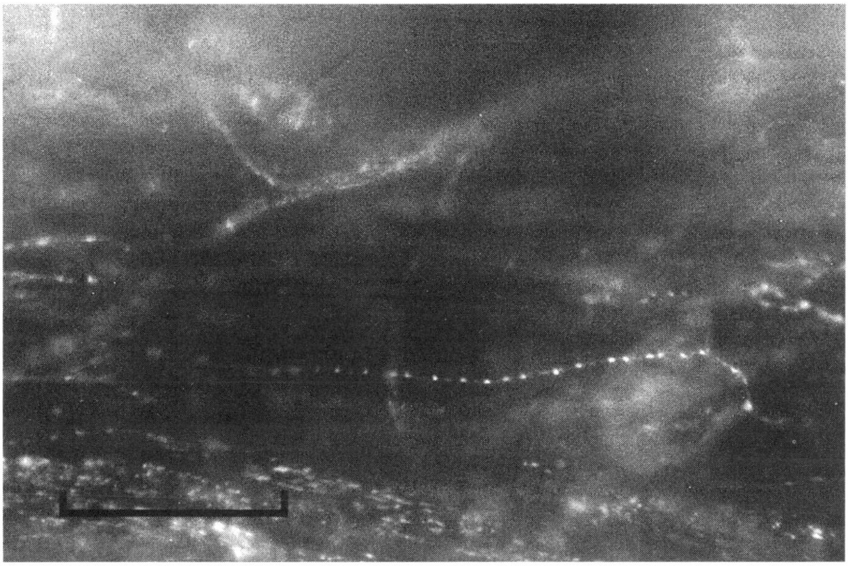
(b)

Fig. 4.20 (a) Cross-section of guinea-pig vas deferens stained by the Falck–Hillarp technique for catecholamines. Note dense innervation throughout the smooth muscle. Scale bar: 1 mm. (b) A beaded varicose axon in the vas deferens. This image was captured with a confocal microscope, and the varicosities are stained with a fluorescent antibody to synaptophysin. Scale bar ≈ 100 μm. Image kindly provided by M. Bennett.

bution of the MEPPs. In the vas deferens, however, it is not possible to establish the relationship between the spontaneous and evoked potential, because of the multiple innervation and electrical coupling between the cells.

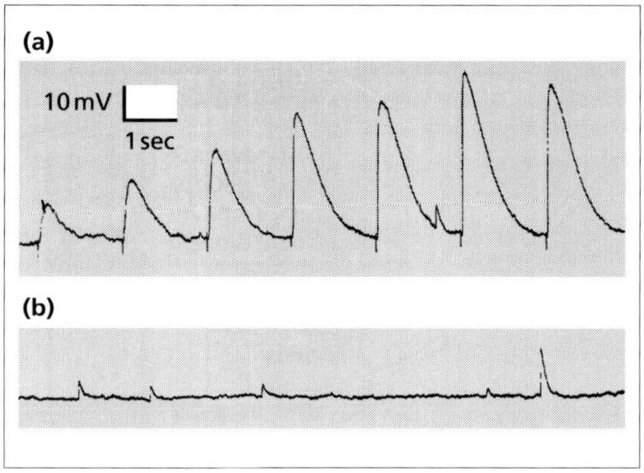

Fig. 4.21 Intracellular recordings of excitatory and spontaneous excitatory junction potentials (EJPs and SEJPs) in the guinea-pig vas deferens. (a) EJPs evoked by a train of seven stimuli at 1 Hz. Note the SEJP that occurs after the fifth EJP. (b) SEJPs in an unstimulated preparation. Note the much briefer time course of the SEJPs compared to the EJPs. Recordings kindly provided by T.C. Cunnane.

Focal extracellular recording

This technique was initially used by Katz at the NMJ (see Katz, 1962), but Cunnane has recently adapted it to studying neuromuscular transmission to the vas deferens and other densely innervated smooth muscles (see Cunnane & Searl, 1994). A small glass pipette with a polished end, filled with physiological saline and connected to an electrode, is applied to the cleaned surface of the tissue, and suction is applied to create a seal resistance between the glass and the tissue. Any current flow into or out of the membranes within this seal will generate a potential difference between the suction electrode and an indifferent electrode outside the electrode. Inward current flowing through channels opened in membranes inside the seal will be associated with a negative potential change in the electrode. Thus, the use of a small suction electrode allows the electrical activity originating from a small population of varicosities and smooth muscle cells located under the electrode to be investigated (Fig. 4.22).

If focal electrodes are applied to the surface of the vas deferens, in the absence of stimulation, occasional spontaneous changes in potential can be recorded, which reflect inward current flow through the smooth muscle membrane. These spontaneous excitatory junction currents (SEJCs) are caused by spontaneous release of quanta of transmitter, and they have characteristics similar to the SEJPs recorded with microelectrodes (Fig. 4.23). The time course of both events is determined by the time course of transmitter action (rather than the passive electrical properties of the membrane, as is the case with the much faster MEPPs at the skeletal NMJ, where the transmembrane voltage changes outlast the current flow). When the hypogastric nerve to the vas deferens is stimulated with single shocks, evoked potentials occasionally occur, and these will reflect excitatory junction currents

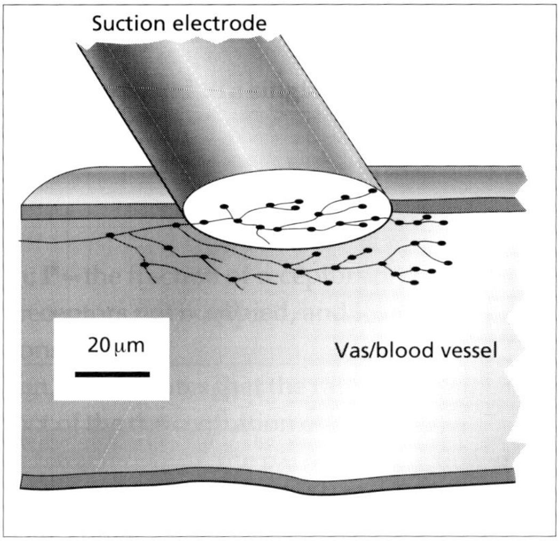

Fig. 4.22 Schematic illustration of extracellular recording using a suction electrode from the surface of the guinea-pig vas deferens. The electrode tip lies over a small population of nerve terminal varicosities and smooth muscle cells. From Brock & Cunnane (1988).

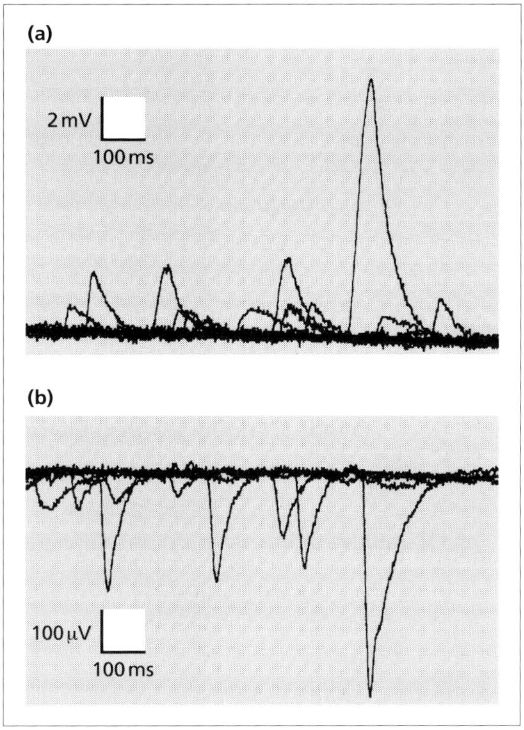

Fig. 4.23 Spontaneous activity recorded with an intracellular microelectrode (a: excitatory junction potentials, SEJPs) and an extracellular suction electrode (b: excitatory junction currents, SEJCs) from the guinea-pig vas deferens. A series of traces is superimposed to show the characteristic features of the events. Note the almost identical time course of the SEJPs and the SEJCs, which is in contrast to the skeletal muscle neuromuscular junction, where the end-plate currents are shorter events than end-plate potentials. From Brock & Cunnane (1988).

(EJCs) flowing in the cells within the seal. The EJCs have roughly the same amplitude and time course as the SEJCs, suggesting that normally only the response to release of a single varicosity is being recorded by the electrode. An EJC does not occur every time the nerve is stimulated, i.e. they are intermittent (Fig. 4.24). Calculating the rough number of varicosities that may be sampled by the focal electrode suggests that the probability of release from a varicosity may be as low as 0.01, i.e. only once every hundred times the nerve is stimulated will a varicosity release a quantum of transmitter. Evoked junctional currents differ from the spontaneous ones in that the evoked EJCs depend on Ca entry, and are abolished when the nerve action potential is blocked with TTX.

This technique also records changes in potential as action potentials invade the nerves under the focal electrode. Thus, one can determine whether the intermittency of release is caused by failure of action potential invasion. It is clear that EJCs were always linked to action potential invasion, but invasion of the action potential also occurred when there was no evoked release, and the size of the invading nerve impulse was unchanged, whether or not it triggered release (Fig. 4.25). The intermittent nature of

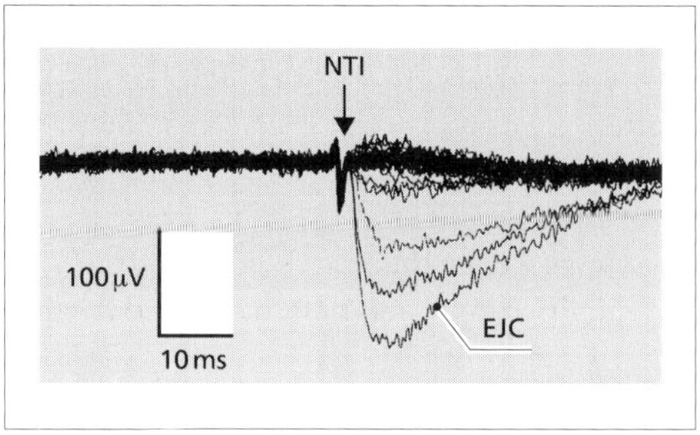

Fig. 4.24 Electrical activity recorded from a surface suction electrode on the guinea-pig vas deferens in response to stimulation of the hypogastric nerve with 25 stimuli and 1 Hz. EJCs were recorded in response to only three of the stimuli at this frequency, i.e. the release is intermittent. From Brock & Cunnane (1987).

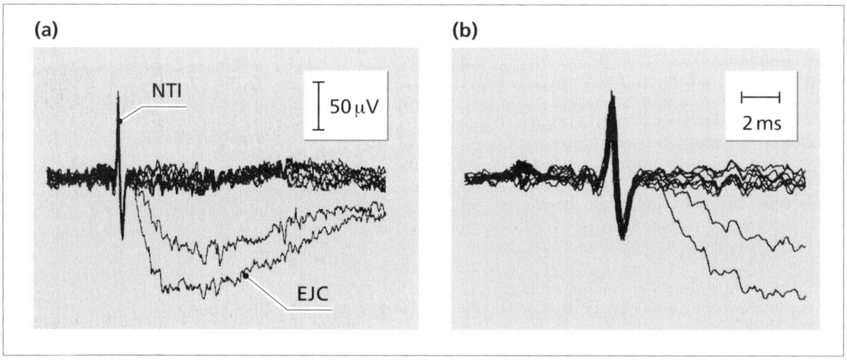

Fig. 4.25 Electrical activity recorded from a surface suction electrode on the guinea-pig vas deferens in response to stimulation of the hypogastric nerve (10 pulses, 0.5 Hz). The electrical activity recorded due to the nerve terminal impulse (NTI) is seen as the brief biphasic response preceding the EJCs in (a) and is shown with an expanded time course in (b). Note that the NTIs occur for every pulse, although they evoke only two EJCs. From Brock & Cunnane (1992).

release is therefore caused by the low probability that an action potential will trigger release, rather than any problems with action potential spread.

Facilitation and auto-inhibition

As stated earlier, the size of the EJP measured with microelectrodes grows with repetitive stimulation (Fig. 4.21). The size of the EJP can also be increased by drugs that block the inhibitory presynaptic action of the released transmitter, and can be reduced by bathing the preparation in low concentrations of the agonist released (or selective agonists of the presynaptic receptors, Fig. 4.26). These latter experiments demonstrate the presence of presynaptic auto-inhibition. Focal recording can throw light on both of these mechanisms. It shows that, with repetitive nerve stimulation, there is no change in the action potential invading the nerves, but that facilitation increases the probability of release from the varicosities (Fig. 4.27). There is no evidence that an individual release site in a varicosity releases a quantum more often; instead, it appears that facilitation involves either recruitment of previously silent varicosities or an increase in the number of functional release sites in the same varicosity. With reference to auto-inhibition, there is no evidence that release of a quantum from one release site affects the probability of subsequent release from the same site. Again, it seems that the effect of released transmitter is to reduce the probability of release from other release sites in its vicinity.

The factors that determine the amount of neurotransmitter secreted are therefore the frequency of nerve impulses in the terminals, with higher frequencies increasing the number of active varicosities, and the lateral spread

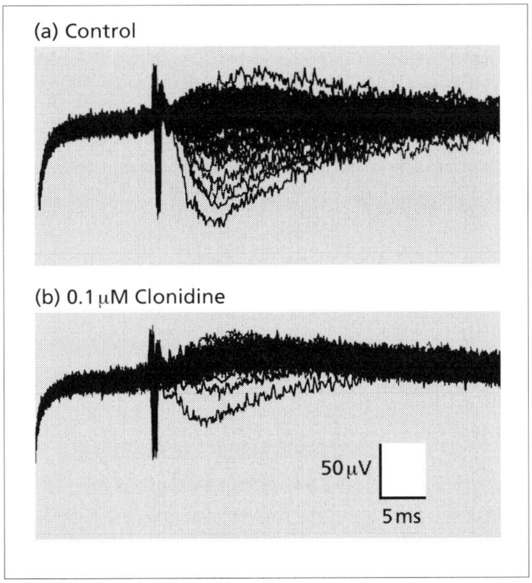

Fig. 4.26 Electrical activity recorded from a surface suction electrode on the guinea-pig vas deferens in response to stimulation of the hypogastric nerve (100 stimuli at 1 Hz). (a) Control and (b) in the presence of clonidine. Clonidine is an α_2 adrenoceptor agonist, and activates the presynaptic α_2 adrenoceptors, reducing the probability of transmitter release. Note that the nerve impulse does not change, showing that clonidine does not affect the impulse propagation. From Brock & Cunnane (1990).

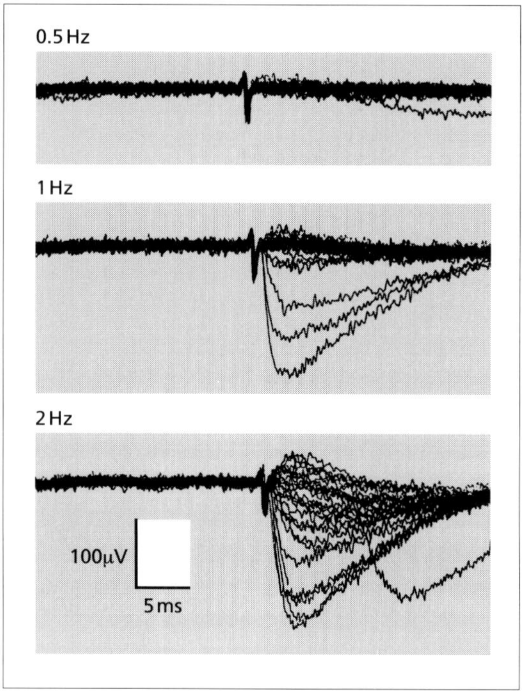

Fig. 4.27 Facilitation of transmitter release from nerve terminals in guinea-pig vas deferens. In each panel the hypogastric nerves are stimulated by trains of 25 impulses at three frequencies. Note the increase in the number of excitatory junction currents as the frequency rises. One spontaneous event is seen at 0.5 Hz and one at 2 Hz. From Brock & Cunnane (1987).

of transmitter that can reduce release. Thus, it is possible to achieve graded responses of smooth muscles by varying the centrally determined pattern of impulse traffic, but this is restrained by auto-inhibition when the release rate is high.

4.7.2 What chemical generates the excitatory junction potential?

Controversy exists over the nature of the neurotransmitter substance producing the EJP in many smooth muscles following sympathetic and parasympathetic nerve stimulation. This is true for both blood vessels and visceral organs. The obvious transmitter candidates – noradrenaline for adrenergic nerves and acetylcholine for cholinergic nerves – may be involved in generating depolarization in some tissues, but in many tissues classical adrenoceptor blockers and antimuscarinic agents, although blocking the effects of bath-applied noradrenaline or acetylcholine, often leave the EJP unaffected. Much recent evidence suggests that, in many tissues, EJPs may be mediated by a second or co-transmitter possibly released from the same nerves – namely the purine, ATP.

Evidence for ATP in sympathetic nerves mediating excitatory junction potentials

The role of ATP in neuro-effector transmission in sympathetic adrenergic nerves has been studied more intensively than its role in cholinergic neuro-

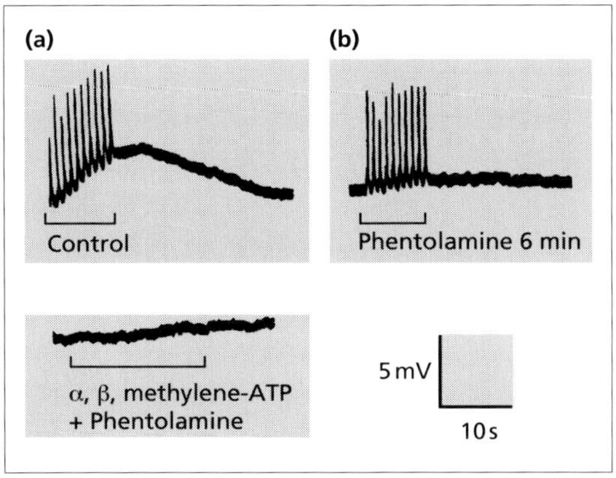

Fig. 4.28 Intracellular microelectrode recording from smooth muscle cells in the rat tail artery. Stimulation of the sympathetic nerves was carried out at 1 Hz during the period indicated by the bars. (a) Control. Each stimulus elicits an excitatory junction potential (EJP), and there is also a slow depolarization of the membrane. (b) In the presence of the α-adrenoceptor antagonist phentolamine, the EJPs are unaffected, but the slow depolarization is nearly abolished. Addition of α,β-methylene ATP, which desensitizes the P_{2X} purinoceptors, abolishes the EJPs. From Sneddon & Burnstock (1984).

transmission. Evidence in favour of its role in generating the EJPs in vas deferens and in several arterial smooth muscles is summarised below.

1 SEJPs and EJPs persist after blockade of postjunctional α- or β-adrenoceptors, but are abolished after desensitisation of P_{2x} purinoceptors by α,β-methylene ATP – indicating that ATP is mediating the response (Fig. 4.28).

2 EJPs are resistant to the actions of reserpine – a drug that blocks uptake of catecholamines but not of ATP into the synaptic vesicles, thus indicating that noradrenaline is not the neurotransmitter generating the EJP.

3 EJPs are abolished by the adrenergic neurone blocking agents bretylium and guanethidine, showing that EJPs are generated by activation of sympathetic neurones.

It therefore seems likely that the ATP in the synaptic vesicles that is released on activation of sympathetic nerves is responsible for generating the EJPs.

Evidence for ATP in other nerves generating excitatory junction potentials

Similar evidence exists for some tissues innervated by parasympathetic nerves, such as the urinary bladder in non-primate mammals. In this case, EJPs elicited by transmural stimulation are not blocked by the muscarinic receptor antagonist atropine or the α-adrenoceptor antagonist phentolamine, but desensitisation of the P_{2x} purinoceptors by α,β-methylene ATP abolishes the EJPs (Fig. 4.29). In parasympathetically innervated tissues, it is less clear whether the ATP is coming from the cholinergic nerves or from a separate population of purinergic nerves, since the right pharmacological

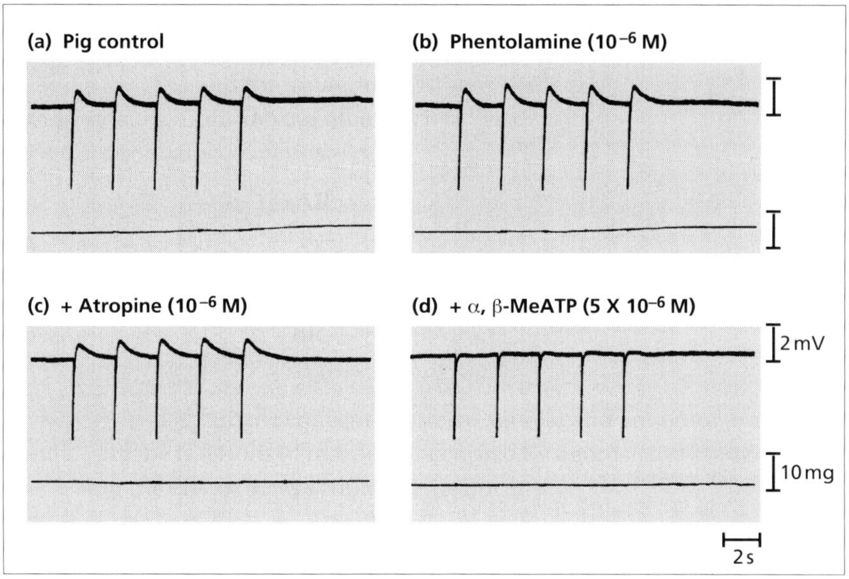

Fig. 4.29 Electrical recording from the smooth muscle cells of the guinea-pig bladder using the double sucrose-gap method. (a) Stimulation of the intrinsic nerves (downward deflections) initiates excitatory junction potentials that are not abolished by the α-adrenoceptor antagonist phentolamine (b), or the muscarinic receptor antagonist atropine (c), but desensitization of the P_{2x} purinoceptors by α,β-methylene ATP (d) abolishes them. From Fujii (1988).

tools are not available. However, it seems likely that again co-release of ATP does occur with acetylcholine in the parasympathetic system.

Role of ATP and classical transmitters in neurogenic contraction

The importance of ATP as a co-transmitter varies widely from tissue to tissue, and in some instances the classical transmitters acetylcholine (Ach) and noradrenaline appear to be solely responsible for both the membrane and contractile responses of the tissues. In general, tissues in which ATP generates EJPs are those in which the nervous system plays a dominant role in initiating contractions of the smooth muscles, rather than just modulating spontaneous activity. Vas deferens and small resistance arteries and arterioles are classic examples. Vas deferens smooth muscle is quiescent unless activated by nerves, and the minute-to-minute smooth muscle tone in the resistance vessels most involved in the baroreceptor reflex control of blood pressure is determined by neural activity. This fast activation of smooth muscle is achieved by action potential initiation, and the most reliable way of triggering an action potential is by membrane depolarization through EJPs. ATP acting through P_{2x} purinoceptors activates directly coupled non-selective ion channels that are ideal for rapid depolarization.

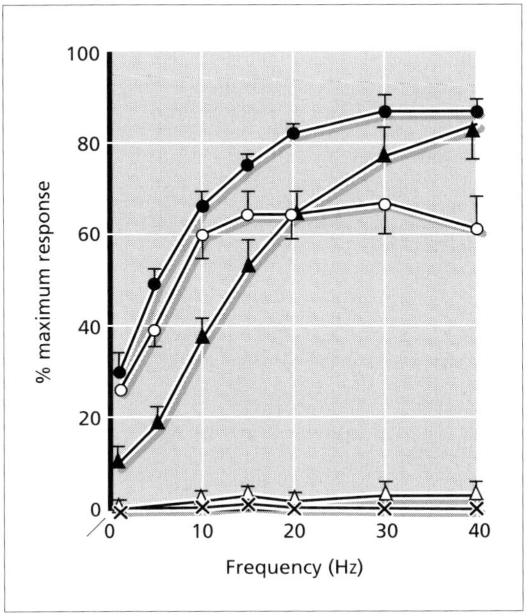

Fig. 4.30 Contractile response of strips of smooth muscle from the guinea-pig bladder to stimulation of their intrinsic nerves at increasing frequencies. The control curve is shown by the solid circles. In the presence of 10^{-6} M atropine (open circles), there is little change at low frequencies, but the contractile response at frequencies above 10 Hz is reduced in size. After desensitization of the P_{2x} purinoceptors by α,β-methylene ATP (3×10^{-5} M) (solid triangles), the responses at all frequencies are reduced, but proportionally the effect is greatest at the low frequencies of stimulation. The contractile responses are abolished in the presence of both drugs (crosses), and also in the presence of tetrodotoxin (2×10^{-7} M) (open triangles). From Brading (1987).

The classic autonomic transmitters produce their effects more slowly via G proteins and second messengers. They can initiate changes in membrane potential, although these are usually slower in onset and longer in duration than the response to ATP, and they can also cause contraction by triggering release of calcium from intracellular stores, by-passing membrane potential changes. Where ATP is important, contractile responses to single nerve stimuli are often predominantly purinergic, but the classical transmitters still have a role in initiating contraction, their influence becoming more prominent when trains of stimuli are given (Fig. 4.30).

Postjunctional receptor specialisation

An additional complexity in the interpretation of results using bath-applied agonists and antagonists of adrenoceptors or cholinoceptors is the recent discovery that postjunctional receptors may have different properties, including affinities for agonists and antagonists, than extrajunctional receptors. Thus, a single agonist on one tissue may activate different synaptic and extrasynaptic receptors, and each may trigger different cellular mechanisms. Even if addition of an agonist produces a response that can be blocked by a specific antagonist, and the response to nerve activation is not blocked by that antagonist, one cannot rule out the possibility that the nerve is still releasing the agonist, since it could be having its effects locally on a different receptor type. In arterioles, for instance, it has been shown by Hirst and Neild (1980) that noradrenaline applied locally to a point distant from a nerve varicosity elicits contraction without depolarization of the arteriole, and that this can be blocked by classical α-adrenoceptor blockers, whereas noradrenaline applied close to a nerve elicits depolarization of the membrane that cannot be blocked by these blockers (Fig. 4.31). This has led to the postulation that a novel class of catecholamine receptors, the γ-receptors, is present postsynaptically and operates through different mechanisms from those of the classical α-adrenoceptors. Similarly, muscarinic receptors in the

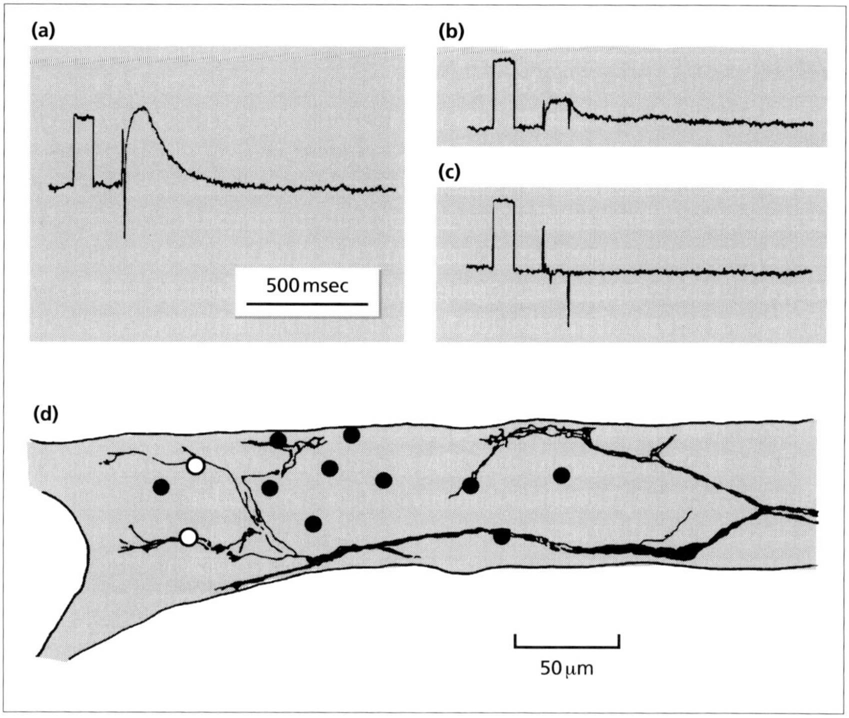

Fig. 4.31 Responses of arterioles to local application of noradrenaline. (a) Response to an iontophoretic injection with the pipette positioned on an open circle of (d), where the membrane is responsive to noradrenaline. (b) Response when pipette positioned over an insensitive area (solid circles) – this is just the response to the iontophoretic current crossing the membrane: when the pipette is moved a little away from the membrane (c), there is no response. From Hirst & Neild (1980). Subsequently, it was shown that noradrenaline applied to a membrane-insensitive site could result in constriction of the arteriole, even in the absence of a membrane response.

heart have been shown to produce slowing of the heartbeat by different mechanisms depending on whether the acetylcholine is working on extra-junctional or postjunctional receptors.

4.7.3 Other possible excitatory transmitters

Although the main excitatory transmitters of the postjunctional nerves seem to be acetylcholine, noradrenaline and ATP, there is evidence to suggest that several other excitatory transmitters may be involved in the activation of particular effectors. A large number of polypeptides have been shown to be present in autonomic nerves, and exogenous application of many of them may have excitatory effects. Examples are substance P, neurotensin, cholecystokinin (CCK) and neuropeptide Y (NPY). Aminergic nerves containing 5-HT and dopamine have also been demonstrated, and these substances may have excitatory effects. It should be remembered, however, that although these substances may be excitatory on some tissues, they may also be inhibitory on others (see below).

4.7.4 Inhibitory innervation

Many smooth muscles are innervated by inhibitory nerves, which can cause relaxation of muscles showing spontaneous or evoked contractions. In some instances, the innervation seems to be mediated by 'classical' autonomic system nerves, as is the case in some parts of the gut, where stimulating postganglionic sympathetic nerves results in relaxations mediated by noradrenaline working on α-adrenoceptors, and in some blood vessels, where stimulating parasympathetic nerves results in relaxation mediated by acetylcholine working on muscarinic receptors (Fig. 4.32). Although in many instances these types of relaxant responses may involve neuronal interactions (presynaptic effects reducing excitatory input from another nerve), the postsynaptic receptors on the smooth muscle also mediate inhibition. Clearly, the receptors are triggering different cellular events from those they trigger to evoke their excitatory responses. Electrophysiological measurements of the membrane potential responses to the inhibitory effects of these 'classical' autonomic system nerves may show only small changes in membrane potential that develop in response to repetitive stimulation, and little evidence of clear inhibitory junction potentials (IJPs) (Fig. 4.33).

There are, however, many more instances in which intrinsic inhibitory nerves are present in a tissue and can be stimulated by transmural stimulation. These nerves often are neither adrenergic nor cholinergic. In the absence of knowledge as to the transmitters involved, these were originally called non-adrenergic, non-cholinergic or NANC inhibitory nerves (there are also NANC excitatory nerves – see above). Activation of these nerves with single shocks leads to large IJPs, normally caused by opening receptor-operated K channels. Repetitive stimulation of the nerves can thus hold the

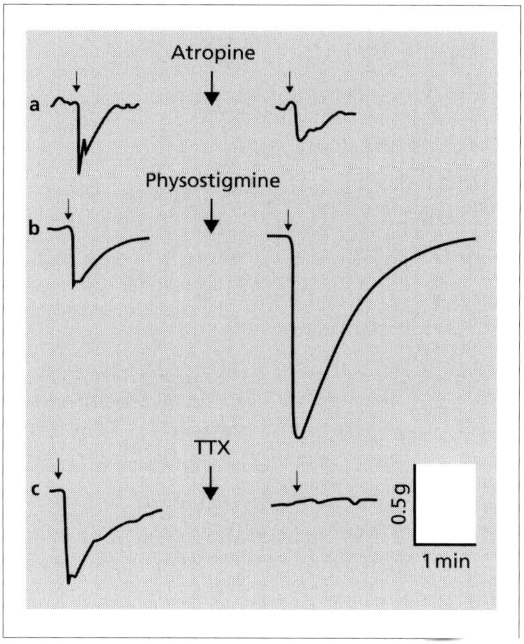

Fig. 4.32 Vasodilation in the rabbit lingual artery evoked by activation of the periarterial nerves. Control responses on the left. (a) Atropine (10^{-7} M) reduced the size of the relaxation. (b) The cholinesterase inhibitor physostigmine (5×10^{-7} M) greatly enhanced the response. (c) Relaxation was abolished by the nerve toxin TTX. Recordings carried out in the presence of guanethidine to block sympathetic nerve activity. From Brayden & Large (1986).

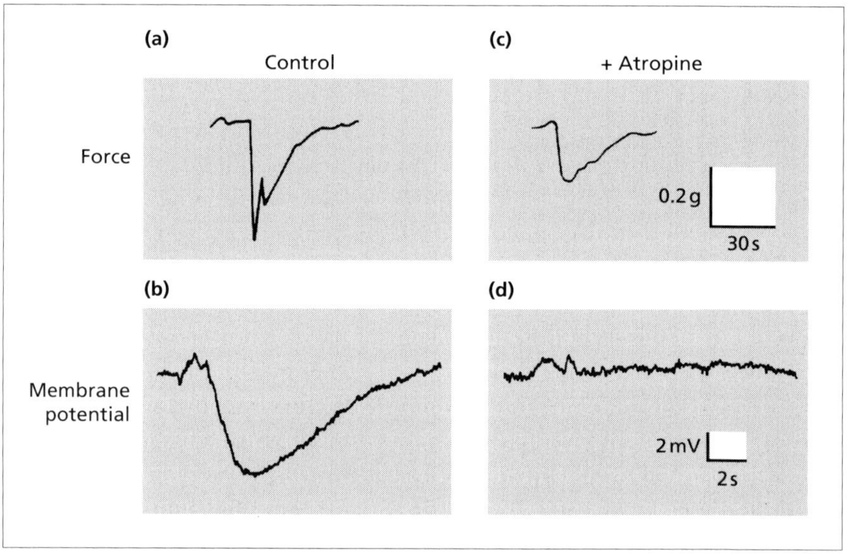

Fig. 4.33 Vasodilation in the rabbit lingual artery evoked by activation of the periarterial nerves. Upper panels show mechanical responses, and lower panels electrical responses. The vasodilation in the control conditions is accompanied by membrane hyperpolarization. In the presence of atropine the hyperpolarization is abolished, and the relaxation reduced. The remaining vasodilation occurs with no change in the membrane potential, and is mediated by a non-adrenergic, non-cholinergic transmitter. Recordings carried out in the presence of guanethidine to block sympathetic nerve activity. From Brayden & Large (1986).

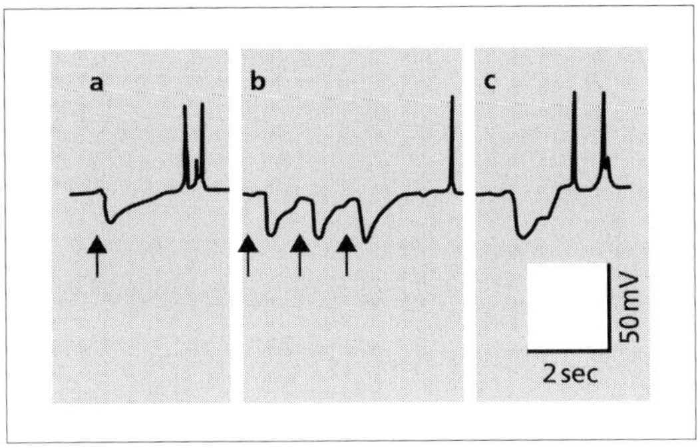

Fig. 4.34 Intracellular microelectrode recording of membrane potential from a smooth muscle cell in the guinea-pig colon. Stimulation of an enteric inhibitory motor neurone. (a) A single pulse gives an inhibitory junction potential. (b) Three successive pulses show little facilitation. (c) Repetitive stimuli (10 Hz) can sustain the hyperpolarization, but it is not larger. Adapted from Furness (1970).

membrane potential well away from the threshold for action potential generation (Fig. 4.34).

In recent years, several possible transmitters have been postulated to mediate the inhibition, and in a few cases the transmitter is pretty well established. The three favoured candidates are the peptide, vasoactive intestinal polypeptide (VIP), the purine ATP and the inorganic molecule NO. 5-HT and substance P also seem to play roles in inhibitory transmission.

Vasoactive intestinal polypeptide (VIP)

Immunohistochemistry can localise VIP in various neurones, and demonstrate its presence in synapses in the peripheral nervous system. It is very common in neurones in the enteric nervous system, and is also frequently found in other tissues with NANC inhibitory innervation. Application of exogenous peptide can mimic neurogenic relaxations in many of these tissues. It has been difficult, however, to obtain conclusive evidence that the peptide is responsible for the neurogenic effects, because of a lack of specific agonists or antagonists. Reduction in the size of the neurogenic inhibitory response on addition of peptidases in some cases provides support for its physiological role. Recently, peptide antagonists have been synthesised that can block both nerve-evoked and exogenous relaxations to VIP, and thus strengthen its claim as an inhibitory transmitter.

Adenosine triphosphate (ATP)

As described earlier, ATP is known to be present in cholinergic and adrenergic nerves, but in these cases it is normally an excitatory co-transmitter, working through activation of directly coupled non-selective cation channels. It has been postulated, however, that there may be exclusively purinergic nerves, and that some of these may be inhibitory. Exogenous ATP can, for instance, mimic the hyperpolarization and relaxation produced by intrinsic nerve stimulation in the gut, through activation of the G-protein-coupled P_{2y} receptors. Unfortunately, the development of specific antagonists has been slow, and evidence for its role as an inhibitory transmitter is still circumstantial.

Nitric oxide (NO)

NO has recently been shown to be a powerful inhibitor of smooth muscle, and to be released from inhibitory nerves, particularly in sphincteric smooth muscles. The case for it is now firmly established. NO is synthesised from L-arginine by an enzyme nitric oxide synthase, which can be shown by immunohistochemistry to be present in nerves and nerve terminals (Fig. 4.35). The enzyme is activated by Ca entry through a Ca–calmodulin-dependent pathway. The free NO molecule seems to be involved, since inhibitory transmission can be suppressed by addition of molecules, such as haemoglobin, which bind avidly to NO. L-Arginine analogues that bind to the enzyme but do not support NO synthesis can be shown to competitively inhibit the effects of stimulating the nerves, and also to reduce the production of NO – an effect reversed by addition of an excess of substrate (Fig. 4.36). The details of the transmission process are not clear, but since the molecule easily permeates membranes, it seems unlikely that release is vesicu-

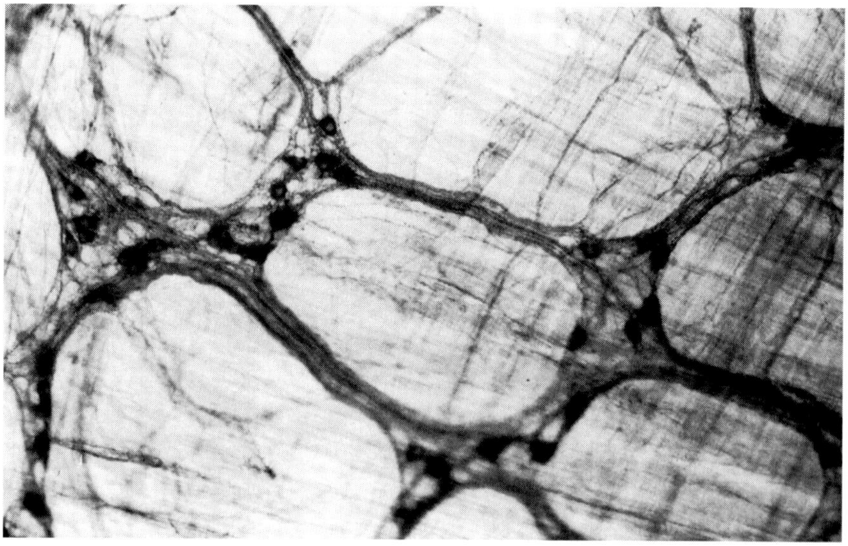

Fig. 4.35 Part of the myenteric plexus of the guinea-pig ileum. A whole mount preparation has been made, and stained for the presence of nitric oxide synthase. This stains a subpopulation of the ganglion cells. Kindly provided by J. Stebbing.

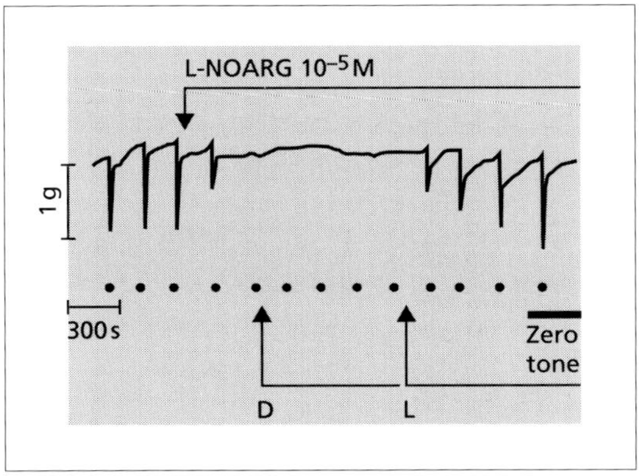

Fig. 4.36 Relaxant responses of the internal anal sphincter to intrinsic nerve stimulation. Relaxant responses are abolished by N-nitro-L-arginine (L-NOARG) which competes with the normal substrate (L-arginine) for the nitric oxide synthase enzyme preventing synthesis of NO. The inhibition can be reversed by increasing the concentration of L-arginine (L), but not D-arginine (D). Adapted from O'Kelly *et al.* (1993).

lar in this instance. The postsynaptic effects are also not mediated by classical receptors, but NO can be shown to activate guanylyl cyclase and elevate the cellular content of cyclic guanosine monophosphate (cGMP), leading to activation of kinases and modulation of cellular processes, including those handling Ca.

5-Hydroxytryptamine (5-HT)

In several smooth muscles, application of 5-HT can cause relaxations that may mimic the neurogenic relaxations, but so far it appears that the majority of these effects are indirect and result from the actions of 5-HT on nerves or neurones, which then presumably liberate the inhibitory transmitter.

Substance P

Substance P is clearly involved in generating vasodilation in response to activating a class of small sensory neurones. Release of the peptide from axon collaterals is responsible for initiating vasodilation in the 'flare' of Lewis's triple response and in axon reflex vasodilation, although it is not certain whether it is the result of the inhibitory transmitter itself or whether it causes release of vasodilator substances from mast cells.

4.8 Autonomic ganglia

The clusters of neurones making up the ganglia in the autonomic nervous system are of many diverse types. There are those of the paravertebral chains, which are part of the sympathetic system, those of the prevertebral ganglia, where the parasympathetic and sympathetic systems may interact, and those in the enteric plexuses, and they all show differences. Preganglionic to postganglionic transmission can involve both convergence and divergence of the incoming signal. In other words, each postganglionic neurone may receive input from many preganglionic neurones, and each preganglionic neurone may innervate many postganglionic neurones. Modulation of the excitability of the postganglionic neurones may also occur. In the prevertebral and paravertebral ganglia, this may occur through interneurones within ganglia, and through collaterals of sensory nerves given off *en route* to the central nervous system, or in the enteric nervous system it may occur via intrinsic modulatory interneurones and sensory neurones.

4.8.1 Fine structure of ganglia

In ganglia of the sympathetic nervous system, where detailed studies have been undertaken, postganglionic neurones may have several main dendrites, each with many branches and dendritic spines. Preganglionic input is largely to the dendritic spines and shafts, and less to the soma (Figs 4.37 and 4.38). A single postganglionic neurone may have several hundred synapses on it from preganglionic neurones. It is not yet known how many synapses on average a single preganglionic neurone makes on each postganglionic one, or how many preganglionic neurones synapse on each postganglionic neurone. The synapses are predominantly asymmetric in electron microscopy. Although both apposed membranes have dense material associated with them, more is associated with the postsynaptic membrane. The presynaptic membrane bears triangular tufts of dense fibrillar material. Vesicles are clustered at this surface. The vesicles in the preganglionic nerve terminals are predominantly small, clear and spherical and about 20–60 nm in diameter; they are presumably cholinergic, although a few large dense-cored vesicles are normally also present. The main transmitter is acetylcholine, activating nicotinic receptors. The nerve terminals also have acetylcholinesterase along their surface membranes.

Ganglia also possess small intensely fluorescent (SIF) cells, which are small cells containing granules with various catecholamines, amines and peptides in them, depending on the species (Fig. 4.39). In many instances, they receive preganglionic synapses (although only a few per cell) and themselves synapse on the postganglionic neurones, and thus are interneurones. Synapses from the SIF cells have small dense-cored vesicles, presumably containing catecholamines. In many of them, the predominant transmitter is dopamine. They are also seen in association with blood vessels, and they may have a paracrine (local endocrine) role (Fig. 4.40). Unmyelinated sensory nerve fibres also send collaterals into the ganglia, which end in varicose branches, synapsing onto the postganglionic

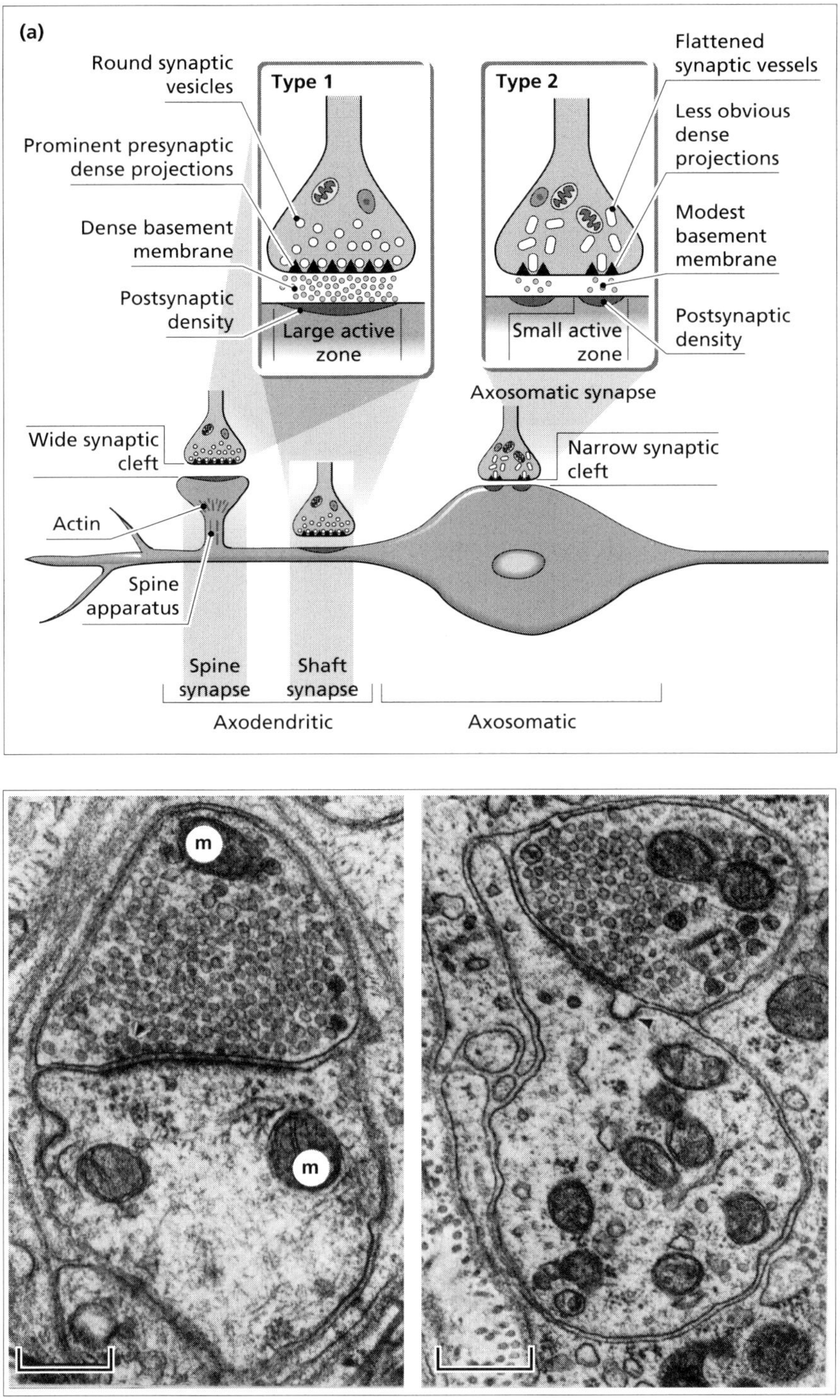

Fig. 4.37 (a) Classification of types of synapse on neurones. The majority of synapses on autonomic neurones are type 1 and occur on the dendritic shafts and spines. (b) Electron micrograph of synapses occurring on a dendritic spine (left) and shaft (right) of a postganglionic neurone in the rat superior cervical ganglion. The synapses contain round clear synaptic vesicles, and are presumptive cholinergic nerve terminals. Some large dense-cored vesicles are also present. Scale bars: 0.5 μm. Kindly provided by M. Matthews.

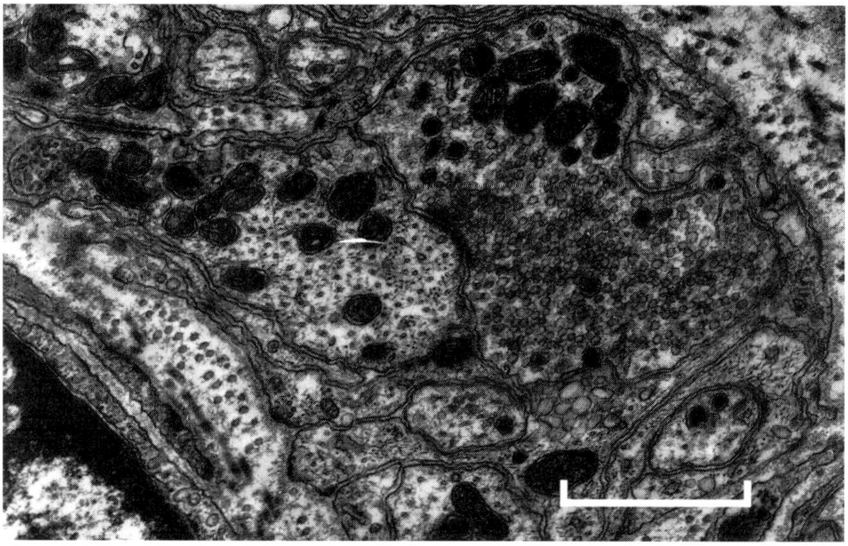

Fig. 4.38 Electron micrograph of a sympathetic ganglion showing a synapse (centre) between an axon (to the right), packed with small agranular vesicles, a few large granular vesicles and mitochondria, and a dendrite (to the left), showing mainly microtubules, neurofilaments, mitochondria and a few elements of smooth endoplasmic reticulum. Scale bar: 1 μm. Micrograph kindly supplied by G. Gabella.

neurones and supplying a small percentage of the incoming synapses, probably using substance P as a transmitter.

In paravertebral ganglia and ganglia in the enteric nervous system, there is a large variety of synaptic profiles, with many different types of vesicle, including large vesicles with cores of different densities, and small, clear, flattened vesicles. Physiological and pharmacological evidence suggests that many non-classical transmitters are employed at these sites.

4.8.2 Ganglionic transmission

Initial experiments on ganglionic transmission used electrical stimulation of nerves innervating ganglia, and extracellular recording of the postganglionic potential changes that resulted. Under these conditions, preganglionic stimulation results in complex postsynaptic potential changes. There is usually a fast excitatory postsynaptic potential that is nicotinic, like the EPSP, but this may be graded in size depending on the number of presynaptic fibres activated, and is usually followed by a series of late potential changes that may be depolarizing or hyperpolarizing, and depend on the strength and frequency of the stimulation parameters of the innervating nerves and which interneurones are present. *In vivo*, the input–output relationship of ganglia may therefore be quite complex, and it can be modulated under different circumstances.

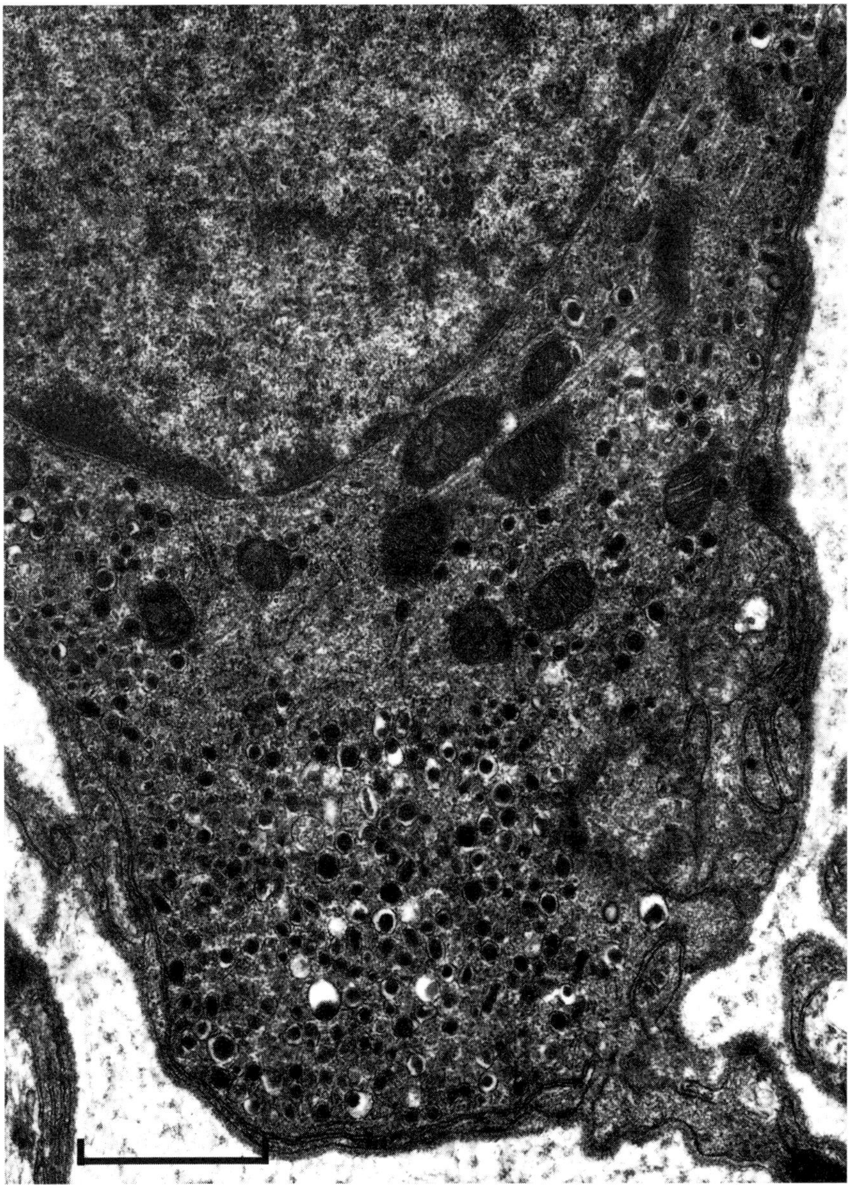

Fig. 4.39 A so-called SIF cell (Small Intensely Fluorescent cell) in an electron micrograph of the pelvic ganglion. The nucleus is at the top left; the whole cell is surrounded by a thin sheath provided by capsule cells (glia). The cytoplasm shows several mitochondria, microtubules, ribosomes and endoplasmic reticulum, and a large number of large granular vesicles, with a dense core. These vesicles store amines in high concentration, which can be secreted in the extracellular space, and they impart to the cell the intense specific fluorescence when the tissue is treated with the appropriate histochemical method. Scale bar: 1 μm. Micrograph kindly supplied by G. Gabella.

Transmission through the ganglia requires initiation of action potentials in the postganglionic neurone, and, as might be expected, this is brought about by the activation of directly coupled ion channels, which mediate inward current flow, depolarize the axon hillock through local circuit currents, and initiate action potentials in the axon. Unlike the NMJ, however, transmission does not seem to be an all-or-none phenomenon here. Neurones signal with repetitive firing, the frequency of the action potentials reflecting the intensity of the input. The dendrites and cell body provide areas at which the presynaptic input can be summed, and the frequency of the action potentials produced at the axon hillock depends on the amount of local current generated and thus the extent of the depolarization produced (see Fig. 3.7).

In the majority of cases, the main transmitter is acetylcholine, working through nicotinic receptors, but there is evidence that there are presynaptic inputs to some ganglia that use 5-HT as a transmitter, working through 5-HT_3 receptors, which are also directly coupled non-selective cation chan-

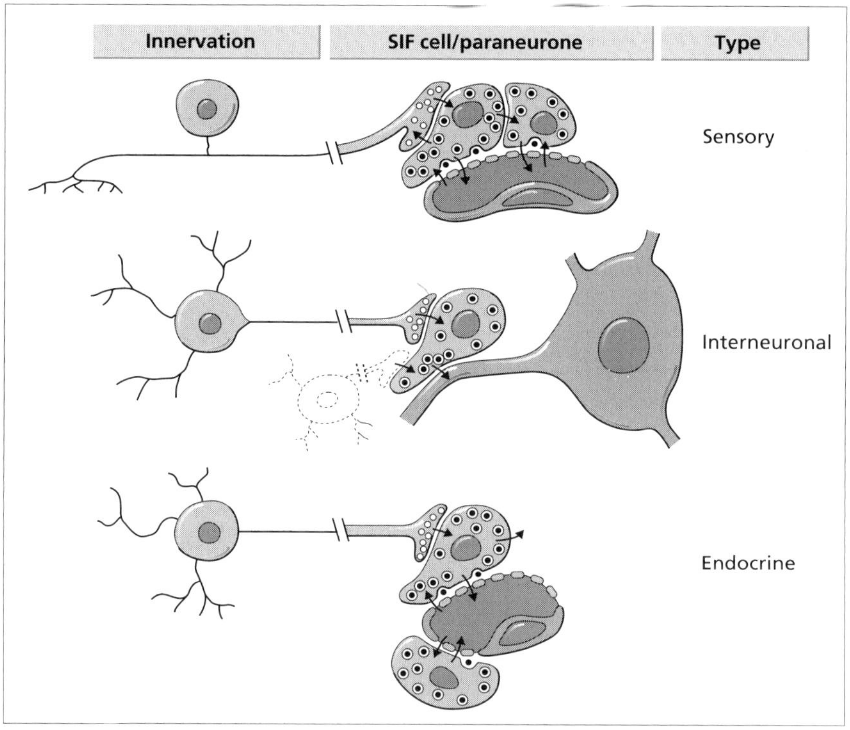

Fig. 4.40 The features and possible roles of SIF cells. The sensory type may be activated by collaterals of sensory nerve fibres, or by blood-borne or humoral stimuli, and may act back on the sensory nerve terminal. The interneuronal type is intraganglionic, and may receive either preganglionic (solid) or postganglionic (dotted) input. These SIF cells then synapse onto the principal neurones of the ganglia. The endocrine type may receive input either from the blood or sympathetic preganglionic fibres. From Matthews (1989).

nels. The ganglionic nicotinic receptors show pharmacological differences from the NMJ nicotinic receptor, and selective ganglionic blockers or activators have been developed, which have little effect at the NMJ. Hexamethonium is a widely used ganglionic nicotinic receptor antagonist, which has been shown to work by blocking the open channel. Dimethylphenylpiperazinium (DMPP) is a specific agonist for ganglionic nicotinic receptors.

4.8.3 Modulation of transmission

As mentioned earlier, the ganglion cells are sites of integration, and the effectiveness of the excitatory presynaptic input can be modulated by activation of other inputs from interneurones or sensory neurones, and also through co-release of peptides or other factors that may have a different pattern of release than the primary transmitter. An important mechanism for modulating the effectiveness of the primary excitatory transmitter is alteration of the resistance of the postjunctional neuronal membrane. This can affect the amount of local circuit current reaching the action-potential initiation region of the axon hillock. Anything lowering the resistance by opening ion channels will reduce the effectiveness of the transmission by providing shunt pathways for the local current flow, whereas anything increasing the resistance, by closing channels, will enhance the effectiveness of the transmission.

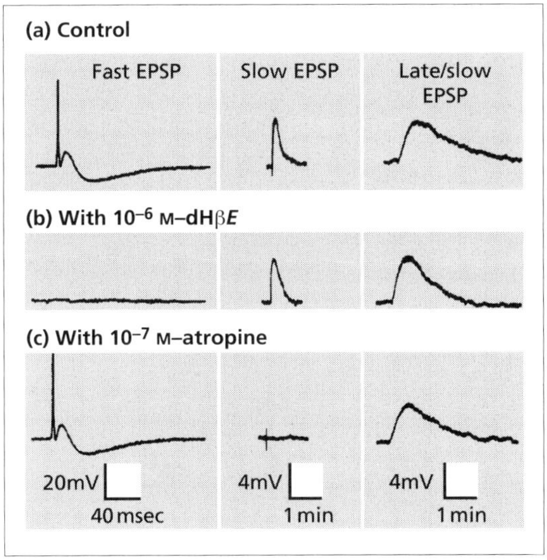

Fig. 4.41 Examples of excitatory postsynaptic potentials (EPSPs) in sympathetic ganglia. Fast EPSPs were initiated by a single stimulus of the preganglionic fibre, and were blocked by the nicotinic blocker dihydro-β-erhthroidine (dHβE), and unaffected by the muscarinic blocker atropine. Slow EPSPs and late slow EPSPs were activated by repetitive stimuli of other inputs. Slow EPSPs were abolished by atropine but not dHβE, and the late slow EPSPs were not affected by either blocker. From Jan & Jan (1982).

Electrophysiologists can detect some interesting changes in ganglion cell membrane properties induced by various patterns of nerve stimulation or application of different agonists, suggestive of physiologically relevant modulation. Often, these stimuli result in slow (seconds) or very slow (minutes) changes in potential (Fig. 4.41). Closing K channels produces depolarization, and is responsible for many slow EPSPs, whereas opening K or Cl channels may hyperpolarize the cells and produce IPSPs.

In many instances, for example in the paravertebral ganglia, it is difficult to activate inputs to ganglion cells selectively to investigate the precise pathways involved in the modulatory responses. Most studies on these

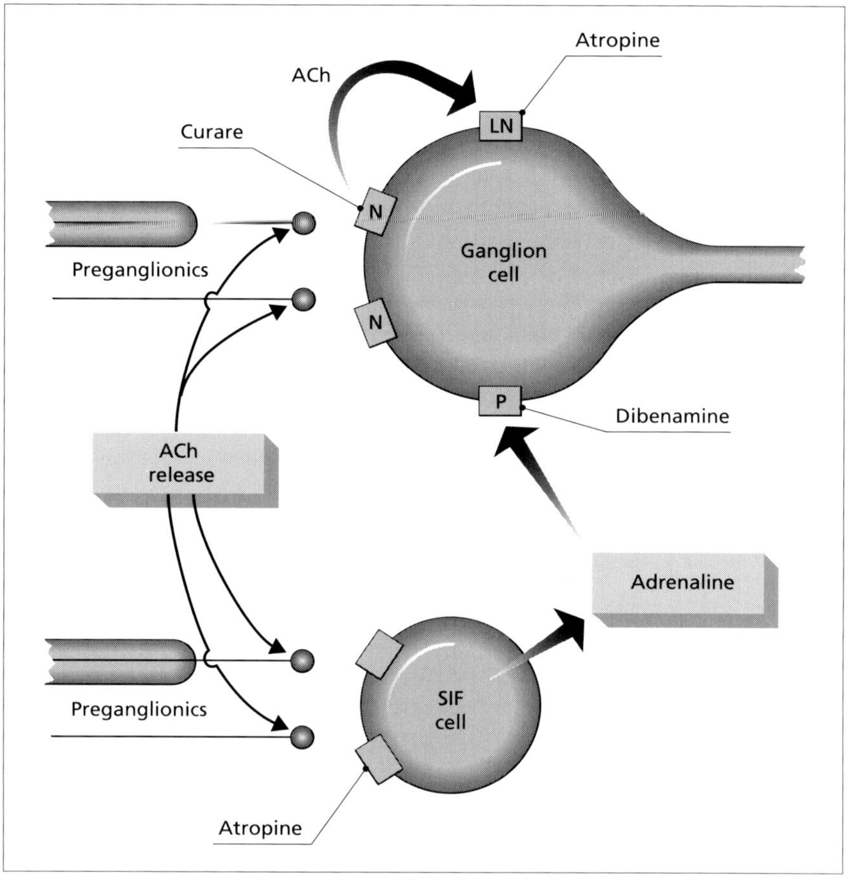

Fig. 4.42 Diagram of proposed arrangement of neurones and nerves in the rabbit superior cervical ganglion. N, LN and P refer to the early negative, late negative and positive waves recorded from the ganglion with extracellular electrodes. Stimulation of the preganglionic nerves activates nicotinic receptors to give a fast excitatory junction potential (N wave). Acetylcholine then diffuses to muscarinic receptors to generate the late negative wave blocked by atropine. Other preganglionic axons innervate the chromaffin cell (SIF cell), which releases a catecholamine acting on adrenergic receptors to give the inhibitory P wave blocked by dibenamine. From Eccles & Libbett (1961).

ganglia have stimulated the main preganglionic input at different frequencies, and dissected the resultant complex postsynaptic membrane potential changes using pharmacological tools. Figure 4.42 shows a scheme proposed by Eccles and Libbett incorporating their results, suggesting the involvement of nicotinic and muscarinic cholinoceptors and α-adrenoceptors.

In the enteric plexuses, the layout of the ganglia allows more precise stimulation of particular inputs to ganglion cells. Extensive work is being carried out on this system (see Chapter 8), and it is now possible to classify the majority of cells in the plexuses in terms of the combinations of transmitters and peptides that can be localised in them. Probably any substance that has been shown to be released from a nerve ending has been identified in neurones somewhere in the enteric nervous system. Examples include peptides – substance P, calcitonin gene-related peptide (CGRP), encephalins, VIP, CCK, gastrin; amines – catecholamines, 5-HT, histamine; and amino acids – glutamate, γ-aminobutyric acid (GABA).

Another mechanism for altering the input–output relationship of the transmission would be to alter the number of synaptic boutons that release transmitter. As mentioned earlier, anatomical evidence shows that each neurone has a large number of synapses on it, probably coming from very many presynaptic neurones. Physiological evidence, however, indicates that only a limited number of inputs are effective, and this suggests that many of the release sites may be inactive. It is thus possible that increased or decreased convergence and divergence could be brought about by mechanisms that 'switched on' or enhanced the probability of release of transmitter from previously silent synapses. Although this is being investigated in central synapses, few studies of this type are being carried out on autonomic ganglion cells. However, the presence of what appear to be synaptic vesicles has been demonstrated in dendrites of ganglion cells, which could be involved in such processes.

Further reading

Bennett, M.R. (1972) *Autonomic Neuromuscular Transmission.* Cambridge University Press, Cambridge.

Ceccarelli, B. & Hurlbut, W.P. (1980) Vesicle hypothesis of the release of quanta of acetylcholine. *Physiol. Rev.* **60**, 396–441.

Cunnane, T.C. & Searl, T.J. (1994) Neurotransmitter release mechanisms in autonomic nerve terminals. *Adv. Second Messenger Phosphoprotein Res.* **29**, 425–59.

Heuser, J.E. (1989) Review of electron microscopic evidence favouring vesicle exocytosis as the structural basis for quantal release during synaptic transmission. *Q. J. Exp. Physiol.* **74**, 1051–69.

Heuser, J.E. & Reese, T.S. (1973) Evidence for recycling of synaptic vesicle membrane during transmitter release at the frog neuromuscular junction. *J. Cell Biol.* **57**, 315–44.

Hirst G.D., Choate, J.K., Cousins, H.M., Edwards, F.R. & Klem, M.F. (1996) Transmission by post-ganglionic axons of the autonomic nervous system: the importance of the specialized neuroeffector junction. *Neuroscience* **73**, 7–23.

Janig, W. & McLachlan, E.M. (1992) Specialized functional pathways are the building blocks of the autonomic nervous system. *J. Auton. Nerv.* **41**, 3–13.

Katz, B. (1962) The transmission of impulses from nerve to muscle, and the subcellular unit of synaptic action. *Proc. R. Soc. Lond.* **B155**, 455–79.

Katz, B. (1966) *Nerve muscle and synapse*. McGraw Hill, New York.

Kuffler, S.W. & Yoshikama, D. (1975) The number of transmitter molecules in a quantum: an estimate from iontophoretic application of acetylcholine at the neuromuscular synapse. *J. Physiol.* **251**, 465–82.

Lundberg, J.M. (1990) Peptide and classical transmitter mechanisms in the autonomic nervous. *Arch. Int. Pharmacodyn. Ther.* **303**, 9–19.

McLachlan, E.M. (ed) (1995) *Autonomic Ganglia.* Harwood Academic Publishers, Luxembourg.

McMahan, U.J. & Kuffler, S.W. (1971) Visual identification of synaptic boutons on living ganglion cells and of varicosities in postganglionic axons in the heart of the frog. *Proc. R. Soc. Lond.* **B177**, 485–508.

References

Almers, W. (1990) Exocytosis. *Ann. Rev. Physiol.* **52**, 607–24.

Boyd, I.A. & Martin, A.R. (1956) The end-plate potential in mammalian muscle. *J. Physiol.* **132**, 74–91.

Brading, A.F. (1987) Physiology of bladder smooth muscle. In: *The Physiology of the Lower Urinary Tract* (eds. M. Torrens & J.F.B. Morrison). Springer Verlag, Berlin.

Bramich, N.J. & Brading, A.F. (1996) Electrical properties of smooth muscle in the guinea-pig urinary bladder. *J. Physiol.* **492**, 185–98.

Brayden, J.E. & Large, W.A. (1986) Electrophysiological analysis of neurogenic vasodilatation in the isolated lingual artery of the rabbit. *Br. J. Pharmac.* **89**, 163–71.

Brock, J.A. & Cunnane, T.C. (1987) Relationship between the nerve action potential and transmitter release from sympathetic postganglionic nerve terminals. *Nature* **326**, 605–7.

Brock, J.A. & Cunnane, T.C. (1988) Electrical activity at the sympathetic neuroeffector junctions in the guinea-pig vas deferens. *J. Physiol.* **399**, 607–32.

Brock, J.A. & Cunnane, T.C. (1990) Transmitter release from sympathetic nerve terminals on an impulse-by-impulse basis and presynaptic receptors. *Ann. N.Y. Acad Sci.* **604**, 176–87.

Brock, J.A. & Cunnane, T.C. (1992) Impulse conduction in sympathetic nerve terminals in the guinea-pig vas deferens and the role of the pelvic ganglia. *Neuroscience* **47**, 185–96.

Dodge, F.A. & Rahamimoff, R. (1967) Co-operative action of calcium ions in transmitter release at the neuromuscular junction. *J. Physiol.* **193**, 419–32.

Eccles, R.M. & Libbett B. (1961) Origin and blockade of the synaptic responses of curarized sympathetic ganglia. *J. Physiol.* **157**, 484–503.

Folkow, B., Haggendal, J. & Lisander, B. (1967) Extent of release and elimination of noradenaline at peripheral nerve terminals. *Acta Physiol. Scand. Suppl.* **307**, 1–38.

Fujii, K. (1988) Evidence for adenosine triphosphate as an excitatory transmitter in guinea-pig, rabbit and pig urinary bladder. *J. Physiol.* **404**, 39–52.

Furness, J.B. (1970) An examination of nerve-mediated, hyoscine-resistant excitation of the guinea-pig colon. *J. Physiol.* **207**, 803–21.

Hall, Z.W. (1992) *An Introduction to Molecular Neurobiology*. Sinauer, Massachusetts.

Heuser, J. (1976) Morphology of synaptic vesicle discharge and reformation at the frog neuromuscular junction. In: *Motor Innervation of Muscle* (ed. S. Thesleff). Academic Press, London.

Hirst, G.D. & Neild, T.O. (1980) Evidence for two populations of excitatory receptors for noradrenaline on arteriolar smooth muscle. *Nature* **283**, 767–8.

Jan, L.Y. & Jan Y.N. (1982) Peptidergic transmission in sympathetic ganglia of the frog. *J. Physiol.* **327**, 219–46.

Kuffler, S.W., Nicholls, J.G. & Martin, A.R. (1984) *From Neuron to Brain*, 2nd edn. Sinauer, Massachusetts.

Kuhne, W. (1887) Neue untersuchungen uber motorische nervenendigung. *A. Biol.* **23**, 1–148.

Liley, A.W. (1956) The quantal components of the mammalian end-plate potential. *J. Physiol.* **133**, 571–81.

Mallart, A. & Martin, A.R. (1967) An analysis of facilitation of transmitter release at the neuromuscular junction of the frog. *J. Physiol.* **193**, 679–94.

Matthews, M.R (1989) Small, intensely fluorescent cells and the paraneuron concept. *J. Electron Microsc. Tech.* **12**, 408–16.

Miller, T.M. & Heuser, J.E. (1984) Endocytosis of synaptic vesicle membrane at the frog neuromuscular junction. *J. Cell Biol.* **98**, 685–98.

O'Kelly, T. Brading, A. & Mortensea, N. (1993) Nerve mediated relaxation of the human internal anal sphincter: the role of nitric oxide. *Gut.* **34**, 689–93.

Rang, H.P., Dale, M.M. & Ritter, J.M. (1995) *Pharmacology*. Churchill Livingstone.

Sneddon, P. & Burnstock, G. (1984) ATP as a co-transmitter in rat tail artery. *Eur. J. Pharmacol.* **106**, 149–52.

Wernig, A. (1975) Estimates of statistical release parameters from crayfish and frog neuromuscular functions. *J. Physiol.* **224**, 207–21.

5 : Recognition Sites in the Autonomic Nervous System

5.1 Introduction

The knowledge that the body produces chemical substances that it uses for communication between cells makes it intuitively likely that the cells will have some recognition site for the chemicals in question. Even before this concept of chemical transmission was accepted, however, the demonstration that applied toxins and chemicals could elicit or inhibit responses from tissues led to the belief that cells must have distinct receptor sites with which such substances bind. The first published suggestion of this probably comes from Langley's paper in the first volume of the *Journal of Physiology* (1878). In a study of the mutual antagonism of atropine and pilocarpine on the secretion of saliva from cat submaxillary glands, he wrote:

> We may, I think, without much rashness, assume that there is some substance or substances in the nerve endings of gland cells with which both atropine and pilocarpine are capable of forming compounds. On this assumption, then, the atropine or pilocarpine compounds are formed according to some law of which their relative mass and chemical affinity for the substance are factors.

However, the receptors involved in Langley's studies – and for that matter any receptors – proved extremely elusive, and nearly 100 years later their isolation and structural identification had still not been achieved. In a review paper in *Nature* in 1971, Rang stated, 'it has not yet been possible to isolate any pharmacological receptor', but he concluded his discussion with the words, 'There seems every reason to hope that studies in progress will lead to successful isolation and characterisation of cholinergic receptors'.

During the century or so between these two reports, binding of other ligands to tissue proteins was studied in more detail by biochemists – such as the binding of substrates to enzymes and of oxygen to haemoglobin. The evidence strongly suggested that receptors were also likely to be proteins. However, the fact that the majority of receptors for endogenous ligands are membrane-bound has made them more difficult to study by several orders of magnitude than the soluble cytoplasmic proteins.

Isolation and characterisation of receptors have nevertheless been achieved in many cases, and the technology is now available not only to isolate receptors, but also to isolate the DNA specifying them. These genes can then be introduced into a suitable cell that can be cultured, with the receptor being expressed in large amounts, greatly enhancing the ease with which the receptor can be isolated and characterised. The amino acid sequences of the proteins can be determined, and hydrophobicity–hydrophilicity plots of the amino acids, combined with studies on the accessibility of various target sequences for modification by extracellularly or intracellularly applied reagents, can lead to predictions about their structure (Box 5.1). However, it is still not possible to define precisely the three-dimensional structure of any membrane-bound receptor, and thus complete knowledge of the molecular interaction between receptors and their ligands, and of the conformational changes that can occur, has not been achieved at the time of writing.

5.2 Definition of receptors

Since there are potentially very many sites in the body to which exogenous or endogenous ligands can bind, it is sensible to define what we mean by receptors in the functional sense. There are several requirements that must be met:

1 the macromolecule must have a binding site or sites for a specific natural endogenous ligand;

2 it must have a genetically determined function;

3 binding of the natural ligand or synthetic agonists must cause a specific perturbation or change in state of the receptor macromolecule or its immediate environment, which initiates a chain of events leading to a response;

4 for the majority of the membrane-bound receptors that mediate responses with magnitudes determined by the ligand concentration, agonist binding must be rapidly reversible, and must not involve making or breaking of covalent bonds.

Thus, we might say that receptors are macromolecules that have evolved with the specific function of binding transiently to endogenous ligands, and mediating changes in cellular function.

5.3 Studies of receptors

It is worth mentioning at the start that the characteristic properties of membrane receptors were initially deduced entirely from the relationship

Box 5.1 Isolation and characterisation of receptors

Isolation of receptors depended initially on finding a good source and being able to label the receptors irreversibly with a radioactive compound. The first receptors to be successfully isolated were the nicotinic receptors from the electric organ of the electric ray *Torpedo marmorata*. The electric organ consists of stacks of flat cells derived from skeletal muscle but lacking contractile machinery. One side of the cell is innervated, and is really a single extensive synapse with the post-synaptic membrane packed full of nicotinic receptors. On simultaneous activation of all the cells in a stack, large extracellular currents can be generated, which can be used by the fish for stunning its prey. This organ thus provides a rich source of nicotinic receptors. A specific irreversible label of the receptors was provided by the venom of a snake, the Formosan banded krait – α-bungarotoxin, known to block transmission at this junction. Receptor isolation from *Torpedo electroplax* using radiolabelled α-bungarotoxin was first reported in *Nature* by Miledi *et al.* in 1971.

In order to purify and characterize receptors they must be isolated from their membranes. Luckily, receptors can be solubilized in a way that allows them to retain their drug-binding ability, so that they can be traced through the various procedures involved. Normally, a crude membrane preparation is made by homogenization and centrifugation, and then the receptors are extracted using mild detergent treatment (e.g. the non-ionic detergent Triton X-100). Purification can be by several different techniques, such as density gradient centrifugation, gel filtration, or more commonly affinity chromatography. In this latter technique, a receptor ligand is bound covalently to an insoluble support such as sepharose, and packed into a column. The crude extract can then be poured through the column, which will retain the receptors through binding to the ligand. After elution, the protein can be run on sodium dodecylsulphate (SDS) electrophoresis to determine its purity and establish the molecular weight. The purified protein can then be analyzed for its amino acid composition and sequenced.

Once the amino acid sequence of a receptor is known, models of its secondary and tertiary structure can be made. One useful technique is to generate a hydrophobicity profile, which can highlight the sequences of the protein that are likely to be in the membrane. To do this, each of the 20 amino acids is allocated a number to represent its hydropathic character (whether its side chains are hydrophobic or hydrophilic), the positive values being hydrophobic, and the negative values hydrophilic. The hydrophobicity of a chain of amino acids from about 7 to 20 is analyzed as a group, and the results plotted in sequence along the protein as shown in Fig. B5.1.1a. Further information about the

Continued

Box 5.1 *Continued*

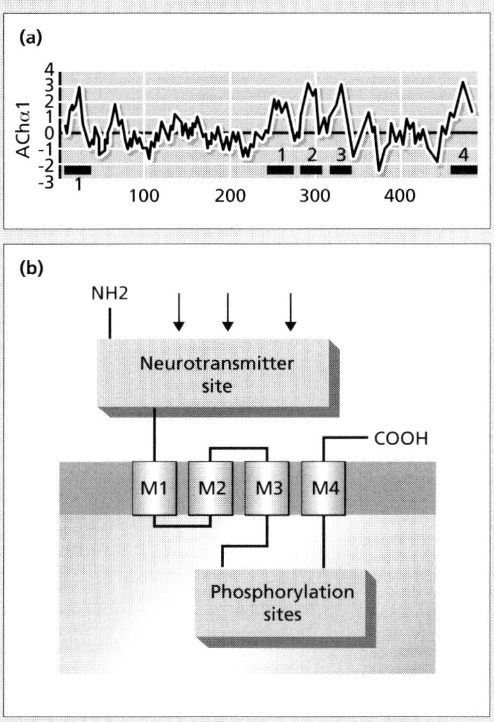

Fig. B5.1.1 A subunit of the nicotinic acetylcholine receptor. (a) Shows a hydrophobicity profile of one subunit of the nicotinic receptor from the *Torpedo* electric organ. The putative transmembrane-spanning hydrophobic segments are indicated by the bars. (b) A model of the subunit organization. From Changeux (1994).

orientation of the protein can be obtained by immunochemical techniques, raising antibodies to groups of amino acids and studying their binding to the intact receptor, or else using photoaffinity labels in a similar fashion. More detailed information can come from cloning receptors and introducing point mutations and studying their functional affects.

Application of these techniques can allow some quite detailed models of individual receptors to be built. The nicotinic receptor has been found to consist of five subunits, each of which is rather similar in structure. It is proposed that each subunit has the amino terminal in the extracellular space, coupled to a large hydrophilic domain, followed by three membrane-spanning segments (M1–M3) connected by short hydrophilic chains, then a large cytoplasmic hydrophilic domain, followed by a fourth membrane-spanning segment (M4) coupled to the extracellular carboxy terminal (Fig. B5.1.1b). The five M2 segments are thought to be involved in lining the channel of the activated receptor and contain negatively charged amino acid side chains which confer the cationic selectivity of the channel.

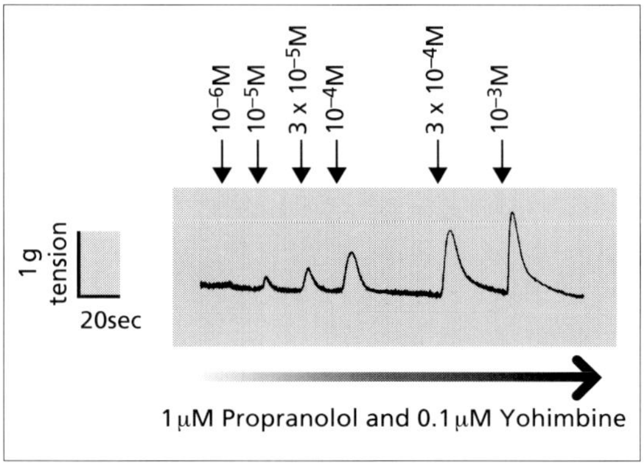

Fig. 5.1 Effects of 20 s applications of increasing doses of the α_1-adrenoceptor agonist phenylephrine on the contractile activity of a circular smooth muscle strip dissected from the pig urethra. The experiment was carried out in the presence of propranolol and yohimbine to prevent activation of β- or α_2-adrenoceptors. Trace kindly supplied by Miss Rachel McCoy.

between the concentration of the drugs applied and the response of the tissue. This meant that, historically, the receptors that were studied at any time were determined to some extent by the ease with which a particular response could be measured. Quantitative studies required responses to be graded with drug concentration, and this limited early work largely to receptors on smooth muscle, heart and glandular tissues. Graded contractions could be evoked and easily measured from smooth muscles, as shown in Fig. 5.1, as could the frequency and contractile force of the heartbeat. Secretions could also be measured from some glands. Thus, the early focus of research was on autonomic receptors, although there were some unusual skeletal muscles (slow fibres), such as the rectus abdominis muscle of the frog and the chick biventer cervicis muscle, which gave graded contractions. All of these responses, however, occurred far downstream from the actual receptor activation, and to some extent limited the amount of information available about the receptor behaviour. In the 1940s, the introduction of microelectrodes allowed another type of response to be measured – the change in membrane potentials. This dramatically shifted the focus of research to the nicotinic receptor in skeletal muscle, allowing depolarisation caused by different concentrations of nicotinic agonists to be measured – a response that was much closer to receptor activation than muscle contraction. Studies on nicotinic receptors dominated pharmacology for the next few decades, until increasing knowledge of second messengers and the development of techniques for measuring their concentration in cells shifted the emphasis back to studies of autonomic receptors and receptors on non-excitable tissues. More recently, the development of brain slice technology has allowed studies of receptors on central nervous system neurones.

5.4 Properties of receptors

There are several properties that all receptors share, and there is a receptor 'terminology' with which a student needs to become familiar (Box 5.2). A 'ligand' is a chemical that binds with a receptor. Receptors show a characteristic 'affinity' for the ligands that bind to them and occupy the receptor. They can be activated by 'agonists', and each has a characteristic 'dose–response relationship'. In response to a high concentration of agonist, receptors show desensitisation, and the total number of receptors in a tissue can vary depending on the frequency with which they are activated *in vivo* (up or down regulation). The responses of a tissue to an agonist can be reduced by 'antagonists', which can be reversible or irreversible, competitive or non-competitive. Ligands for a particular receptor can vary not only

Box 5.2 Definitions

Affinity. The affinity of a receptor for the ligand is the reciprocal of the equilibrium constant (Box 5.3). The higher the affinity of the receptor for the ligand, the lower the concentration necessary to occupy it, and the smaller the equilibrium constant.

Occupancy. This is the fraction of the total number of receptors present that is bound to a ligand at any instant of time in the steady state.

Agonist. A molecule that can bind to a receptor and activate it.

Antagonist. In general terms, this is a molecule that prevents the response to an agonist. Since this could equally well apply to an agonist that initiated an opposite response (physiological antagonism) or to a molecule that blocked some part of the receptor effector coupling beyond the receptor, it is often useful to define a specific 'receptor antagonist' as a molecule that binds to a receptor and prevents the agonist from activating it. In this framework, a 'competitive' antagonist will bind to the same site on the receptor as the natural agonist, and may bind either reversibly or irreversibly. It is competitive because when both the agonist and the antagonist are added together, they will compete for occupancy of the receptor. A 'non-competitive' antagonist will bind to some other site on the receptor to prevent its activation by the agonist. It could stabilise the inactive conformation of the receptor, or could block an effector site on the receptor (e.g. the ion channel of a directly coupled receptor, or the G protein-binding site – see below).

Efficacy. This describes the extent to which a population of receptors can be activated by bound ligand. The efficacy of an antagonist is zero.

Spare receptors. Most natural ligands can initiate a maximal functional response of a tissue while only occupying a fraction of the total number of available receptors. The ones left over are the 'spare receptors'.

in their affinity for the receptor, but also in their ability to activate the receptor. This latter property of the ligand is known as 'efficacy'. Antagonists have zero efficacy.

5.5 Properties of agonists

5.5.1 Dose–response relationship

This relationship is normally saturating, and rather similar in shape to a rectangular hyperbola (Fig. 5.2). It is often more convenient to express the relationship in terms of a log dose–response (DR) curve, where the response is plotted against the logarithm of the drug concentration. This gives a sigmoid curve, with a significant linear segment in the middle. It allows easier comparison of curves, and is particularly useful when comparing agonists or looking at the effects of antagonists on the relationship.

The agonists for a particular receptor can be divided into full agonists and partial agonists. All full agonists of a particular receptor elicit log DR curves that have approximately identical slopes and maxima, but may occur at different positions along the x axis (Fig. 5.3). Partial agonists are never able to elicit the full response of the tissue, and thus show a shallower curve – although the position of the curve along the x axis can also vary, and

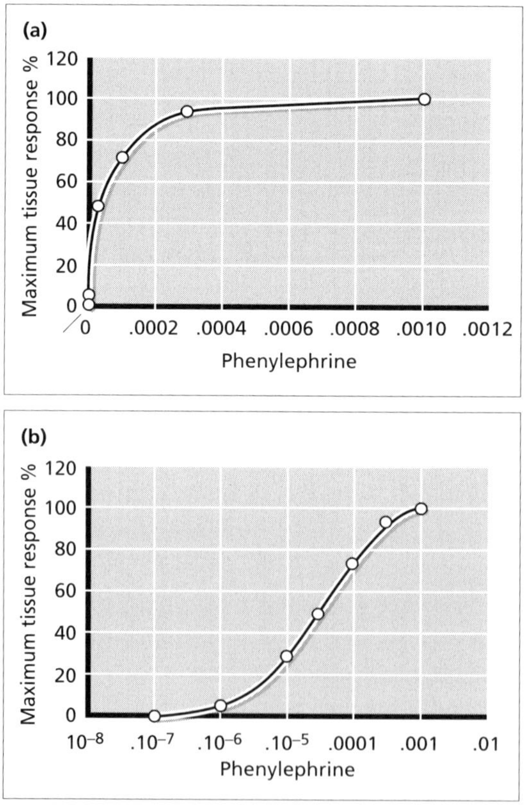

Fig. 5.2 Dose–response curves of a strip of urethral circular smooth muscle to 20 s applications of the α_1-adrenoceptor agonist phenylephrine. Points taken from the trace shown in Fig. 5.1. Concentrations expressed as M. (a) Dose–response curve plotted on linear co-ordinates. (b) Log dose–response curve. The concentration is plotted using a logarithmic scale. The dose–response curve spans about four log units. Kindly supplied by Miss Rachel McCoy.

if the response is expressed as a percentage of its own maximum, the curve will usually have the same shape as that of the full agonists.

Students should be aware that the shapc of a dose–response relationship is determined by an often long and complex sequence of events that intervenes between receptor occupancy and the tissue response – the process of *receptor–effector coupling* that is unique for each receptor and tissue. This accounts for the identical shape of the curves for full agonists acting on the same receptor on the same tissue. Some dose–response curves have a sigmoid shape even when plotted on a non-logarithmic scale, suggesting that there must be *co-operativity* in the interaction (Fig. 5.4). This could be

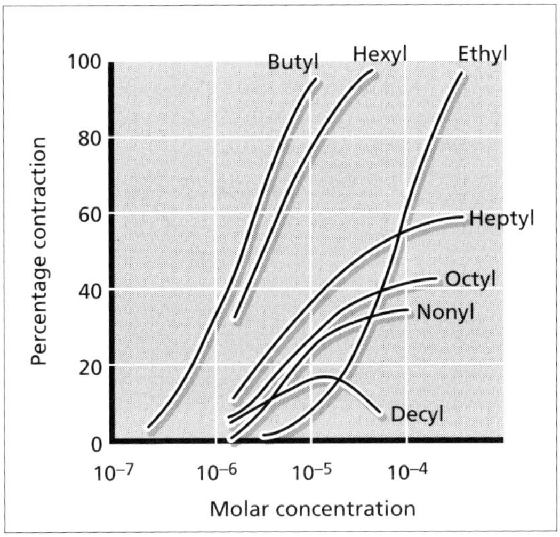

Fig. 5.3 Full and partial agonists. This figure shows log dose–response curves of strips of guinea-pig ileum to a series of alkyltrimethylammonium compounds. The butyl-, hexyl- and ethylammonium compounds are all full agonists, note similar slopes and maxima, although their positions along the x axis are different. The other four compounds are partial agonists, and will clearly not elicit a full response whatever concentration is used.

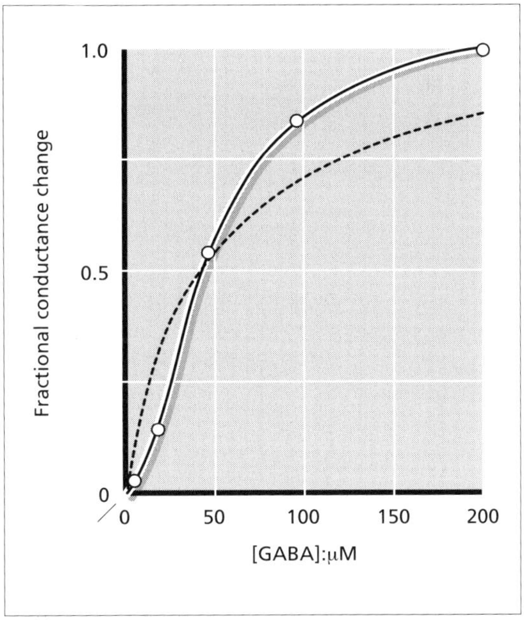

Fig. 5.4 Dose–response curve for the conductance change caused by application of GABA on to a crustacean neuromuscular junction. The curve is plotted on linear co-ordinates. Note the sigmoid shape of the curve (open symbols and solid line). The dotted line is the curve expected from the Langmuir equation with the same equilibrium constant. The sigmoid shape of the DR curve is probably due to the fact that the receptor has several binding sites for GABA, and the probability that the channel opening increases as more agonist molecules bind to the receptor.

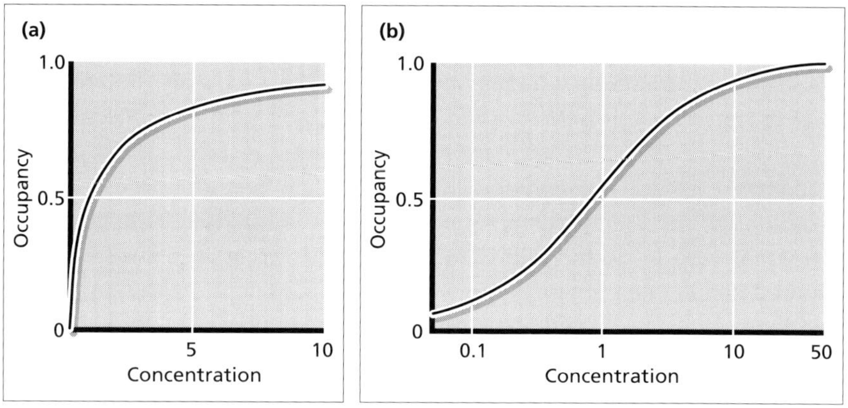

Fig. 5.5 Theoretical relationship between fractional receptor occupancy and drug concentration according to the Langmuir equation. (a) Plotted on linear co-ordinates, (b) plotted logarithmically. Concentration is expressed as a multiple of the equilibrium constant for the drug (concentration at which 50% of the receptors are occupied).

due, for instance, to the necessity for binding of more than one ligand molecule to a receptor in order to activate it, or might result from co-operative interactions downstream from receptor activation.

DR curves on their own can give very little information about the behaviour of the receptors. Nevertheless, early pharmacologists, who knew nothing of the intervening mechanisms, produced theoretical models that speculated about the relationship between occupancy of the receptor by an agonist and the response. The first step in such an analysis is to consider the factors determining the occupancy of the receptor by the ligand. This can be defined in terms of the laws of mass action, an extremely fruitful approach probably initiated by A.V. Hill and refined by A.J. Clark. Receptors are considered as identical and non-interacting. As shown in Box 5.3, one can derive the relationship between receptor occupancy and drug concentration and express it as the Langmuir equation. The relationship is a rectangular hyperbola, as shown in Fig. 5.5.

The simplest theory relating ligand binding to effect is 'occupancy theory'. This theory assumes that the response of a tissue is a function of the number of receptors occupied by the agonist. The function is not specified, and the DR curve would only be described by the Langmuir equation if there were a linear relationship between all the steps linking occupancy to response.

5.5.2 Determinants of potency

Using simple occupancy theory and the assumption that a 100% response only occurs with 100% occupancy, the potency of an agonist and thus the position of the DR curve on the x axis would be uniquely determined by its affinity for the receptors and the equilibrium constant of the reaction. The

Box 5.3 Derivation of the Langmuir equation

Consider a population of receptors exposed to a single drug that combines reversibly with them:

$$\underset{X}{\text{Drug}} + \underset{(1-P)}{\text{Receptor}} \underset{k_2}{\overset{k_1}{\rightleftharpoons}} \underset{P}{\text{DR}}$$

where X = drug concentration; P = the fraction of receptors occupied by drug; (1 – P) = the fraction of receptors not occupied; and k_1 and k_2 are forward and backward rate constants.

From the law of mass action, which states that the rate of a chemical reaction is given by the product of the concentration of reactants, multiplied by a rate constant characteristic of the particular reaction, the forward reaction rate = $k_1X(1-P)$ and the backward reaction rate = k_2P. At equilibrium, the two rates are equal

$$\therefore\ k_1X(1-P) = k_2P \quad (1)$$

and $$\frac{k_2}{k_1} = \frac{X(1-P)}{P}$$

$$\frac{k_2}{k_1} = K, \text{ the equilibrium constant}$$

If a drug concentration is used that causes 50% occupancy,

$$K = \frac{X(1-0.5)}{0.5}$$

$$\therefore\ K = X$$

The equilibrium constant is numerically equal to the concentration of the drug required to occupy one half of the receptors.

The Langmuir equation is derived from equation (1) above:

$$P = \frac{X}{X+K}$$

This is the fundamental binding equation for a saturable system. It can also be written

$$P = \frac{X/K}{X/K+1}$$

demonstration that ligands can have different efficacies introduces further complications. Evidence strongly suggests that the efficacy of a ligand is a separate attribute to its affinity, and that some full agonists can elicit a maximal response whilst occupying only a small fraction of the available pool, while others (partial agonists) can never produce maximal effects even when their concentration is high enough to produce maximal occupancy (Fig. 5.6). It would be theoretically possible to have ligands with

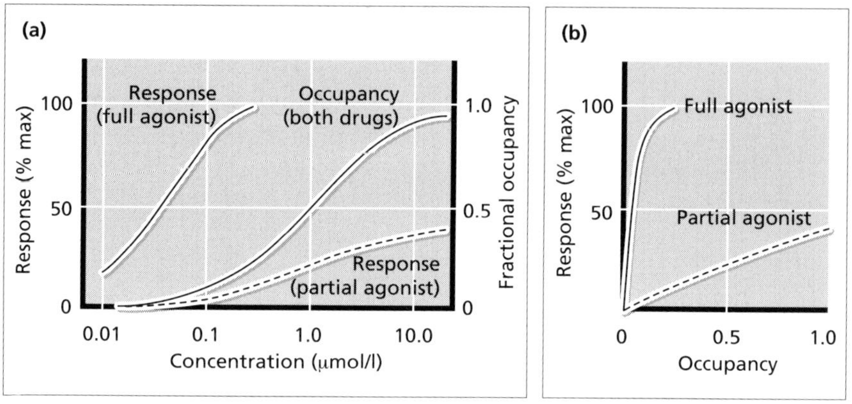

Fig. 5.6 Theoretical occupancy and response curves for full and partial agonists. (a) The middle curve shows the relationship between occupancy (right-hand ordinate) and concentration for both the full and partial agonist. A maximum response is produced by the full agonist at low occupancy, whereas maximum occupancy results in only a small response to the partial agonist. (b) Relationship between fractional occupancy and response for the two drugs.

identical affinities for the receptor, but quite different efficacies. There thus appears to be spare receptors in many tissues, particularly with respect to bath-applied agonists.

The potency of an agonist is therefore affected both by its efficacy and its affinity for the receptor. For antagonists, the situation is easier, since the efficacy for an antagonist is zero and potency is therefore more closely related to affinity. It should be remembered, however, that the potency of a drug is also determined by the concentration of the drug that reaches the receptors, and this may not be the same as the concentration the tissue is exposed to, particularly in the case of exogenous application of natural agonists, where the body is likely to have a powerful mechanism for removing the agonist, which may result in a much lower concentration actually reaching the receptors. Obvious examples of this are the presence of acetylcholinesterase at the neuromuscular junction and of uptake mechanisms on nerve terminals for catecholamines.

5.5.3 Efficacy

It is not at present entirely clear what the efficacy of a drug depends on. Theoretically, efficacy and occupancy theory would only be compatible if a single receptor could undergo different degrees of activation. This seems unlikely to be the case for those receptors for which the activated state is an open ion channel, since the single-channel conductance does not seem to vary with the agonist that activates it. Instead, the duration of the active state (in this case open channel) varies, as shown in Fig. 5.7 (see also Box 5.5). Thus, for these receptors, it seems more likely that efficacy represents

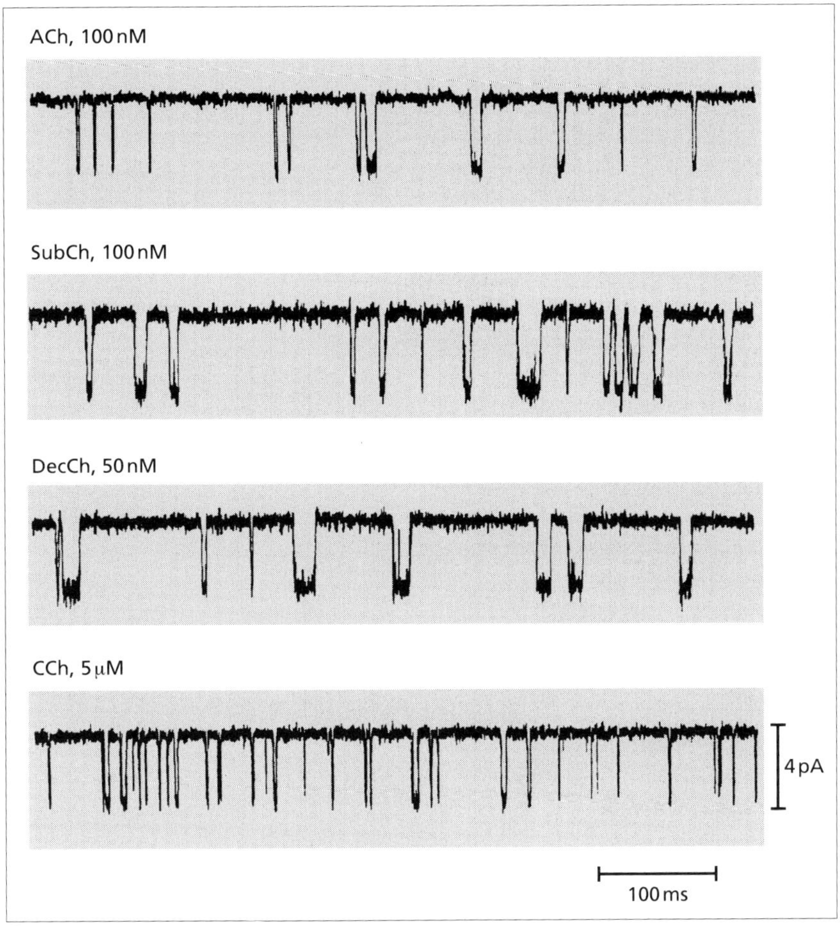

Fig. 5.7 Single-channel currents recorded from the frog neuromuscular junction, showing the different mean channel open times that different nicotinic agonists induce from the end-plate receptors. The traces show channel openings (downward deflections) in response to acetylcholine (ACh), suberyldicholine (SubCh), dicarboxylic acid dicholine ester (DecCh) and carbachol (CCh). Note similar amplitude of currents in response to each of the agonists, but different durations. From Colquhoun & Sakmann (1985).

the chance that a receptor with ligand bound will take on the active configuration. This will be determined by k_3 and k_4 in the equation below:

$$D + R_i \underset{k_2}{\overset{k_1}{\rightleftharpoons}} DR; \underset{k_4}{\overset{k_3}{\rightleftharpoons}} DR_a$$

where R_i is the inactive form of the receptor and R_a the active form. The position of an agonist DR curve on the x axis is thus determined both by the affinity and by the efficacy of a ligand. In this case, the response would be a function not of the receptor occupancy, but of the number of receptors in the active state.

5.5.4 Desensitization

Experimentally, if a receptor is exposed to a high agonist concentration, then after wash-out, a low dose that was previously active may now initiate a smaller response, and time is necessary before recovery occurs (Fig. 5.8a). This type of desensitization usually recovers relatively rapidly, and does not seem to involve withdrawal of receptors from the membrane. It involves some sort of uncoupling of the receptor from the effector system. Desensitization can be homologous (involving the response to only a single type of receptor), as is often the case for receptors that are ion channels, or heterologous, in which case the response to several receptors may be diminished by exposure to only one ligand. In the latter case, it is likely that

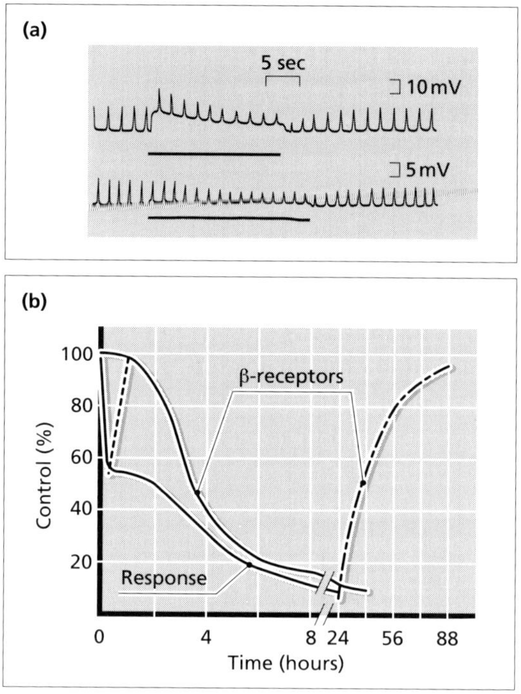

Fig. 5.8 Desensitization. (a) Depolarizing potentials recorded from the end plates of two frog striated muscle fibres in response to brief iontophoretically applied pulses of acetylcholine. The interval between stimuli is initially long enough for recovery from any desensitization. During the long bars additional acetylcholine was applied continuously. This causes the responses to the short pulses to decline with a time constant of about 20 s. Discontinuing the steady application allows recovery of the response to short pulses with a similar time course. (b) The effect of 1 μM isoprenaline on the adenylyl cyclase activity (lower line) and β-adrenoceptor number (upper line) of tissue cultured rat glioma cells. The response drops off rapidly initially without any loss of receptors (true receptor desensitization), and then declines more slowly concomitantly with a drop in the β-adrenoceptor number (receptor downregulation). The dotted lines show a relatively rapid recovery of the response on washing off the agonist in the initial phase, and a slow recovery of receptor number in the late phase (note change in time scale). (a) From Katz & Thesleff (1957), (b) from Perkins (1981).

uncoupling occurs downstream from the receptor, and involves some common step in the receptor–effector mechanisms. Often this is caused by phosphorylation of one of the proteins involved. Longer exposure to agonists can lead to internalization of receptors and a reduction in the number of functional receptors (down-regulation, see Fig. 5.8b).

5.6 Properties of antagonists

5.6.1 Reversible competitive antagonists

These are considered to bind reversibly to the same site on the receptor as its natural ligand, although they do not activate the receptor. When agonists and antagonists are present together, they compete for occupancy of the ligand-binding site. This allows the use of the mass action equations to calculate the occupancy of the receptors by an agonist in the presence of a competitive antagonist (Box 5.4).

If a log dose–response curve is constructed in the absence and then in the presence of increasing concentrations of a reversible competitive antagonist, a parallel shift to the right of the curve is found experimentally (Fig. 5.9).

On the assumption that equal occupancies of the receptors by the agonist produce equal response, the Schild equation (Box 5.4) predicts this parallel shift using simple mass action assumptions. It also predicts that the dose ratio (the concentration of the drug needed to produce a certain response in

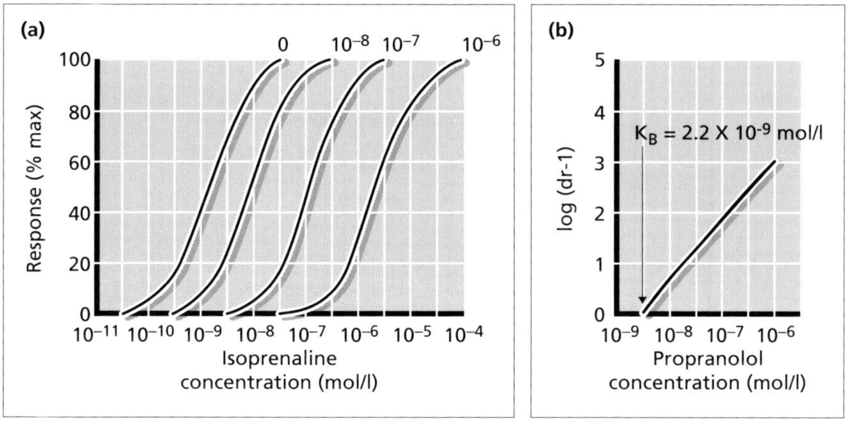

Fig. 5.9 An example of the effects of a competitive antagonist. (a) Log dose–response curves of the effect of isoprenaline on the isolated guinea-pig atrium in the absence and presence of increasing concentrations of the competitive antagonist propranolol. Note the parallel shift to the right of the log dose–response curve. (b) Schild plot of the results. Log (dr–1) is plotted against the log of the antagonist concentration (where dr is the dose ratio). The intercept on the abscissa gives the antagonist equilibrium constant K_B. Results from Potter (1967).

Box 5.4 Competitive antagonism

The agonist (A) and the antagonist (B) are competing for the same receptor sites. Considering them each in turn.
For the agonist

$$\underset{X_A}{A} \quad + \quad \underset{(1-P_A-P_B)}{R} \quad \underset{k_2}{\overset{k_1}{\rightleftharpoons}} \quad \underset{P_A}{AR}$$

For the antagonist

$$\underset{X_B}{B} \quad + \quad \underset{(1-P_A-P_B)}{R} \quad \underset{k_4}{\overset{k_3}{\rightleftharpoons}} \quad \underset{P_B}{BR}$$

where X_A and X_B are the concentrations of agonist and antagonist, and P_A and P_B are the fractions of receptors occupied by agonist and antagonist.

Using the law of mass action, at equilibrium:

$$k_1X_A(1-P_A-P_B) = k_2 P_A \tag{2}$$

$$k_3X_B(1-P_A-P_B) = k_4 P_B \tag{3}$$

$$\frac{k_2}{k_1} = K_A \text{ and } \frac{k_4}{k_3} = K_B$$

From equation (3) $P_B = \dfrac{(1-P_A)X_B/K_B}{X_B/K_B+1}$

Inserting P_B into equation (2) and solving for P_A

$$P_A = \frac{X_A/K_A}{X_A/K_A + X_B/K_B + 1}$$

This is called the competitive equation.

If one assumes that equal occupancies of the receptor by the drug produce equal responses, then:

initially $P_A = \dfrac{X_{A1}/K_A}{X_{A1}/K_A+1}$ (Langmuir equation)

and finally $P_A = \dfrac{X_{A2}/K_A}{X_{A2}/K_A + X_B/K_B + 1}$ (competitive equation)

Equating these:

$$\frac{X_{A1}/K_A}{X_{A1}/K_A+1} = \frac{X_{A2}/K_A}{X_{A2}/K_A + X_B/K_B + 1}$$

or

$$\frac{1}{1+K_A/X_{A1}} = \frac{1}{1+(X_B/K_B+1)/(X_{A2}/K_A)}$$

Inverting:

Continued

Box 5.4 *Continued*

$$\frac{1+K_A}{X_{A1}} = \frac{1+K_A(X_B/K_B+1)}{X_{A2}}$$

hence $\frac{X_{A2}}{X_{A1}} = \frac{X_B}{K_B} + 1$

By definition $\frac{X_{A2}}{X_{A1}}$ = dose ratio (dr)

$$dr - 1 = \frac{X_B}{K_B} \quad \text{(Schild equation)} \qquad (4)$$

This equation can be written:

$\log(dr - 1) = \log X_B - \log K_B$

the presence of a reversible competitive antagonist divided by the concentration needed to produce the same response in its absence) should be independent of the agonist used, and depend only on the concentration (X_B) and equilibrium constant (K_B) of the antagonist; and that the dose ratio should increase in a linear fashion with the antagonist concentration. The slope of the plot of (dr−1) against X_B should be equal to $1/K_B$. This is important, since it gives an easy method of estimating the equilibrium constant for the antagonist. Using the logarithmic expression of the Schild equation (Box 5.4), a plot of log (dr−1) against log X_B gives a straight line of unity slope with an intercept on the abscissa of log K_B. This is called a Schild plot.

5.6.2 Reversible non-competitive receptor antagonists

These bind reversibly to the receptor in a manner that may not prevent agonist binding, but prevents receptor activation. Log DR curves in the presence of increasing concentrations of such antagonists have reduced maxima and shallower slopes (Fig. 5.10), since the antagonists are effectively reducing the number of receptors available for activation. There is thus no competition between agonists and antagonists, and increasing the concentration of the agonist cannot surmount the antagonist effect. In fact, in the case of receptors that are ion channels, antagonists that block ion permeation through the open channel actually become more effective with increased agonist concentration, since the channel blockers bind preferentially to the active receptor (open channel).

5.6.3 Irreversible antagonists

These bind to the receptors but dissociate from them very slowly, or not at all. If a certain amount of such an antagonist is added to an organ bath con-

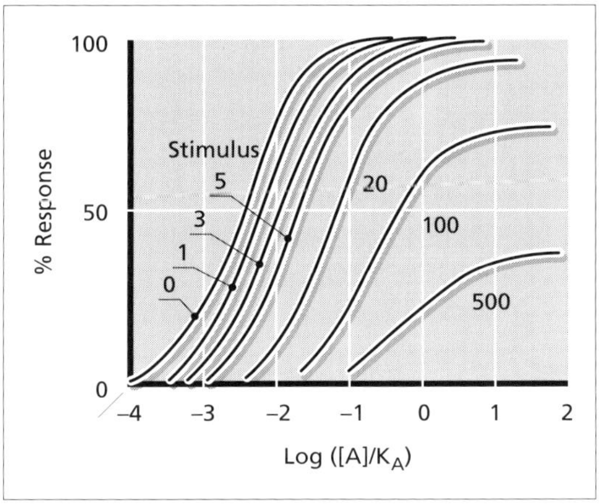

Fig. 5.10 Theoretical effects of increasing concentrations (from 1–500) of a non-competitive reversible antagonist on the log dose–response curves of a tissue to an agonist (the agonist concentration is normalized by dividing it with the equilibrium constant K_A). In this example, the curves are shifted to the right at low antagonist concentrations, because the agonist has a relatively high efficacy and can produce a maximum effect when occupying a small proportion of the receptors. At higher concentrations, the curves are further shifted to the right and have a suppressed maximum.

taining a tissue with the appropriate receptors, progressive occupancy of the receptors will occur with time, either until all the available antagonist is bound, leaving no free drug but a fraction of unoccupied receptors, or until all the receptors present are bound to antagonist, and there is still free drug present in the solution. To study the effect of irreversible antagonists on DR curves in steady state, the antagonist is applied first for a short time, and washed out. The tissue will now contain a smaller population of unbound receptors. If there are no longer enough activatable receptors left to produce a maximum tissue response, the log DR curve will now have a lower maximum and a shallower slope than in the absence of antagonist (Fig. 5.11). It should be noted that, in many tissues, even with a significant proportion of the receptors removed, a maximum physiological response can be achieved, albeit at a higher agonist concentration. Thus, there is often an initial parallel shift of the dose–response curve before the maximum is suppressed. This indicates that there are normally more receptors present than are required for a full effect, and that the tissue possesses 'spare receptors'.

Irreversible antagonists can be competitive, in the sense that they can bind to the same site as the agonist, or non-competitive, if they bind to another site. Both will have similar effects on DR curves, but the two can be distinguished if the irreversible antagonist is initially applied in the presence of the agonist. In this case, if the drug is competitive, the agonist will reduce the amount of antagonist binding in unit time, because of the time it will spend occupying the receptors. Non-competitive irreversible antago-

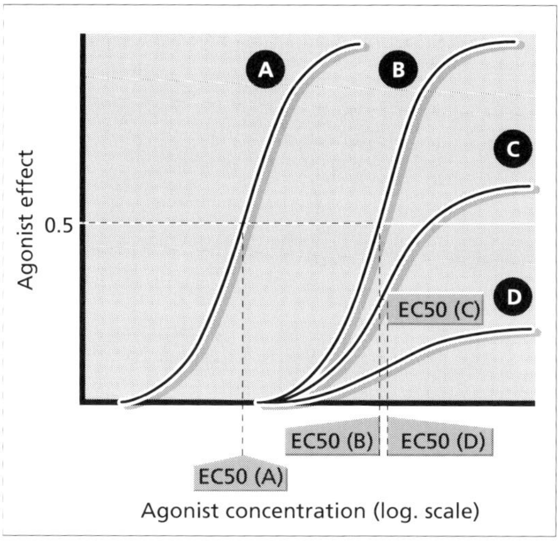

Fig. 5.11 Effect of treating the tissue with increasing concentrations of an irreversible antagonist on the log dose–response curve of the tissue to an agonist. The irreversible antagonist is applied and then washed out before the agonist dose–response curve is obtained. The irreversible antagonist will then have eliminated some of the receptors from activation by the agonist. Curve A is the curve in the absence of antagonist. Curves B–D are with increasing numbers of receptors eliminated. There are sufficient spare receptors to allow a maximum response to be generated in curve B with a higher concentration of agonist (larger EC50 value), but for curves C and D there are not enough to generate the maximum response. With a competitive irreversible antagonist, when the EC50 values remain the same even with greater elimination of receptors, this value theoretically will approximate to the equilibrium constant for the agonist.

nists will, on the other hand, inactivate receptors at the same rate, whether or not agonist is present.

5.7 Types of receptor

A sufficient number have now been isolated to make it clear that there are several distinct types of receptor, as shown in Fig. 5.12. For membrane-bound receptors, one can define three classes: ion channels, G protein-linked receptors and enzymes. Lipid-soluble ligands, such as steroids, bind to intracellular receptors.

5.7.1 Receptor-operated (directly coupled) ion channels

These receptors are oligomers, usually of four or five rather similar protein subunits, which in the absence of bound ligand exist in the closed configuration, but when the right number of ligand molecules occupies the binding sites can flip transiently into a configuration containing an open ion channel. The subunits characteristically each have four membrane-

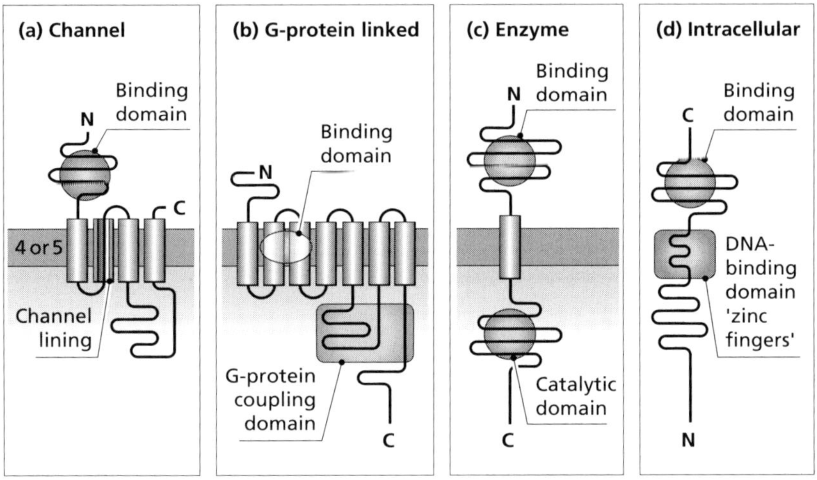

Fig. 5.12 General structure of four receptor families. (a) Directly coupled receptor-operated ion channels. This shows a representative structure of a single subunit of the channel. It contains an agonist binding domain, four membrane-spanning hydrophobic domains, one of which probably forms part of the channel lining, and a cytoplasmic loop which may be involved in regulation by intracellular systems of the channel function. Each channel will have four or five of these subunits. (b) G-protein linked receptors. These typically have seven transmembrane domains, with the agonist binding site involving more than one of these, and an intracellular domain involved in coupling to G-proteins. (c) Receptors that are enzymes. These are usually tyrosine kinases, and have a single membrane-spanning domain, linking the binding and catalytic domains. (d) Intracellular receptors. These are mainly steroid receptors, and have a steroid binding domain, and a domain for interaction with the cellular DNA. From Rang *et al.* (1995).

spanning alpha helices. At present, five types of endogenous ligand have been identified, which activate distinct channels: acetylcholine, the excitatory amino acids (glutamate and aspartate), the inhibitory amino acids (γ-aminobutyric acid (GABA) and glycine), serotonin and adenosine triphosphate (ATP). The channels may differ in their ionic selectivity, numbers of ligand-binding sites and kinetics. Activation of these channels causes a rapid increase in membrane conductance, and the functional response is normally the rapid change in membrane potential that results from movement of ions down their electrochemical gradients through the channels. Channels normally show a relatively unselective permeability to either cations or anions. Cation-selective channels are excitatory, mediating depolarization of the cell membrane (end-plate potentials, excitatory junction potentials, etc.), whereas anion-selective channels are inhibitory, either through hyperpolarization (if net Cl movement is inward), or by stabilising the membrane near to the equilibrium potential for Cl. It seems likely that this class of receptor has evolved more recently than the others, since it is mainly used in excitable tissues to initiate or inhibit the production of action potentials.

It is interesting to note that the properties of these receptors can be studied in considerable detail with the technique of patch clamp recording (Box 5.5), in which it is sometimes possible to isolate a single receptor and measure current flowing through the channel as it opens and closes (Fig.

Box 5.5 Patch clamp recording

The conductance of individual ion channels is so great that quite large currents can pass through them when the correct electrochemical gradients exist. The development of good amplifiers has allowed the currents flowing through single channels to be resolved, if they can be isolated. The patch clamp technique was developed by Neher and Sakmann in 1976. It is really a method of voltage clamping a small patch of membrane. A fine glass pipette with a polished end of about 1–5 μm in diameter filled with an isotonic conducting solution is pushed gently against the cleaned surface of a cell, effectively isolating a patch of membrane. The isolation of the patch was improved later by Neher, who used gentle application of negative pressure to suck the membrane into the orifice of the pipette, resulting in the sealing of the membrane to the glass with a leak resistance to the extracellular fluid of some 100 gigaohms. An electrode connects the inside of the pipette and the extracellular solution, and current is passed between them to hold the patch of membrane at the desired potential. The resistance of the patch is infinitely large compared with the resistance of the rest of the cell membrane, and thus almost all of the voltage drop occurs across the patch. If a channel in the isolated patch opens, the current flowing through it can be detected in the voltage-clamp feedback circuitry. This methodology allows the opening and closing of channels to be monitored. It is worth emphasising that this elegant, yet remarkably simple, technique allows the behaviour of a single protein molecule to be followed in real time, something which no other technique, however sophisticated, can achieve. With reference to directly coupled ion channel receptors, if low concentrations of an agonist are included in the pipette solution, the activation of individual receptors can again be followed. This is illustrated in Fig. B5.5.1.

This technique can be modified to produce several useful applications. If the patch is pulled gently away from the cell, the membrane seals round to form a small vesicle in the pipette tip. The outer aspect of this vesicle can be broken by exposure to air, resulting in an inside-out membrane patch. This configuration is very useful for examining the effects of intracellular ligands on channels. If a strong pressure is applied to the pipette in the cell-attached state, the patch of membrane can be ruptured, connecting the inside of the pipette to the

Continued on p. 152

Box 5.5 *Continued*

cell interior. This is called the whole cell configuration, and allows a low resistance access to the cell, enabling voltage clamping of the whole cell membrane to be achieved in cells that are short in relation to their length constant (important for ensuring a uniform voltage). After the whole cell configuration has been achieved, if the pipette is pulled gently away from the cell, the membrane fuses over to create an outside-out patch, which is particularly useful for examining the effects of different concentrations of ligands on receptor-operated channels. This outside-out patch has an additional use, since it can be used as a 'sniffer' to detect the release of transmitters from nerve endings.

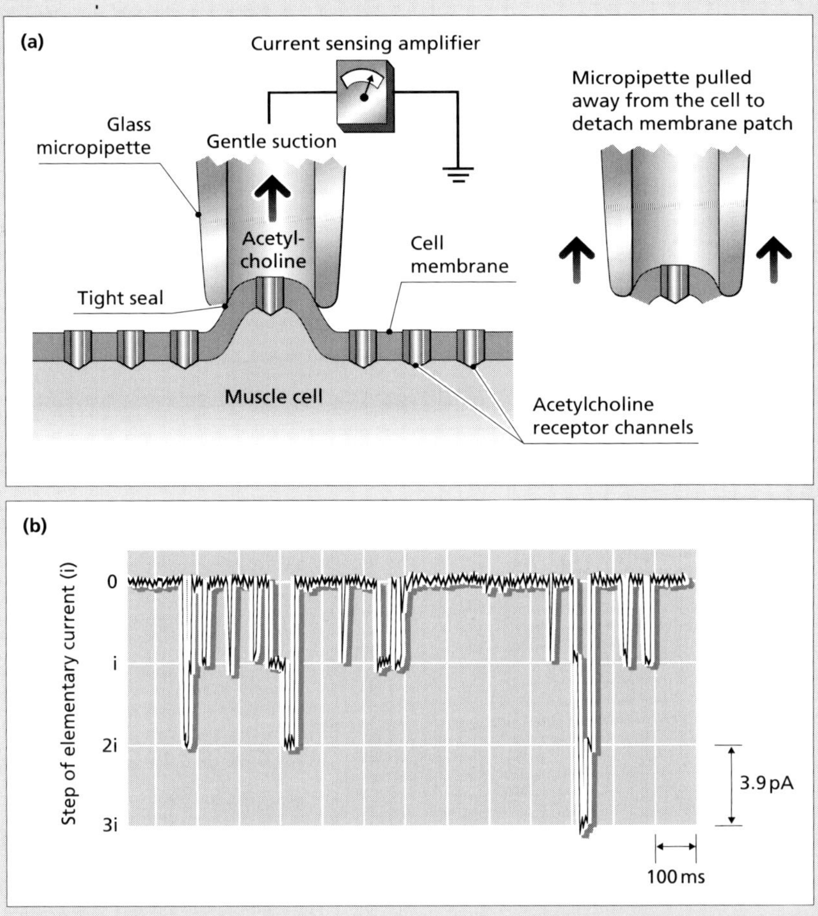

Fig. B5.5.1 Patch clamp technique. (a) A pipette is placed against the clean cell membrane and gentle suction applied to generate a tight seal between the membrane and the electrode glass. Current flowing through any channel within the seal can be monitored. On the left, an isolated patch of membrane has been pulled from the cell. (b) Recording of currents from a membrane patch. This membrane must have at least three channels in it, since there are three different current levels apparent (i, 2i and 3i).

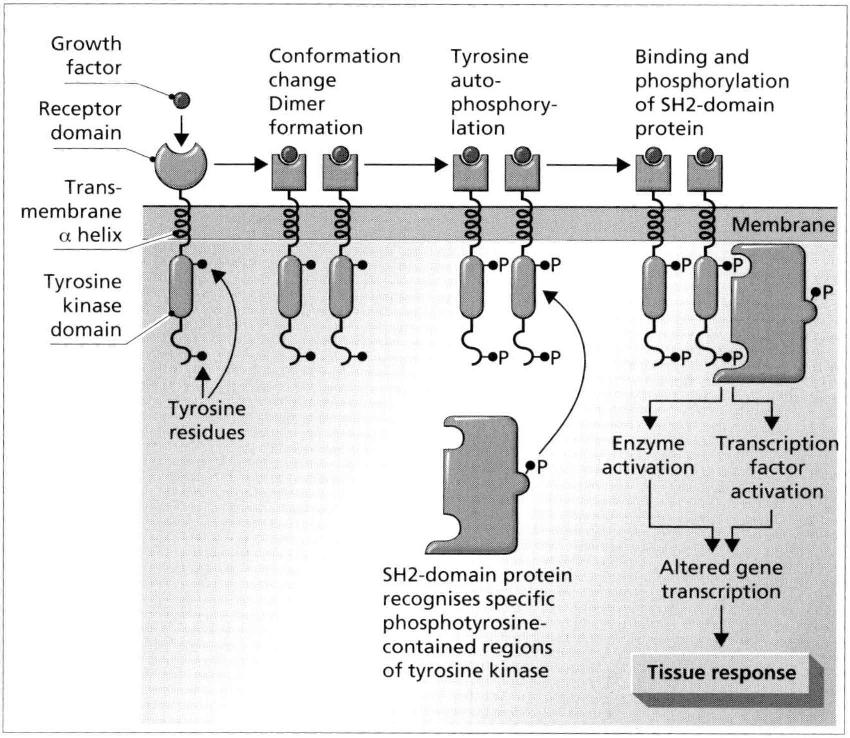

Fig. 5.15 Diagram of events occurring after activation of a tyrosine kinase receptor with its agonist (a growth factor). The first step is dimer formation, followed by autophosphorylation. This then allows interaction with intracellular proteins and a cascade of further interactions leading to the tissue response. From Rang *et al.* (1995).

Other enzyme receptors are guanylyl cyclases, such as the receptor for the atrial natriuretic factor; or phosphatases, such as the receptors for protein ligands produced during inflammatory responses. Again, activation of these receptors results in complex sequences of cellular events and second-messenger production.

5.7.4 Intracellular receptors

Cytoplasmic guanylyl cyclase (as opposed to the membrane-bound variety) may be considered an intracellular receptor that can be activated by NO to produce moderately fast responses through alterations in the second-messenger cyclic guanosine monophosphate (cGMP) levels.

Steroid receptors are large intracellular proteins, which are often stabilised in an inactive conformation by binding to other specific proteins, such as heat-shock proteins. The lipid-soluble ligand diffuses through the membrane and binds to the receptor, which then dissociates its stabilising proteins, and diffuses through the pores in the nuclear envelope to alter

DNA transcription, either directly through interaction with regulatory sequences of DNA, or indirectly through interaction with various transcription factors. Tissue responses result from the alterations in protein production, and are thus slow in onset, and often long-lasting.

5.8 Classification of receptors

Historically, the classification of receptors was initially in terms of their natural ligand, and the two most studied receptors in the early days of pharmacology were therefore acetylcholine receptors (cholinoceptors) or catecholamine receptors (adrenoceptors). This major classification has been preserved for other naturally occurring ligands. Early subclassification began when agonist compounds were found that distinguished different types of receptor. For instance, nicotine and muscarine were shown to activate only non-overlapping populations of cholinoceptors, and noradrenaline and adrenaline were shown to have a different relative potency on certain populations of adrenoceptor. Thus, the first subclasses were muscarinic and nicotinic acetylcholine receptors, and α and β catecholamine receptors.

Increasing knowledge of receptors makes it clear that different classes or subclasses of receptor must have differences in their structures. In the absence of any techniques for looking directly at receptor structure, the best probe for this is ligand affinity. If two identical receptors occur in two different tissues, then one might expect any ligand to have an identical affinity and thus equilibrium constant for both. It is difficult to actually measure equilibrium constants experimentally, and the best indicator of receptor structure comes from antagonist potency, since this is probably better correlated with affinity than agonist potency, which is also affected by efficacy and tissue factors that can reduce agonist concentration near the receptor (see p. 142). Nowadays, a receptor is therefore normally classified in terms of the potency of competitive antagonists. A β-adrenoceptor is one that is blocked by a β-blocker.

It is interesting that the early classes of receptor that were described clearly had different physiological functions, and were also different types of receptor (the nicotinic receptor being a directly coupled ion channel, and the other three being G protein-coupled, but preferentially activating different classes of G proteins). However, since then, ever-growing numbers of receptor subclassifications are being proposed from antagonist potency ratios. This process has largely been led by the search for tissue-specific drugs, since it is becoming extremely important for drug companies to develop selective drugs to treat clinical conditions. If there are small differences in the receptor structures of different cells, then it may be possible to design drugs that can selectively affect them.

During the course of evolution, it seems that, for many receptors, gene replication and gene shuffling has occurred, so that there may be multiple copies of the gene for the receptor of a particular natural ligand, and these may occur on different chromosomes. These separate genes can undergo mutations, and provided the mutation does not prevent activation of the receptor by its natural ligand (i.e. is neutral or beneficial in its effect), this could lead to functionally identical receptors, but with subtle differences in structure that result in different antagonist affinities. Over time, this might also lead to preferential coupling to particular G proteins, and changes in function. A well-studied example is the muscarinic receptor. Five distinct genes for muscarinic receptors occur in the human genome, and four of these match with four subclasses of muscarinic receptors identified functionally and by antagonist potency ratios. There is evidence that the M_1 and M_3 receptors couple preferentially to G proteins, activating production of one type of second messenger (increased IP_3 levels, see Section 6.2.3), and that the M_2 and M_4 receptors couple to G proteins, leading to a reduction in cyclic adenosine monophosphate (cAMP) levels. So far, no M_5 receptor has been found to occur naturally.

How important is it for students to learn the subclassifications of different receptors? With the increasing use of molecular biological techniques, it seems likely that the growth in knowledge may lead to a considerable simplification of the situation in the near future. It is perhaps useful for students to be aware of the subclasses of receptors for a particular ligand that have distinct physiological functions and mechanisms – such as the directly coupled channels as opposed to the G protein-coupled receptors, but students should realise that a great deal of research into receptor subtypes is carried out on animals, and although it may in time be possible to trace the evolution of different receptors within the animal kingdom, it is highly unlikely that a receptor will have survived unchanged in humans and animals. Unless a career in veterinary science is anticipated, there seems little value in learning receptor subtypes in species other than humans, and it is really only in pharmacological research that detailed knowledge of the minor subclassifications of receptors will be important.

5.9 Important receptors in the autonomic nervous system

The classic description of the autonomic nervous system transmitters and receptors states that the presynaptic neurones release acetylcholine, which acts on nicotinic receptors at ganglia, and the postsynaptic neurones release either acetylcholine, acting at muscarinic receptors (parasympathetic and some sympathetic), or noradrenaline, acting at α-adrenoceptors. Although this is an oversimplification, as we have seen, these transmitters and receptors are nevertheless of considerable importance in the autonomic nervous system. Apart from these, amino acids, serotonin, purines and peptides probably all play a role as transmitters and neuromodulators in the

Table 5.1 Some important receptors in the autonomic nervous system.

Receptor	Receptor type	Natural ligand	Effectors	Response
Nicotinic				
Neuronal	Channel (cation)	Acetylcholine	Neurones	Excites
Muscarinic				
M_1	G-protein linked	Acetylcholine	Stomach	Acid secretion
M_2	"	"	Heart	Slows rate
M_3	"	"	Smooth muscle	Contracts
Adrenoceptors				
α_1	G-protein linked	Noradrenaline/	Smooth muscles	Contracts/relaxes
α_2	"	adrenaline	Nerve terminals	Inhibits release
β_1	"	"	Heart	Rate/force increase
β_2	"	Adrenaline/	Smooth muscles	Relaxes
β_3	"	noradrenaline	Brown fat	Lipolysis/thermogenesis
Purinoceptors				
P_{2X}	Channel (cation)	ATP	Smooth muscles	Depolarizes
P_{2Y}	G-protein linked	ATP	Smooth muscles	Relaxes
Tachykinin receptors				
NK_1	G-protein linked	Substance P	Smooth muscles	Contracts/vasodilates
GABA receptors				
$GABA_A$	Channel (chloride)	GABA	Neurones	Inhibits
5-HT receptors				
5-HT_3	Channel (cations)	Serotonin	Neurones	Excites
5-HT_2	G-protein linked	"	Smooth muscles	Contracts/relaxes
5-HT_1	G-protein linked	"	Blood vessels	Dilated (via endothelium)
NPY receptors	G-protein linked	NPY	Sympathetic transmission	Enhances
Opioid receptors				
μ	G-protein linked	Metenkephalin	Gut	Constipation
Eicosinoid receptors				
EP_3	G-protein linked	PEG2	Uterus	Contraction
Histamine receptors				
H_1	G-protein linked	Histamine	Smooth muscles	Contracts/vasodilates
H_2	"	"	Stomach	Acid secretion

Note that this is only a small selection both of receptors and also of their action. The same receptor can mediate different effects on different tissues. Many different classes of G-protein are involved in mediating the actions of the G-protein linked receptors.

autonomic nervous system. The more common receptors present in the autonomic nervous system are shown in Table 5.1, and the release of transmitters is considered in Chapter 4. The mechanisms involved in receptor–effector coupling are described in Chapter 6, and the innervation and control of various autonomic effector systems in Chapters 8, 9 and 10.

Further reading

Changeux, J.P. (1987) The nicotinic acetylcholine receptor: molecular architecture of a ligand-regulated ion channel. *TIPS* **8**, 459–65.

Colquhoun, D., Ogden, D.C. & Mathie, M. (1987) Nicotinic acetylcholine receptors of nerve and muscle: functional aspects. *TIPS* **8**, 465–72.

Dani, J.A. & Mayer, M.L. (1995) Structure and function of glutamate and nicotinic acetylcholine receptors. *Current Opinions Neurobiol.* **5**, 310–17.

Findlay, J. & Eliopoulos, E. (1990) Three-dimensional modelling of G protein-linked receptors. *TIPS* **11**, 492–9.

Hamill, O.P., Marty, A., Neher, E., Sakmann, B. & Sigworth, F.J. (1981) Improved patch-clamp techniques for high-resolution current recording from cells and cell-free membrane patches. *Pflugers-Arch* **391**, 85–100.

Hucho, F., Tsetlin, V.I. & Machold, J. (1996) The emerging three-dimensional structure of a receptor. The nicotinic acetylcholine receptor. *Eur. J. Biochem.* **239**, 539–57.

Hulme, E.C. (1990) Muscarinic acetylcholine receptors: typical G-coupled receptors. *Symp. Soc. Exp. Biol.* **44**, 39–54.

Kenakin, T.P. (1997) *Molecular Pharmacology: A Short Course.* Blackwell Science, Oxford.

Linden, J. & Delahunty, T.M. (1989) Receptors that inhibit phosphoinositide breakdown. *TIPS* **10**, 114–20.

Miledi, R., Moinoff, P. & Potter, L.T. (1971) Isolation of the cholinergic receptor protein of Torpedo electric tissue. *Nature* **229**, 554–7.

Rang, H.P., Dale, M.M. & Ritter, J.M. (1995) Chapter 1. *Pharmacology,* 3rd edn, pp. 3–21. Churchill Livingstone, Edinburgh.

Rang, H.P. (1973) Receptor mechanisms: Fourth Gaddum Memorial Lecture. *Br. J. Pharmac.* **48**, 475–95.

Strange, P.G. (1996) The energetics of ligand binding at catecholamine receptors. *TIPS* **17**, 238–44.

Unwin, N. (1993) Neurotransmitter action: opening of ligand-gated ion channels. *Cell* **72** **(**Suppl**)**, 31–41.

White, M.F. (1991) Structure and function of tyrosine kinase receptors. *J. Bioenerg. Biomembr.* **23**, 63–82.

References

Changeux, J.P. (1994) Functional architecture and dynamics of the nicotinic acetylcholine receptor: an allosteric ligand-gated channel. *Fidia Research Foundation Neuroscience Award Lecture*, 21–168. Raven Press, New York.

Colquhoun, D. & Sakmann, B. (1985) Fast events in single-channel currents activated by acetylcholine and its analogues at the frog muscle end-plate. *J. Physiol.* **369**, 501–57.

Katz, B. & Thesleff, S. (1957) A study of the 'desensitization' produced by ACh at the motor end-plate. *J. Physiol.* **138**, 63–80.

Langley, J.N. (1878) On the physiology of the salivary secretion. Part II. On the mutual antagonism of atropin and pilocarpin, having especial reference to their relations in the sub-maxillary gland of the cat. *J. Physiol.* **1**, 339–69.

Miledi, R., Molinoff, P. & Potter, L.T. (1971) Isolation of the cholinergic receptor protein of Torpedo electric tissue. *Nature* **229**, 554–7.

Neher, E. & Sakmann, B. (1976) Single channel currents recorded from membranes of denervated frog muscle fibres. *Nature.* **260**, 799–802.

Perkins, J.P. (1981) Catecholamine-induced modification of the functional state of β-adrenergic receptors. *Trends in Pharmacol. Sci.* **2**, 326–8.

Potter, L.T. (1967) Uptake of propranolol by isolated guinea-pig atria. *J. Pharmacol. Exp. Ther.* **155**, 91–100.

Rang, H.P. (1971) Drug receptors and their function. *Nature* **231**, 91–6.

Rang, H.P., Dale, M.M. & Ritter, J.M. (1995) *Pharmacology*. Churchill Livingstone.

6: Postjunctional Mechanisms of Transmitters

6.1 Introduction

Modulation of the behaviour of the target cells of autonomic neurones occurs through mechanisms triggered by the interaction of the transmitters with specific postsynaptic membrane receptors. In this chapter, we will consider the mechanisms by which activation of the receptors can lead to the effects seen in the target cells.

Synaptic interactions can occur at many different sites in the autonomic nervous system, and the important effects that are produced in the various locations and that should be considered are as follows:

Postganglionic and enteric neurones Initiation of action potentials, increase or decrease of excitability, presynaptic modulation of transmitter release.

Smooth muscle Contraction, relaxation, alteration in the pattern of activity, changes in the sensitivity of the tissue to other inputs.

Heart muscle Changes in the frequency and force of contraction, changes in the conduction velocity in the propagating tissues.

Epithelia and glands Secretion of products or fluids, suppression of secretion, reabsorption of fluids, suppression of reabsorption.

Brown fat Alterations in the metabolism.

The interaction of the transmitters with the receptors can affect the behaviour of the whole cell. How does activation of these often precisely localised and superficial receptors lead to this? It is possible to define two main routes, depending on the initial events. The first one is through changes in the electrical properties of the cell membranes, which can, for example, initiate or modulate the production of action potentials in the target cell, and thus the sequence of events leading to contraction or secretion. This route is characteristically used for the more rapid signalling events. The second route is electrically silent, involving activation of enzymes that have intracellular effects, and may mediate rather more long-term events (Fig. 6.1). The two routes interconnect at many points. For example, products of the enzyme-mediated reactions may result in alterations of the electrical properties of the cells, and changes in the intracellular ionic environment secondary to ion flow through membrane channels may activate some enzymes. A large number of receptors may use both routes at the same time.

In either case, the initial event normally results in the alteration of the concentrations of intracellular second messengers – ions or molecules that can trigger or suppress the cellular events. The most common second mes-

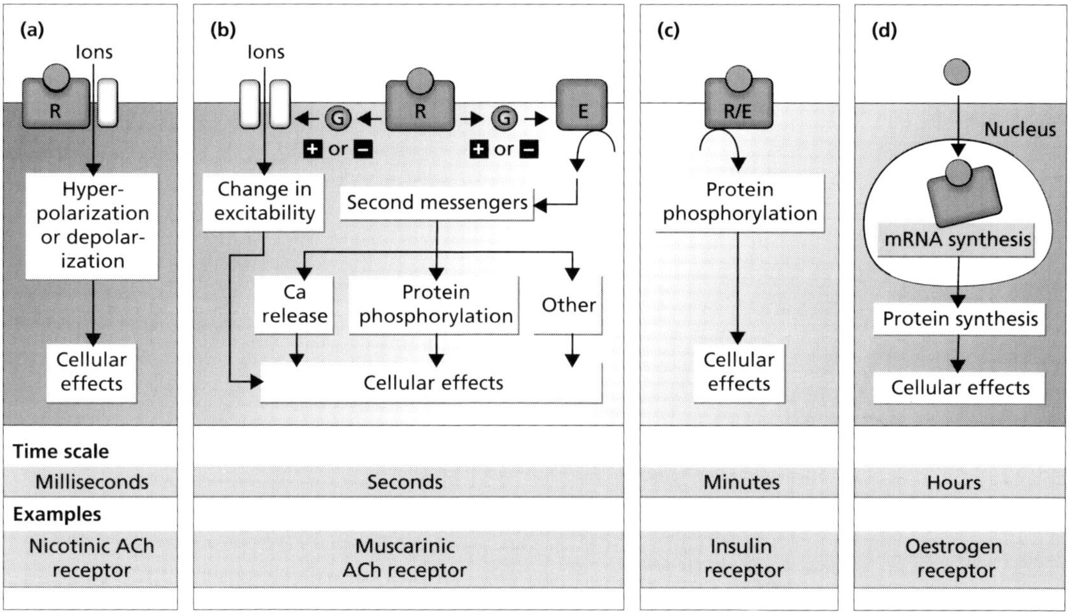

Fig. 6.1 Diagram showing various types of receptor–effector coupling. (a) Activation of the receptor directly opens or closes an ion channel. (b) G-protein linked pathway. The activated receptor interacts with a G-protein which can then have several effects. (c) The receptor is an enzyme that can directly control protein phosphorylation. (d) The receptor is intracellular, and activation can lead to control of DNA transcription. R, receptor; G, G-protein; E, enzyme. From Rang *et al.* (1995).

sengers are cyclic nucleotides – both cyclic guanosine monophosphate (cGMP) and cyclic adenosine monophosphate (cAMP); the products of metabolism of the membrane lipid, phosphatidylinositol – myo-inositol 1,4,5-trisphosphate (IP_3) and diacylglycerol (DAG); and Ca^{2+} ions. More recently, cyclic adenosine diphosphate (cADP)-ribose has been proposed as a second messenger.

In this chapter, we will first consider how drug–receptor interaction can lead to the generation of second messengers. We will then examine how receptor activation can result in changes in the electrical properties of the cell membrane, or trigger the electrically silent pathways; and finally we will consider how these events link to trigger the changes in cellular activity.

6.2 Generation of second messengers

Although direct evidence is hard to obtain, indirect evidence makes it practically certain that receptor activation involves a conformational change in the receptor protein, triggered by binding of the drug to a specific site on the receptor molecule. Some receptors have evolved into very complex macromolecules that incorporate both agonist binding sites and ion channels, as will be discussed later, but, for the majority of receptors functioning in the autonomic nervous system, the conformational change occurring on receptor activation enables the receptor to interact with one or more members of another family of proteins, the G proteins.

6.2.1 G-proteins

G proteins are so called because they bind to guanine nucleotides and are guanosine triphosphatases (GTPases). Many different G-proteins have been identified, and they have been classified into four subfamilies (G_s, G_i, G_q, G_o), largely based on the properties of their α subunits. They are all trimers, consisting of α, β and γ subunits. In the inactivated state, the subunits are associated, and the α subunit is bound to guanosine diphosphate (GDP) through a high-affinity binding site. As shown in Fig. 6.2, an activated drug receptor can interact with G-proteins of one or more type, and this triggers a conformational change that results in the dissociation of the α subunit from the β and γ subunits (which remain associated), and an alteration in the affinity of the nucleotide binding site. The affinity of the site for GDP is decreased, and that for guanosine triphosphate (GTP) is increased. When bound to GTP, the α subunit is active and can then interact with other proteins and initiate a series of events, frequently by activating enzymes. The activation of the α subunit ends when it hydrolyses its GTP, and the G-proteins can then reassociate. It has recently been established that the $\beta\gamma$ subunits on their own may also be involved in initiating some cellular events. A large number of isoforms of each of the subunits have been identi-

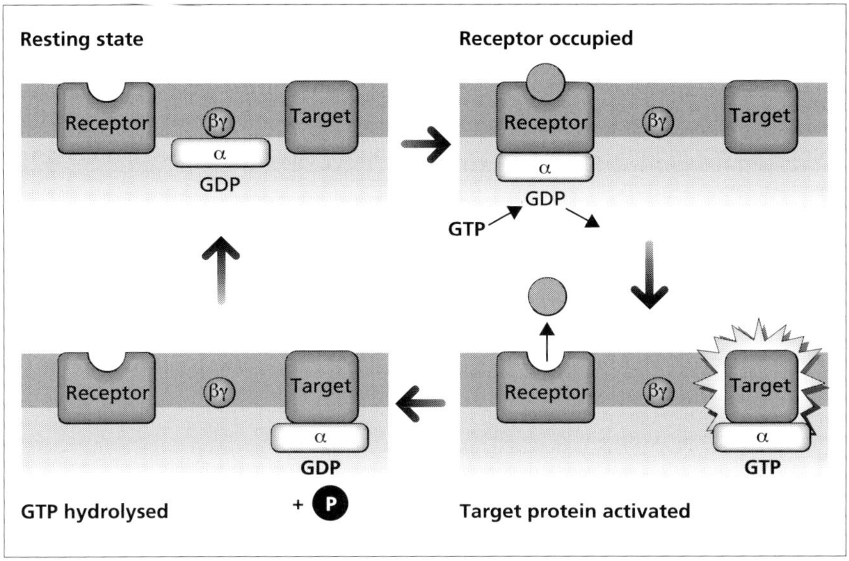

Fig. 6.2 G-protein function. Activation of the receptor allows it to interact with G-proteins, leading to dissociation of the βγ subunits, and a change in the affinity of the α subunit. This leads to release of GDP and association with GTP. The α subunit with GTP attached is active, and can interact repetitively with target proteins until hydrolysis of GTP. After this the subunits reassociate. From Rang *et al*. (1995).

fied, meaning that there is a vast number of potential trimeric structures, each with unique characteristics.

6.2.2 Cyclic nucleotides

cAMP

Cyclic nucleotides were the first organic second messengers to be identified. The best known is cAMP (cyclic adenosine-3′,5′-monophosphate). This molecule is formed from adenosine triphosphate (ATP) by the action of the membrane-bound enzyme adenylyl cyclase. It was initially discovered as the second messenger mediating the effects of β-adrenoceptor activation, and is now known to be involved in many different receptor-activated pathways. One of the family of G-proteins (G_s) has adenylyl cyclase as its target enzyme. The enzyme is a tetramer with two regulatory and two catalytic subunits. Activation of this enzyme leads to the formation of cAMP, as shown in Fig. 6.3. Another G-protein, G_i, can interact with and inhibit adenylyl cyclase. If the cAMP levels have already been increased through the G_s pathway, stimulation of G_i can lower the cAMP levels in the cell. cAMP is metabolised in the cell by a phosphodiesterase to 3′AMP. cAMP can activate protein kinase A (PKA), which can phosphorylate a number of

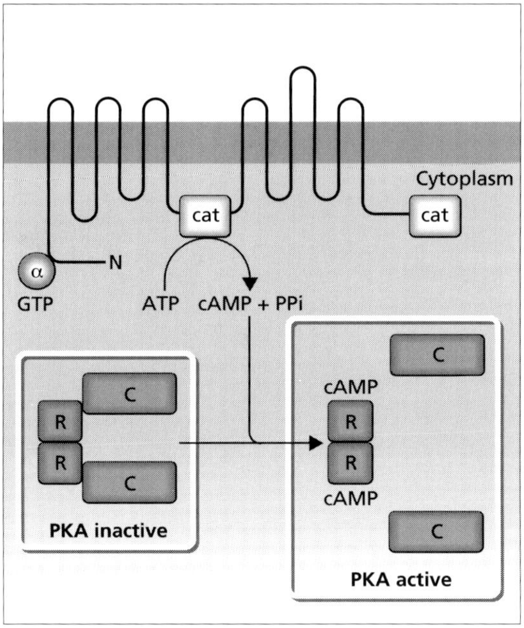

Fig. 6.3 Adenylyl cyclase and protein kinase A. Adenylyl cyclase is a membrane-bound glycoprotein, with two intracellular catalytic subunits (cat). It is activated by the α subunit of the G protein G_s, and catalyses the formation of cAMP from ATP. cAMP then activates protein kinase A, allowing its catalytic subunits (C) to split off from the regulatory subunits (R) and phosphorylate target proteins. From Nicholls (1994).

cellular proteins. The molecule may also directly interact with and modulate membrane channels without the involvement of phosphorylation.

cGMP

This may also act as a second messenger in some systems. Cells possess both membrane-bound and soluble forms of guanylyl cyclase, and activation of these enzymes results in the synthesis of cGMP from GTP. The membrane form may be activated through receptors and G-proteins, whereas the soluble enzyme is activated by NO, which is an inhibitory transmitter and can also be produced by many other cells (for instance the endothelium derived relaxing factor in blood vessels is NO; Fig. 6.4). A well-studied example of cGMP as a second messenger is in the rods and cones of the retina. Here, the G-protein involved is called transducin, and is switched on by activation of the sensory receptor by light. Transducin then activates a membrane-bound phosphodiesterase, which can lower the free cGMP levels in the cell. cGMP can directly interact with membrane channels or activate a cGMP-dependent protein kinase.

cADP-ribose

cADP-ribose has been found in many different cells, and shown to be a potent activator of the ryanodine receptor. The ryanodine receptor is a complex protein present in the sarcoplasmic or endoplasmic reticulum of muscle and non-muscle cells, incorporating a Ca^{2+} channel, and involved in

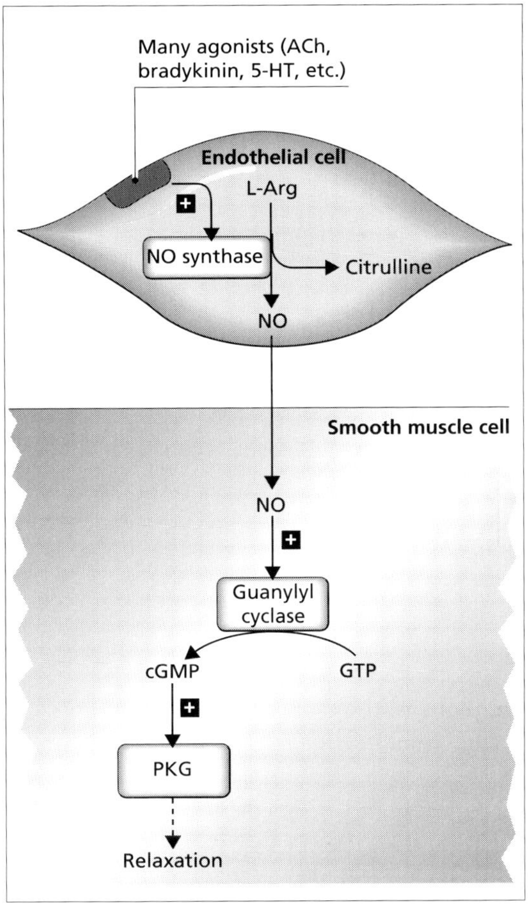

Fig. 6.4 Production of nitric oxide (NO) by the endothelial cells, and its mechanisms of action on vascular smooth muscle. The endothelial cell possesses many different receptors which, on activation, can result in stimulation of nitric oxide synthase (through elevation of intracellular Ca^{2+}). NO diffuses into the smooth muscle cell, where it activates soluble guanylyl cyclase. The cGMP produced then activates a cGMP-dependent protein kinase (PKG).

Ca^{2+} release from intracellular stores. In smooth muscle, cardiac muscle and several non-muscle cells, ryanodine receptors are responsible for triggering Ca^{2+}-activated Ca^{2+} release. cADP-ribose is postulated to be the endogenous ligand which can modulate these receptors, in much the same way as IP_3 is the endogenous ligand for the IP_3 receptor (see below), although it probably acts by binding to a modulatory protein rather than directly to the ryanodine receptor; (Fig. 6.5). ADP-ribosyl cyclase catalyses the formation of cADP-ribose from NAD^+, and it seems likely that modulation of this enzyme's activity may result from activation of receptors in some tissues, although this remains to be established.

6.2.3 Products of phosphatidylinositol metabolism

The two most important second messengers produced by this pathway are inositol 1,4,5-trisphosphate (IP_3) and diacylglycerol. Phosphatidylinositol is a membrane lipid, coupled through a phosphate link with inositol. It exists

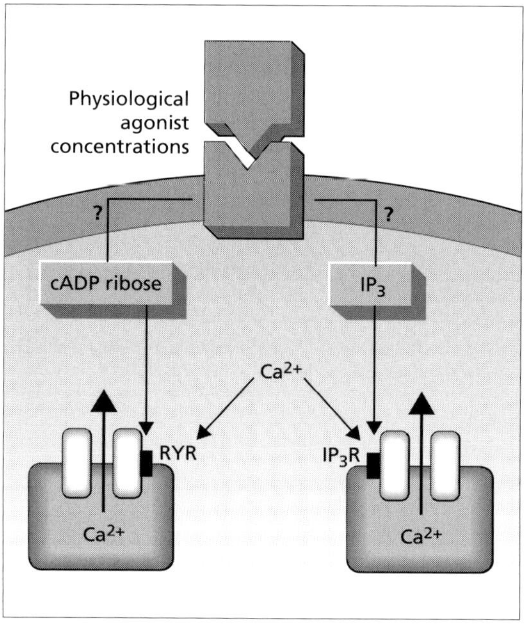

Fig. 6.5 Diagram illustrating possible modulation of Ca^{2+} release from internal stores through production of cADP ribose or inositol tris phosphate (IP_3). These molecules modulate opening of different Ca channels in the walls of the intracellular calcium stores (the ryanodine receptor (RYR) and the IP_3 receptor (IP_3R), respectively).

in the membrane in the unphosphorylated, monophosphorylated and bisphosphorylated forms (PI, PIP and PIP_2). Activation of receptors, again through the mediation of a G-protein, leads to activation of an enzyme, phospholipase C. This enzyme cleaves the phosphate link from the lipid chains of the PIP_2, releasing IP_3 into the cytoplasm, and leaving diacylglycerol in the membrane (Fig. 6.6). IP_3 may be further phosphorylated in the cell and metabolised through several possible intermediates. The most common route for metabolism involves dephosphorylation, catalysed by phosphatases to IP_2, IP_1 and inositol. The last dephosphorylation step is blocked by lithium ions, which reduce the production of inositol in the cell. Resynthesis of PI occurs relatively slowly from diacylglycerol and inositol using cytosolic enzymes, with subsequent phosphorylation. IP_3 binds to and activates Ca^{2+} channels in the membranes of intracellular Ca^{2+} stores, causing the release of intracellular Ca^{2+} ions. Diacylglycerol remains in the membrane and can activate protein kinase C, leading to phosphorylation of many substrate proteins.

6.2.4 Calcium ions

Ca^{2+} ions by virtue of their small size and high charge density can interact with many binding sites, and thus act as important second messengers. Changes in the concentration of Ca^{2+} ions in the cytoplasm can be produced by alterations in the passage of Ca^{2+} ions across the plasma membrane, or through release or uptake of Ca^{2+} by intracellular binding sites or storage organelles.

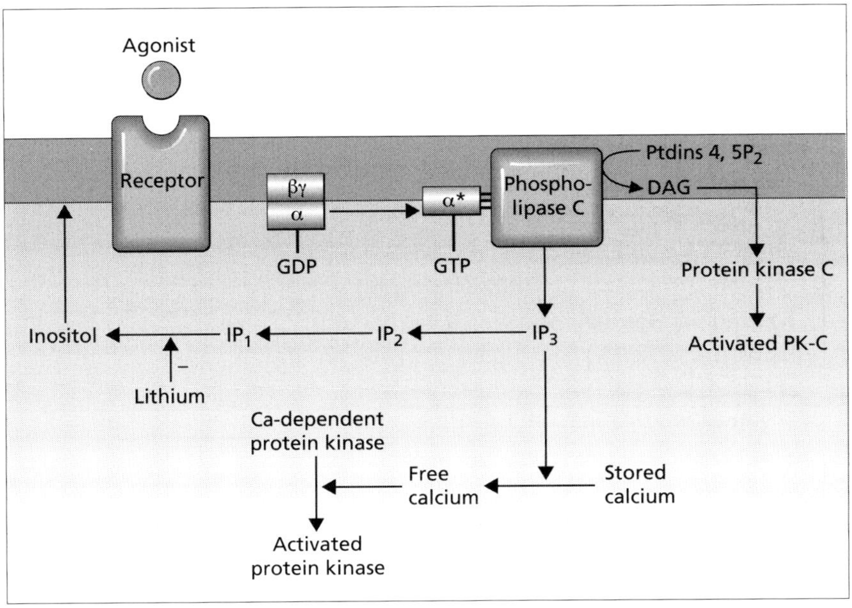

Fig. 6.6 Phospholipase C activation and its effects. Drug–receptor interaction leads via activation of a G-protein to activation of phospholipase C. This enzyme results in the breakdown of the membrane lipid, phosphatidylinositol 4,5-bisphosphate (Ptdins4,5P_2). The products of this breakdown, diacylglycerol (DAG) and inositol trisphosphate (IP_3), are involved in further cellular interactions, IP_3 through release of intracellular calcium and DAG through activation of protein kinase C. Metabolism of IP_3 to inositol can be inhibited by lithium, which can thus reduce the resynthesis of Ptdins4,5P_2.

Ca^{2+} homeostasis

The intracellular Ca^{2+} ion activity in resting cells is very low, usually in the region of 100–200 nmol/l, about 10 000 times lower than the concentration in the extracellular fluid. There is thus a very large electrochemical gradient favouring Ca^{2+} entry into the cytoplasm. The passive permeability of resting cell membranes to calcium ions is, however, very small, and there is little leak of calcium into inactive cells. Extrusion of calcium out of cells must occur against both the electrical and the chemical gradients, and requires energy expenditure. Two mechanisms exist, as shown in Fig. 6.7: Ca^{2+} pumps (Ca^{2+}-ATPases), which use the energy from ATP hydrolysis, and Na^+–Ca^{2+} exchange, which uses the potential energy of the Na^+ gradient to expel Ca^{2+} from the cell by linking the entry of 3 Na^+ to the extension of 1 Ca^{2+} ion. The Na^+ entering is then pumped out on the Na^+ pump (Na^+,K^+-ATPase). If the total cellular calcium content of cells is measured, it is found to be in the order of millimoles per litre of cell volume – in other words, to account for the very low free Ca^{2+} ion concentration, a large amount of Ca^{2+} must be bound. Ca^{2+} ions are bound to many intracellular proteins and membranes, and are also accumulated into intracellular organelles. The most important of these for the regulation of the free

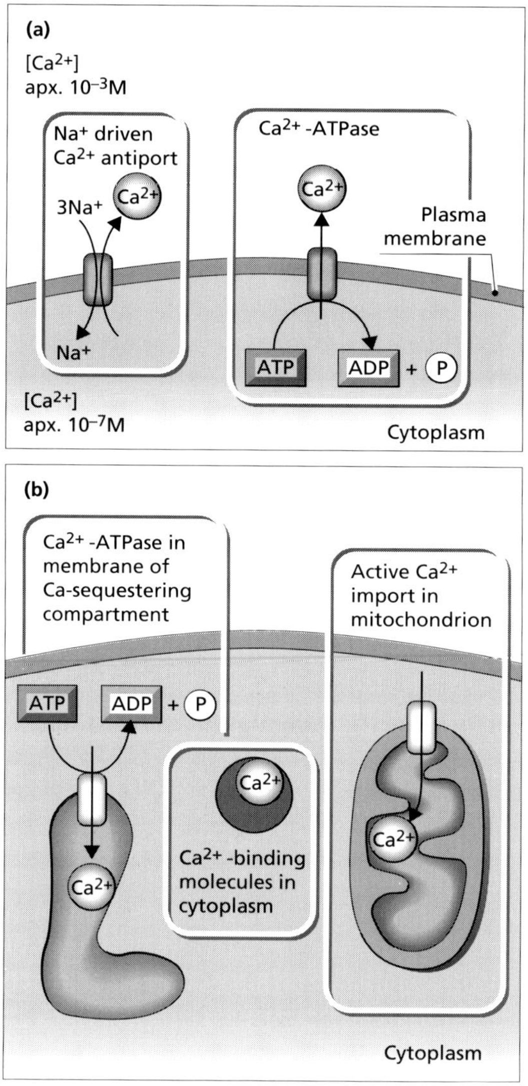

Fig. 6.7 Cellular calcium homeostasis. (a) Two mechanisms which mediate extrusion of Ca^{2+} from the cell: Na/Ca exchange and Ca ATPase. (b) Intracellular mechanisms for reducing free [Ca^{2+}] in the cell: uptake into the endoplasmic reticulum, binding to macromolecules, and uptake in mitochondria.

Ca^{2+} levels is the endoplasmic reticulum (called sarcoplasmic reticulum in muscle cells). Ca^{2+} ions are taken up into the membrane-bound intracellular stores against an electrochemical gradient by a Ca^{2+}-ATPase (SRCA), which may have characteristic differences from the plasma membrane pump, and may be associated with a regulatory protein, phospholamban.

Regulation of Ca^{2+} entry across the plasma membrane

Receptor activation can increase Ca^{2+} entry either by opening channels with a high Ca^{2+} permeability (receptor-operated channels), or by causing a depolarization of the cell membrane, leading to opening of voltage-sensitive Ca^{2+} channels (Fig. 6.8). There is at present no known example of a

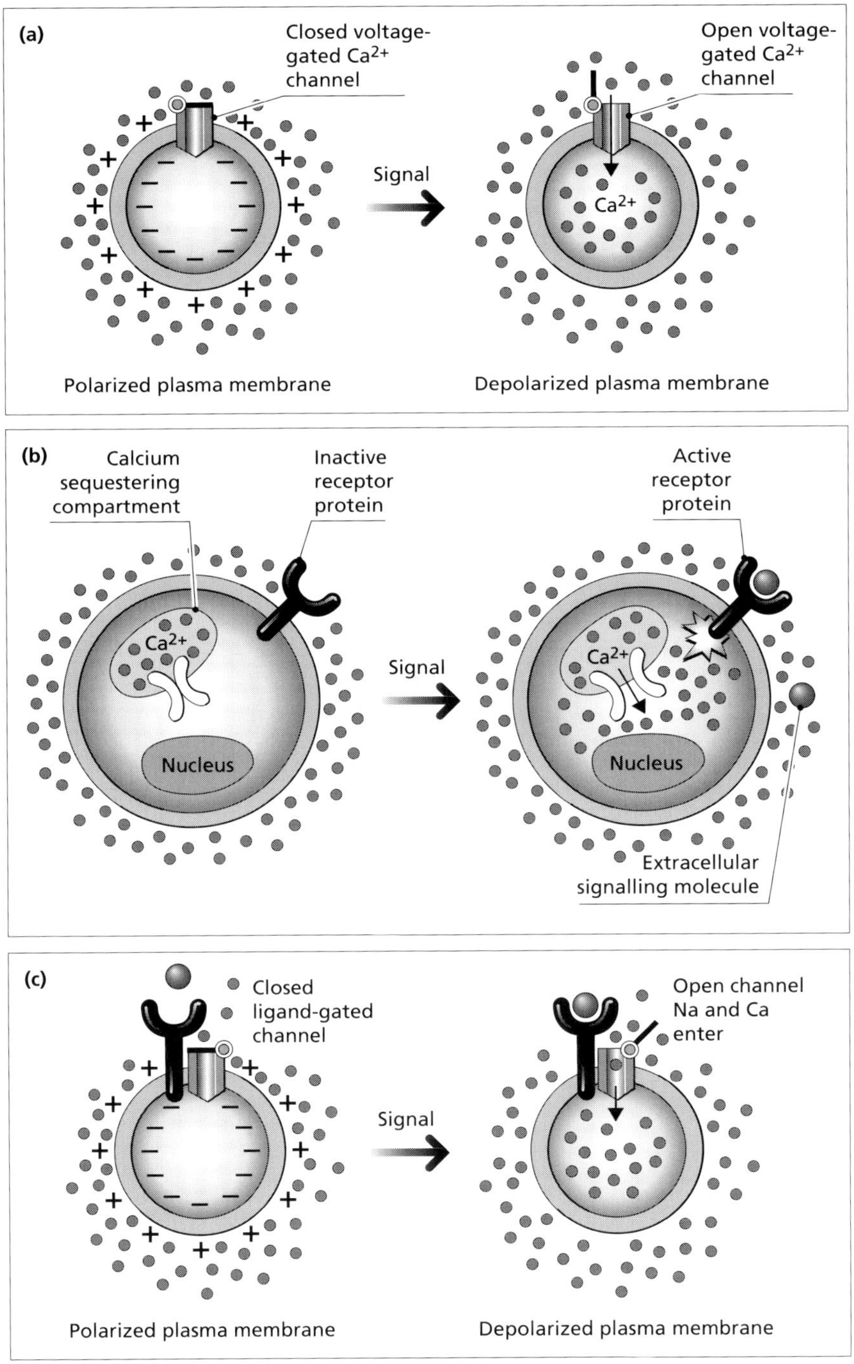

Fig. 6.8 Mechanisms for increasing intracellular Ca^{2+}. (a) In the normal state the membrane is polarized, and the voltage-gated Ca^{2+} channels closed. A stimulus that depolarizes the membrane opens these channels, and allows Ca^{2+} entry. (b) A signal interacting with a receptor causes release of second messenger molecules that trigger release of calcium from an intracellular compartment. (c) A signal interacts with a directly operated non-selective cation channel and opens it. Na^{+} and Ca^{2+} enter depolarizing the membrane and raising intracellular Ca^{2+}. This may result in secondary increases in the opening of voltage-sensitive Ca^{2+} channels and further entry.

receptor-operated divalent cation-selective channel, although some of the non-selective cation channels have a significant Ca^{2+} permeability. Emptying of Ca^{2+} from internal stores is, however, thought to release a second messenger, which can activate Ca^{2+} channels and trigger Ca^{2+} entry into the cell. Most commonly, Ca^{2+} entry is through voltage-sensitive Ca^{2+} channels secondary to the depolarization induced by opening non-selective cation channels. The L-type Ca^{2+} channels may begin to activate at potentials around –50 mV, and in non-excitable cells the Ca^{2+} channels may be open continuously over a range of membrane potentials, although they will inactivate if the membrane is depolarized too far. In excitable cells that have Ca^{2+}-based action potentials, depolarization may trigger action potentials, or increase their frequency, and the Ca^{2+} will enter carrying the inward current.

Regulation of intracellular Ca^{2+} stores

Ca^{2+} can be released from intracellular stores by several mechanisms, which involve the opening of Ca^{2+} channels in the store membrane. There are at least two types of Ca^{2+} channel, both very large and complex proteins incorporating a channel which can be activated by specific intracellular ligands (Fig. 6.9). The ryanodine receptor (so called because the plant alkaloid from *Ryania speciosa* binds to these channels specifically, holding them in a partially open configuration) is activated by an increase in free Ca^{2+} and is responsible for Ca^{2+}-activated Ca^{2+} release. Thus, in tissues with Ca^{2+}-dependent action potentials, such as smooth and cardiac muscle, the rise in $[Ca^{2+}]_i$ close to the plasma membrane with each spike triggers Ca^{2+} release from superficial stores. cADP-ribose is also a potent activator of these channels. In striated muscle cells, ryanodine receptors form permanent connections to voltage-sensitive Ca^{2+} channel proteins in the T tubules in the structures known as 'end feet', and these connections through an electromechanical coupling mediate Ca^{2+} release from the terminal cisternae of the sarcoplasmic reticulum (Fig. 6.10). The second Ca^{2+} channel is the IP_3 receptor, structurally similar to the ryanodine receptor, but activated by IP_3. Free Ca^{2+} can also enhance channel opening, but only in the presence of IP_3.

It seems clear that the Ca^{2+} channels involved in Ca^{2+} release are separate from the Ca^{2+}-ATPase mediating Ca^{2+} uptake, and also that they may have quite complicated properties. Drug–receptor interaction may also lead to alterations in the Ca^{2+} pump activity. Enhanced pumping either into the endoplasmic reticulum or across the plasma membrane will lower the free intracellular calcium ion concentration.

Other mechanisms

Ca^{2+} binding to other Ca^{2+} buffers may be affected by receptor activation, for instance alterations of the conformation of membrane proteins may cause release or uptake of Ca^{2+} ions onto binding sites.

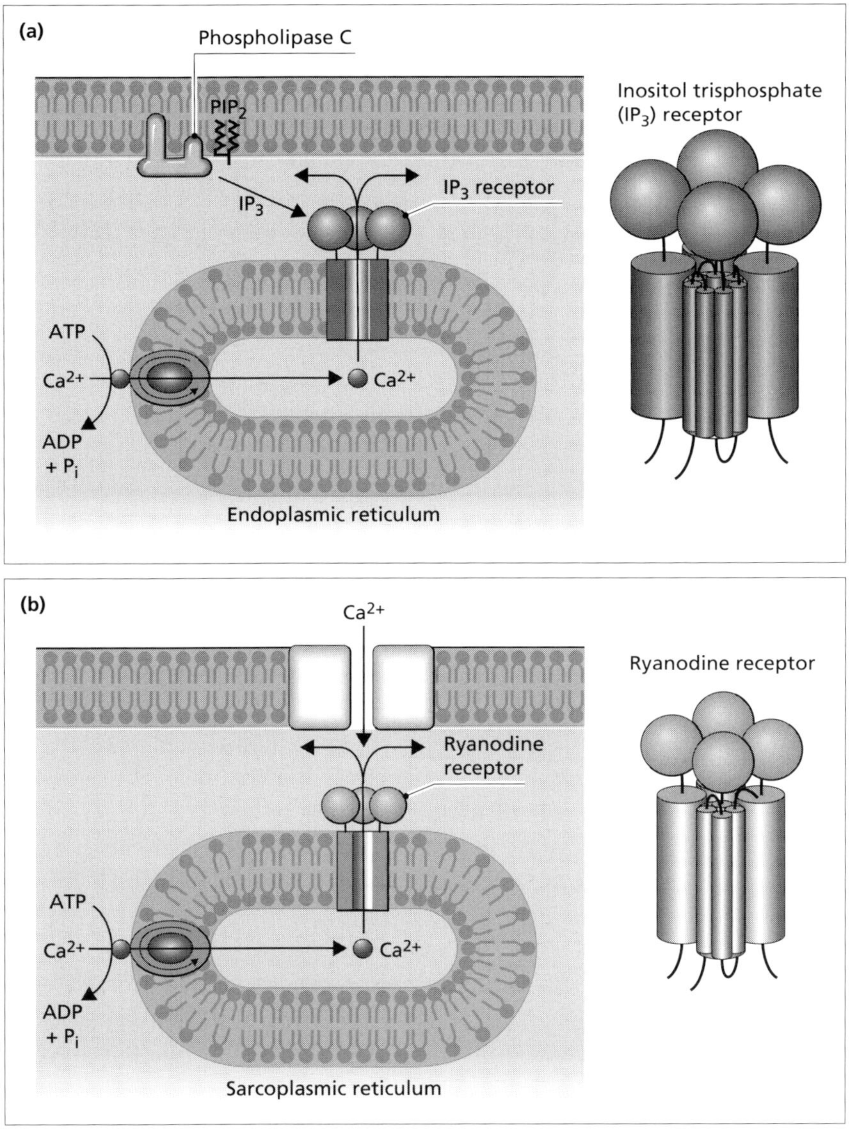

Fig. 6.9 Ca release from intracellular stores. The IP_3 receptor and the ryanodine receptor are both calcium channels, with similar structures. They are both tetramers, although the subunits of the IP_3 receptor are thought to have seven transmembrane domains, and the ryanodine receptors only four. The IP_3 receptor is activated by inositol trisphosphate liberated by the actions of phospholipase C on a membrane lipid. The ryanodine receptor is activated by Ca which normally enters through voltage-sensitive Ca^{2+} channels.

6.3 Receptor activation and electrical properties of the membrane

6.3.1 Ion channel properties

Drugs alter the electrical properties of cell membranes by opening or

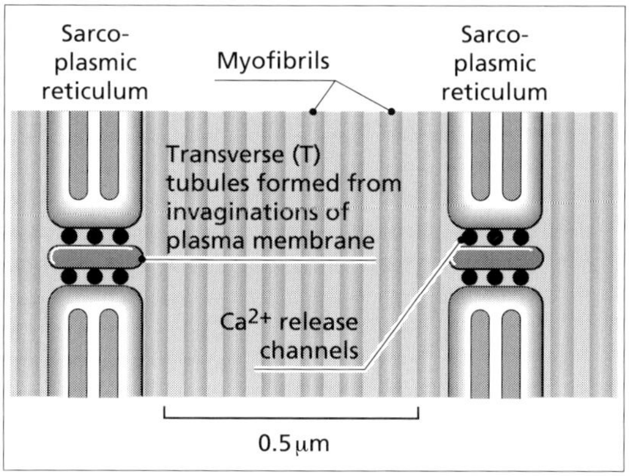

Fig. 6.10 Arrangement of 'end feet' in skeletal muscle. The end feet link the 'T' tubules with the terminal cisternae of the sarcoplasmic reticulum. The feet are composed of 'dihydropyridine receptors' in the 'T' tubular membrane (these are modified L-type calcium channels) and ryanodine receptors in the sarcoplasmic reticulum membrane. Depolarization alters the conformation of the dihydropyridine receptors and this results in activation and thus opening of the calcium channels of the ryanodine receptors.

closing ion channels. This changes the membrane resistance and may result in current flow.

An open channel will have current flowing through it if there are net driving forces on the ions that can penetrate the channels (this is determined by the difference between the membrane potential and the equilibrium potential for the channel). For example, if K^+ is the only ion present that can move through the channel, then the 'reversal potential' for the channel (the potential at which opening or closing the channel generates no current flow) will be the equilibrium (or Nernst) potential for K^+ ions (E_K, see Section 3.2.4). This is negative to the normal range of membrane potentials, and opening the K^+ channels will allow current to flow outward. Outward current will leave the inside of the cell more negative, hyperpolarizing the cell and moving the membrane potential towards E_K. Figure 6.11 shows the driving forces on all the common ions. Reference to this figure will show that opening Na^+ or Ca^{2+} channels will generate inward (depolarizing) current. Opening Cl^- channels may generate inward, outward or no current, depending on the Cl^- equilibrium potential.

In the case of channels permeant to a single ionic species, the reversal potential of the channel is equal to the Nernst potential for the ion in question. However, many channels are permeant to more than one of the ions present. In this case, the reversal potential of the channel will be determined by the relative permeability of the penetrating ions, the concentration of the ions and the driving forces operating on them. An example is the ion channel responsible for the end-plate potential, which is a cation-selective channel, permeable to both Na^+ and K^+ ions, with a reversal potential between 0 and −10 mV.

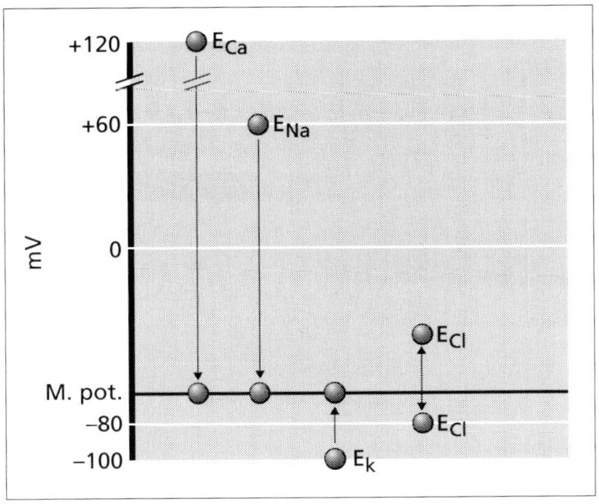

Fig. 6.11 Diagram to show the driving forces operating on ions in a typical cell. The driving force can be estimated as the difference between the membrane potential and the equilibrium potential for the ion in question. Note that the chloride equilibrium potential may vary in different cells. Opening a channel selective to a particular ion will result in movement of that ion along its driving force, thus generating a current. Na and Ca will move into the cells, and generate inward current. K ions will flow out generating outward current. Cl ions may flow into the cell (outward current), out of the cell (inward current), or not move, depending on how they are distributed across the membrane in the resting state.

If the reversal potential of a channel is equal to the membrane potential, then no currents will flow when the channels are opened or closed, but there will be changes in the membrane resistance. This can be significant since, if the membrane resistance is decreased, then, by Ohm's law ($V = IR$), any net current flowing through another channel will be less effective at changing the membrane potential, and if the membrane resistance is increased, currents through other channels will be more effective.

In summary:

opening an ion channel may lead to:

1 generation of an inward current, leading to depolarization;

2 generation of an outward current, leading to hyperpolarization;

3 no generation of current, but an increased conductance, which will result in stabilisation of the membrane potential.

Closing an ion channel may lead to:

1 switching off an inward current, leading to hyperpolarization;

2 switching off an outward current, leading to depolarization;

3 no change in current, but reduced conductance, which will result in increased sensitivity of the cell to other currents.

6.3.2 Coupling of receptors to channels

Receptor activation can lead to opening or closing of ion channels through several methods. These will be discussed with reference to the three main types of channel affected:

1 directly coupled channels;
2 second-messenger-activated channels;
3 G-protein-activated channels.

Directly coupled channels

The directly coupled, receptor-operated channels are a family of proteins that have many features in common (Fig. 6.12). They are oligomeric structures, typically five subunits, which may have evolved by gene replication. The macromolecule is both the receptor and the channel. Typically, each subunit has four membrane-spanning segments, a long extracellular N-terminal segment and an intracellular loop between the third and fourth transmembrane segments. Several of the subunits may carry the receptor binding sites, and activation of the receptors results in a conformational

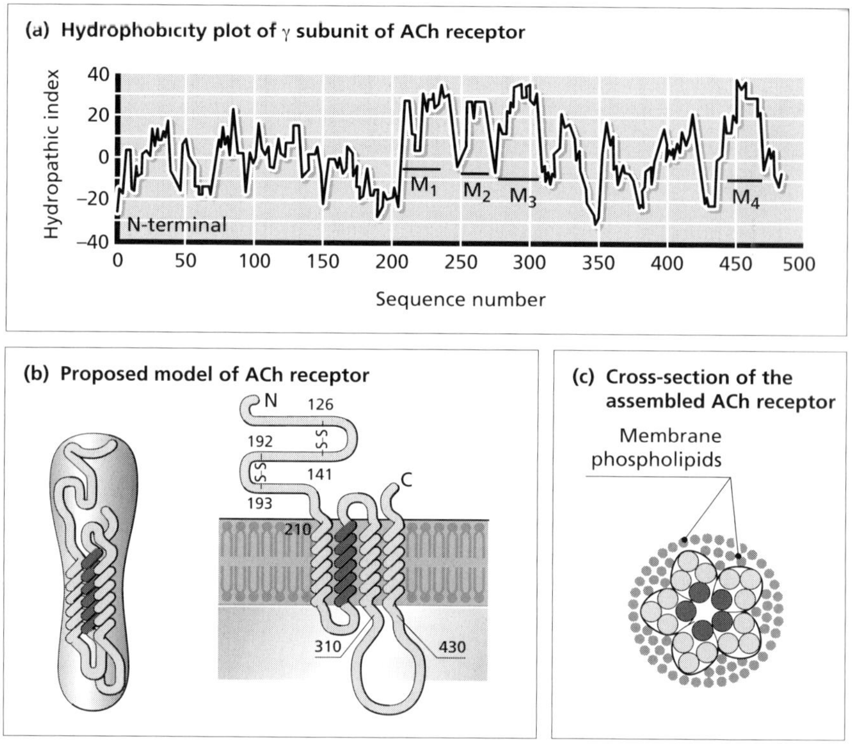

Fig. 6.12 The molecular arrangement of a directly coupled, receptor-operated channel. In this figure the structure of the nicotinic receptor is featured. (a) Shows a plot of the hydrophobicity index of the amino acids making up the γ subunit, with the four putative membrane-spanning units M1–M4 indicated. (b) Illustrates the arrangement of the amino acids in one subunit. (c) Shows the arrangement of the subunits in the channel. From Hall (1992).

change that creates an ion channel running between the membrane-spanning segments.

The properties of the channel depend on the amino-acid residue sequences of the transmembrane segments of the subunits that line the channel. If these are positively charged at cellular pH (such as the basic amino acids, arginine and lysine), then the channel will select for anions, and if the channel is lined with negatively charged acidic amino acids (for instance, glutamate and aspartate), the channel will be a cation channel. The dimensions of the channel will determine its relative permeability to ions.

Directly coupled ion channels are involved in the rapid excitatory and inhibitory signalling between cells, and are thus most common on neurones and the skeletal neuromuscular junction. Examples of excitatory transmitters working through directly coupled ion channels are acetylcholine, through the nicotinic receptor; glutamate, through a family of glutamate receptors (*N*-methyl-D-aspartate (NMDA), AMPA and kainate receptors); ATP, through the P_{2x} purinoceptor and 5-hydroxytryptamine (5-HT), through the 5-HT_3 receptor. These excitatory channels are relatively non-selective, with reversal potentials near 0 mV. They usually show co-operativity in their activation, desensitise rapidly, and have relatively little voltage sensitivity. Inhibitory transmitters include glycine and γ-aminobutyric acid ($GABA_A$ receptors). They activate Cl^- or K^+ channels, with reversal potentials near or negative to the membrane potential.

In the autonomic nervous system, these directly coupled channels are found predominantly on the ganglion cells. Nicotinic receptors mediate transmission between preganglionic and postganglionic neurones in the sympathetic and parasympathetic divisions, and nicotinic receptors are also present in the enteric nervous system. In this latter system, 5-HT is also an excitatory ganglionic transmitter, and GABA is present in some of the enteric neurones, GABA receptors playing a role in neural inhibitory pathways. However, evidence has recently been accumulating that ATP may be operating through directly coupled receptors on smooth muscles. It is thought to mediate inhibitory junction potentials in the gut, and excitatory junction potentials in some vascular smooth muscles and in the urogenital tract.

Channels activated by second messengers

Ion channels can be opened or closed as a result of direct interaction with second messengers, or through phosphorylation of channel proteins triggered by second messengers. For example, there are many channels with an open probability that is very low in the resting cells, but increases in response to a rise in intracellular free calcium ions. Examples are the Ca^{2+}-activated K^+ channels and Ca^{2+}-activated Cl channels. Binding of Ca^{2+} ions can also lead to inactivation of some channels, as for instance occurs with some of the voltage-sensitive Ca^{2+} channels, in which Ca^{2+} ions have a negative feedback role. Other second messengers that have been demonstrated to modulate ion channels by acting as an internal ligand are the cyclic nucleotides. For instance, cGMP binding opens cation channels in the rods and cones of the retina, and cAMP has a similar effect in olfactory neurones. It is interesting to note that these channels are very similar to the directly coupled channels described earlier, except that the receptors on the channel are intracellular, and the ligand is produced indirectly as a result of receptor activation.

The other way in which second messengers can lead to channel opening or closing is through binding to allosteric sites, or initiating phosphorylation of the channel protein, leading to alterations in its behaviour. An example of the former is the effect of cAMP on the cardiac I_f channel, shifting its voltage sensitivity, and an example of phosphorylation is the effect of β-adrenoceptor activation on the voltage-dependent Ca^{2+} channels in the heart. Activation leads to an increase in cAMP, which, through activation of protein kinase A, results in phosphorylation of the channel protein and an increase in the number of channels opening in response to depolarization. Another enzyme involved in channel phosphorylation is protein kinase C, activated by diacylglycerol as a consequence of receptor activation of PIP_2 metabolism.

In the autonomic nervous system, it is very common to find membrane potential or resistance changes resulting from activation of the myriad different receptors present on the effector organs. However, the time course of these changes suggests that the channel modulation is brought about predominantly through second-messenger-operated channels. The precise details involved have not been elucidated in many systems, and there are enormous tissue-to-tissue and interspecies variations in the responses to different transmitters. Nevertheless, it is becoming clear that there are families of receptors or receptor subtypes that normally use particular second-messenger pathways. For example, β-adrenoceptor activation, wherever it occurs, seems to involve cAMP as a second messenger, whereas the α_1-adrenoceptor does not, and uses Ca^{2+} and possibly IP_3. Acetylcholine muscarinic receptors (M_1, M_3 and M_5) also use IP_3 and intracellular Ca^{2+} for their effects. α_2-Adrenoceptors and muscarinic receptors both may activate the inhibitory G-protein G_i, and switch off cAMP production.

Channels activated by G-proteins

It has recently been shown that G-proteins may have as their targets not only enzymes, but also ion channels. Thus in the heart, β-adrenoceptor stimulation as well as activating G_s, also leads to the activation of a class of G-proteins which can directly interact with, and open K^+ channels. This all occurs within the plasma membrane, and does not involve cytoplasmic second messengers. Recent evidence suggests that in some cells Ca^{2+} channels may be modulated by G-proteins without phosphorylation, and also a similar route may be involved in opening the non-selective cation channels in response to muscarinic receptor activation.

6.4 Electrically silent pathways

The electrically silent pathways involve the activation of enzymes by the second messengers, and direct activation of pathways by calcium ions. At present it is believed that the majority of the enzymes activated are kinases, which initiate the cellular responses by phosphorylating substrate molecules to activate cellular processes. The target enzymes of the second messengers have not all been identified, and although many substrates for the kinases have been demonstrated *in vitro*, the physiological significance of these steps is still unclear in the majority of cases. The following section outlines the known properties of the better understood kinases and their relevant functions, and discusses some of the other effects of calcium.

6.4.1 Protein kinase A

This enzyme is activated by cAMP. It is a tetrameric protein, consisting of two catalytic subunits and two regulatory subunits. Each regulatory subunit has two binding sites for cAMP, and activation by cAMP shows cooperativity. Binding of three or four molecules of cAMP causes dissociation of the regulatory from the catalytic subunits. The catalytic subunits can now catalyse phosphorylation of substrate proteins (Fig. 6.13).

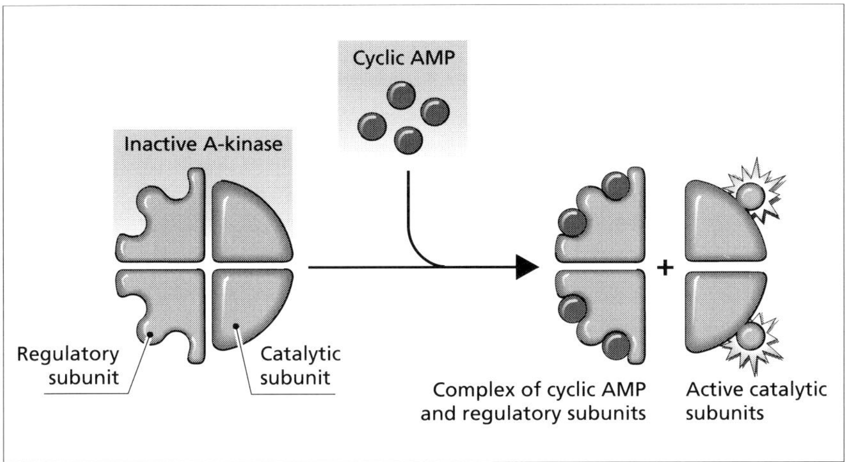

Fig. 6.13 Activation of cAMP-dependent protein kinase A. The kinase is composed of two catalytic and two regulatory subunits. Each regulatory subunit has two binding sites for cAMP, and binding of three or four cAMP molecules causes dissociation of the catalytic subunits, and their activation. From Alberts (1994).

Metabolic effects

Substrates phosphorylated include enzymes that are important regulators of the metabolic pathways of the cell. Glycogen synthase is phosphorylated, and this inhibits the enzyme, preventing laying down of glycogen. Phosphorylase kinase is another substrate. It is activated by phosphorylation, and in its turn activates glycogen phosphorylase, resulting in the production of glucose-6-phosphate from glycogen (Fig. 6.14). Triglyceride lipase is also a substrate, and its activation can result in the release of fatty acids from fat cells. Thus, for example, β-adrenoceptor stimulation can prepare tissues for activity, and increase the circulating glucose and fatty acids to provide energy for working tissues.

Alterations in Ca^{2+} sensitivity

Other substrates for the catalytic subunit of protein kinase A are enzymes that can bind Ca^{2+}. For instance, myosin light chain kinase and troponin are both substrates, and when phosphorylated undergo a reduction in their affinity for Ca^{2+}. Ca^{2+} pumps (Ca^{2+}-ATPases) are also substrates in many

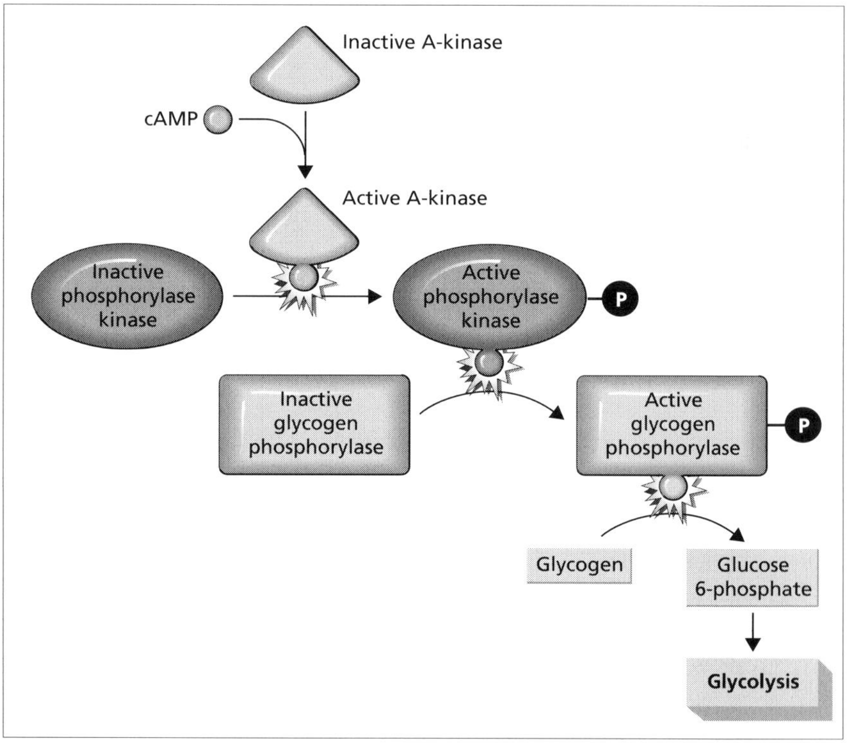

Fig. 6.14 Diagram of pathway involved in cAMP-induced stimulation of glycogen breakdown. From Alberts (1994).

cells. In the heart, the Ca^{2+} pump of the sarcoplasmic reticulum is regulated by an accessory protein, phospholamban, which on phosphorylation increases the affinity of the pump for Ca^{2+}, and enhances Ca^{2+} uptake into the sarcoplasmic reticulum. In smooth muscle, the plasma membrane Ca^{2+} pump is similarly affected, enhancing transport of Ca^{2+} out of the cells. These processes can result in relaxation of smooth muscles. In the heart, the extra Ca^{2+} available for release from the sarcoplasmic reticulum results in an enhancement in the force of contraction (positive inotropic effect), with a shortening of the contraction mediated by the faster removal of Ca^{2+} by the sarcoplasmic reticulum pumps and the lower affinity of troponin for it.

6.4.2 Protein kinase C

This enzyme contains a single polypeptide chain, and in its active form it is tightly bound to phosphatidylserine molecules in the plasma membrane. It is activated by Ca^{2+} ions. The affinity of the binding site for Ca^{2+} is greatly increased by diacylglycerol, so that it can be activated in the physiological range of cell Ca^{2+} concentrations. Thus, diacylglycerol produced from PIP_2 in response to receptor activation can act as a membrane-bound second messenger to trigger protein kinase C activation. This enzyme has provoked much interest, since it is directly activated by the tumour-producing phorbol esters. It is thought to be involved in feedback regulation of many of the processes initiated by receptor activation, including modulation of ion channels, as discussed earlier. Proteins known to be substrates include one of the myosin light chains, filamin and vinculin, which suggests that the enzyme may be involved in regulation of smooth muscle activation. Also, the epidermal growth factor receptor and tyrosine hydroxylase have been shown to be substrates. Studies on the effects of the activation of protein kinase C by phorbol esters can reveal some of the effects of the enzyme. Such studies have shown that it may evoke or potentiate the secretion of hormones and neurotransmitters, and that it can stimulate ion pump activity.

6.4.3 Kinases activated by Ca^{2+}–calmodulin

Many of the effects of raised intracellular Ca^{2+} are mediated through calmodulin. This is a highly conserved protein of 148 amino acid residues, with four Ca^{2+} binding sites (Fig. 6.15). On binding to calcium, the molecule undergoes a conformational change, exposing a hydrophobic site that allows it to interact with a complementary hydrophobic site on inactive calmodulin acceptor proteins, resulting in activation. Many of these acceptor proteins are kinases.

Myosin light chain kinase is an important example. This is responsible for the phosphorylation of the myosin light chains in smooth muscle, which activates the actomyosin ATPase and allows cross-bridge cycling to occur,

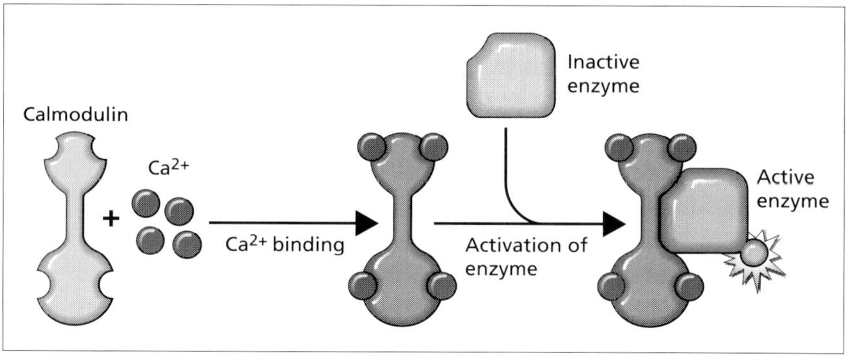

Fig. 6.15 Ca^{2+}, calmodulin and enzyme activation. Calmodulin contains four binding sites for Ca^{2+}. With these sites occupied, calmodulin can then interact with and activate some enzymes.

and contraction. It is activated by Ca^{2+} calmodulin, and confers the Ca^{2+} sensitivity to smooth muscle contraction. Another Ca^{2+}–calmodulin-dependent kinase is responsible for phosphorylating the protein synapsin I, which is found in nerve terminals associated with the external face of synaptic vesicles. This may play a role in exocytosis. Other kinases include phosphorylase kinase, NAD kinase, and glycogen synthase kinase.

Other calmodulin-activated enzymes

Ca^{2+}–calmodulin can also have many effects through modulating the enzymes involved in the metabolism of other second messengers, such as the cyclic nucleotides. Adenylyl cyclase, guanylyl cyclase and various cyclic nucleotide phosphodiesterases are all substrates. This may lead to complicated changes in the concentrations of second messengers in response to receptor activation. The membrane ATPases responsible for ionic regulation are also substrates, as are various phospholipases and protein phosphatases.

6.4.4 Ca^{2+} effects on other regulatory proteins

The role of Ca^{2+} as a trigger for contractile processes often involves Ca^{2+} binding to regulatory proteins. A good example is Ca^{2+} binding to troponin, which triggers contraction in striated muscles. Troponin has a great structural similarity to calmodulin. Another regulatory protein, which it has recently been suggested may be involved in the regulation of smooth muscle contraction, is caldesmon, which binds Ca^{2+}–calmodulin, and may be involved in a thin filament regulatory system in smooth muscles. Both Ca^{2+}–calmodulin and actin can bind caldesmon, and an increase in free calcium may result in the movement of caldesmon away from the actin filaments to bind with calmodulin, thus altering the contractile activity of the cell.

6.4.5 Arachidonic acid

Arachidonic acid, a 20-carbon atom unsaturated fatty acid, is the precursor of a family of active compounds, the eicosanoids, which can have marked effects on cells through their own receptors. The eicosanoids include prostaglandins, leukotrienes and thromboxanes, compounds involved in the control of many physiological processes and also involved in inflammatory responses. Arachidonic acid is not stored in the cells, but is found as part of the structure of membrane phospholipids. It can be liberated in response to a wide range of different stimuli, including activation of receptors, antigen–antibody reactions and general cell damage. Once liberated, it is metabolised into the various eicosanoids through various lipoxygenase and cyclo-oxygenase enzymes.

Arachidonic acid can be liberated through various pathways involving different phospholipase enzymes. It can be split off from phospholipids in a single step using phospholipase A_2, a membrane-bound enzyme that can be activated through G-proteins. It can also be liberated in two-step processes. One of these involves first phospholipase C to form diacylglycerol, and then diacylglycerol lipase, which splits the molecule into arachidonate and glycerol (Fig. 6.16). Thus, activation of receptors coupled to the phosphatidylinositol pathway can also result in the formation of prostaglandins, thromboxanes and leukotrienes.

Many of the responses of tissues such as smooth muscles to receptor

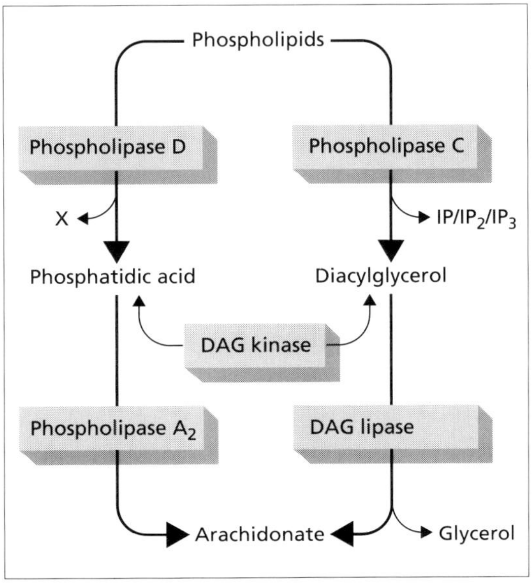

Fig. 6.16 Two-step processes for arachidonic acid formation from membrane phospholipids.

activation are quite complex, due to the secondary effects that follow liberation of arachidonic acid. These actions often appear as 'off responses' on washing off the primary agonist. Involvement of these pathways can be assessed if synthesis of the eicosanoids is prevented, for instance by the use of non-steroidal anti-inflammatory drugs.

6.5 Receptor-mediated changes in cellular activity

A consideration of the above phenomena will lead to a realisation of the enormous complexity that is possible. Activation, inhibition or modulation of ongoing cellular activity initiated by the actions of a hormone or transmitter on its target cell inevitably involves a large number of processes. This is true even in the simplest example of nicotinic receptor activation on the ganglion cells. In this case, directly coupled non-selective cation channels are opened, leading to an excitatory postsynaptic potential and action potentials in the neurones. When they reach the nerve terminals, these action potentials activate voltage-sensitive Ca^{2+} channels, and Ca^{2+} enters the cell and triggers vesicle release. The mechanisms involved in this step are far from clear, but it is known that Ca^{2+} is acting as a second messenger. It is likely that Ca^{2+} calmodulin-dependent kinases are activated, and possibly interaction of Ca^{2+} with regulatory proteins, which results in fusion of vesicles with the plasma membrane and movement of vesicles towards the release sites on the prejunctional terminal. Cellular processes will also be activated that result in retrieval of vesicle membrane and re-formation and filling of vesicles.

When the transmitters are activating muscle or glands, the initial receptor activation will trigger multiple pathways in the cell. In almost every instance, changes in the membrane potential or membrane conductance will occur, and alterations in the cellular free Ca^{2+} concentration, as well as activation of G-proteins and production of organic second messengers, with consequences determined by the substrates present for the various enzymes and regulatory proteins affected.

The changes in intracellular calcium can be very complicated. In many instances, there will be a rapid transient increase in free Ca^{2+} caused either by Ca^{2+}-activated Ca^{2+} release from the endoplasmic reticulum, or by IP_3-stimulated release. This rise in calcium, or the production of other second messengers, may then alter the properties of membrane channels and cause depolarization, triggering sustained Ca^{2+} entry through voltage-sensitive Ca^{2+} channels. The emptying of sarcoplasmic reticulum stores is also thought to promote Ca^{2+} entry from the extracellular space, possibly by an unknown second messenger and opening of a special Ca^{2+} channel. The second messengers may also change the sensitivity of Ca^{2+} regulatory proteins, so that even if free Ca^{2+} levels fall, their effects may continue. It is well documented, for instance, that in smooth muscles, different agonists may cause the same elevation in tension with quite different changes in free intracellular Ca^{2+} levels.

In Chapters 8, 9 and 10, more specific examples of the pathways involved in regulating particular organs in the autonomic nervous system will be discussed.

Further Reading

Berridge, M.J. (1984) Cellular control through interactions between cyclic nucleotides and calcium. *Adv Cyclic Nucleotide Protein Phosphorylation Res* **17**, 329–35.

Galione, A. (1994) Cyclic ADP-ribose, the ADP-ribosyl cyclase pathway and calcium signalling. *Mol Cell Endocrinol* **98**, 125–31.

Hughes, A.R., Horstman, D.A., Takemura, H. & Putney, J.W. Jr. (1990) Inositol phosphate metabolism and signal transduction. *Am Rev Respir Dis* **141**, S115–18.

Kikkawa, U. & Nishizuka, Y. (1986) The role of protein kinase C in transmembrane signalling. *Ann Rev Cell Biol* **2**, 149–78.

Lapetina, E.G. & Michell, R.H. (1973) Phosphatidylinositol metabolism in cells receiving extracellular stimulation. *FEBS Lett* **31**, 1–10.

Lee, H.C. (1994) Cyclic ADP-ribose: a new member of a super family of signalling cyclic nucleotides. *Cell Signal* **6**, 591–600.

Matthews, G. (1991) Ion channels that are directly activated by cyclic nucleotides. *Trends Pharmacol Sci* **12**, 245–7.

Meissner, G. (1994) Ryanodine receptor/Ca2+ release channels and their regulation by endogenous effectors. *Ann Rev Physiol* **56**, 485–508.

References

Alberts, B. (1994) *Molecular Biology of the Cell*, 3rd edn, Garland, New York.

Berridge, M.J. (1981) Phosphatidylinositol hydrolysis: a multifunctional transducing mechanism. *Mol Cell Endocrinol* **24**, 115–40.

Hall, Z.W. (1992) *An Introduction to Molecular Neurobiology*. Sinauer, Massachusetts.

Nicholls, D.G. (1994) *Proteins, Transmitters and Synapses*. Blackwell Science, Oxford.

Petersen, O.H. (1995) Inositol trisphosphate and cyclic ADP ribose as long range messengers generating local subcellular calcium signals. *J Physiol* (Paris) **89**, 125–7.

Rang, A.P., Dale, M.M. & Ritter, J.M. (1995) Section 1: General Principles. In: *Pharmacology*, 3rd edn, pp. 3–97. Churchill Livingstone, Edinburgh.

7 : Properties of Effectors

The postganglionic nerve fibres of the autonomic nervous system synapse with a variety of effectors. In this chapter, we will discuss the properties of the various effector systems, including smooth muscle, cardiac muscle, glandular tissue, endothelia and brown fat.

7.1 Smooth muscle

7.1.1 Function of smooth muscles

Smooth muscles serve many varied functions in the body. They are most often arranged around hollow organs, and their function is usually to control the volume and pressure of the space they surround. They are therefore often involved in developing pressure gradients that control or lead to the movement of the contents of the organs. Contractions are much slower and less precise than in striated muscles. The rapidity of action of the skeletal muscles and the precise synchronisation necessary in the cardiac muscles for the heart to function are not required. Contractions need to be more sustained and variable depending on local conditions, and many smooth muscles can generate tension for long periods with minimal energy use.

Smooth muscles, although sharing some features, nevertheless display a surprisingly wide range of different basic properties and patterns of innervation. This diversity ensures that they are exquisitely suited for the different functions they perform. The greatest amount of smooth muscle is in the gut, but within the gastrointestinal tract the properties of the smooth muscles will differ both along the length and across the width of the gut, with the different layers of smooth muscle often having different properties. This diversity allows the gut contents to be ingested, mixed, and exposed to the digestive juices and absorptive epithelia for the appropriate lengths of time, with the remains finally being expelled as faeces. The urinary tract is well supplied with smooth muscle, and again, adjacent areas such as the smooth muscle in the walls of the ureters, the bladder and the urethra differ markedly in their properties to allow delivery, storage and expulsion of urine. The smooth muscles of the genital system include the vas deferens in the male and the uterus in the female, with their specific reproductive functions. In the lung, air flow is controlled by the smooth muscles of the trachea, bronchi, bronchioles and alveolar sphincters. Perhaps one of the most important classes of smooth muscle is that of the vascular and lymphatic systems, again showing remarkably different properties from vessel to vessel, and responsible for maintaining the blood pressure and the correct perfusion of the various organs as required by their needs. Other smooth muscles include the muscles of the iris of the eye, the ciliary muscles controlling the diameter of the lens and the smooth muscles of the hair follicles. The details of the control of the various organ systems will be given in Chapters 8–10. Here we will consider the common properties of smooth muscle cells.

7.1.2 Properties of smooth muscles

Size, shape and structure of the cells

Histologically, all mammalian smooth muscle cells look very similar, regardless of their source, an exception being arterial smooth muscle cells, which are irregular in outline. Successfully isolated smooth muscle cells are instantly recognisable as such, but even experts would have difficulty in guessing the tissue they came from (Fig. 7.1). They are very much smaller than skeletal muscle fibres, and the cells have a cross-sectional area that is even smaller than most cardiac muscle cells, although they may be considerably longer. The cells are normally very long, thin spindles with single centrally placed nuclei and a diameter rarely more than 6 μm in the widest part of the cell. The cells range in length between 30 μm in small arterioles to 400 μm, for instance in the vas deferens, the majority being on the longer side. Figure 7.2 shows a cross-section of the longitudinal muscle of the taenia of the guinea-pig caecum (very like the human taenia coli muscles). As a matter of interest, the section of muscle shown, which contains more than 1500 smooth muscle profiles, has a width of 120 μm and would contain only two average-sized skeletal muscle fibres.

One of the important consequences of this cell size is the enormous surface area–volume ratio of the cells. In the taenia illustrated in Fig. 7.2, the cells have 1.5 μm^2 of membrane for every 1 μm^3 volume, and in smooth muscles with smaller cells the ratio can be as much as 2.7 : 1. This means that none of the cell contents are very far from the membrane, and the cells are more vulnerable than their larger striated relations to changes in intracellular composition. Alterations in membrane permeability, extracellular composition and transmembrane transport processes can readily lead to changes in the intracellular concentrations of small solutes. For instance,

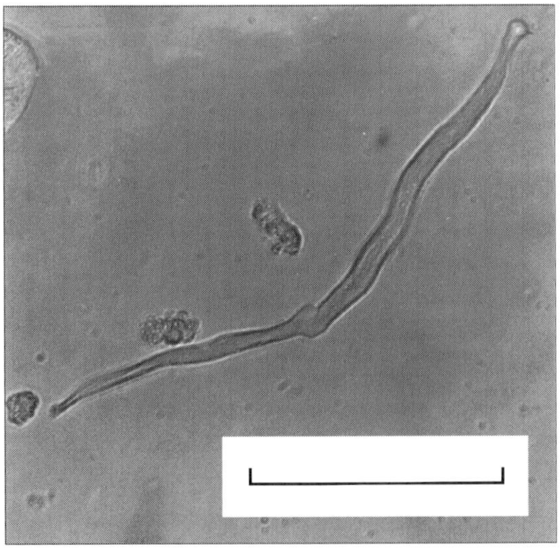

Fig. 7.1 Light micrograph of a single smooth muscle cell isolated from guinea-pig bladder. Scale bar 100 μm.

Ca^{2+} ions entering the cell membrane are more likely to elevate the free intracellular Ca^{2+} significantly than in either skeletal or cardiac muscle.

Smooth muscles possess a sarcoplasmic reticulum, although it only occupies about 1–5% of the cell volume, and is not as regularly organised as in skeletal muscle. There are no 'T' tubules present, and often many of the elements of the reticulum are situated close to the surface of the cell. In some smooth muscle cells (for instance, in arterial smooth muscle) deeper elements are also present. Another feature of the cell membrane in smooth muscles is the presence of caveolae – flask-shaped indentations 70 × 120 nm in dimension that are often found grouped in rows parallel to the long axis

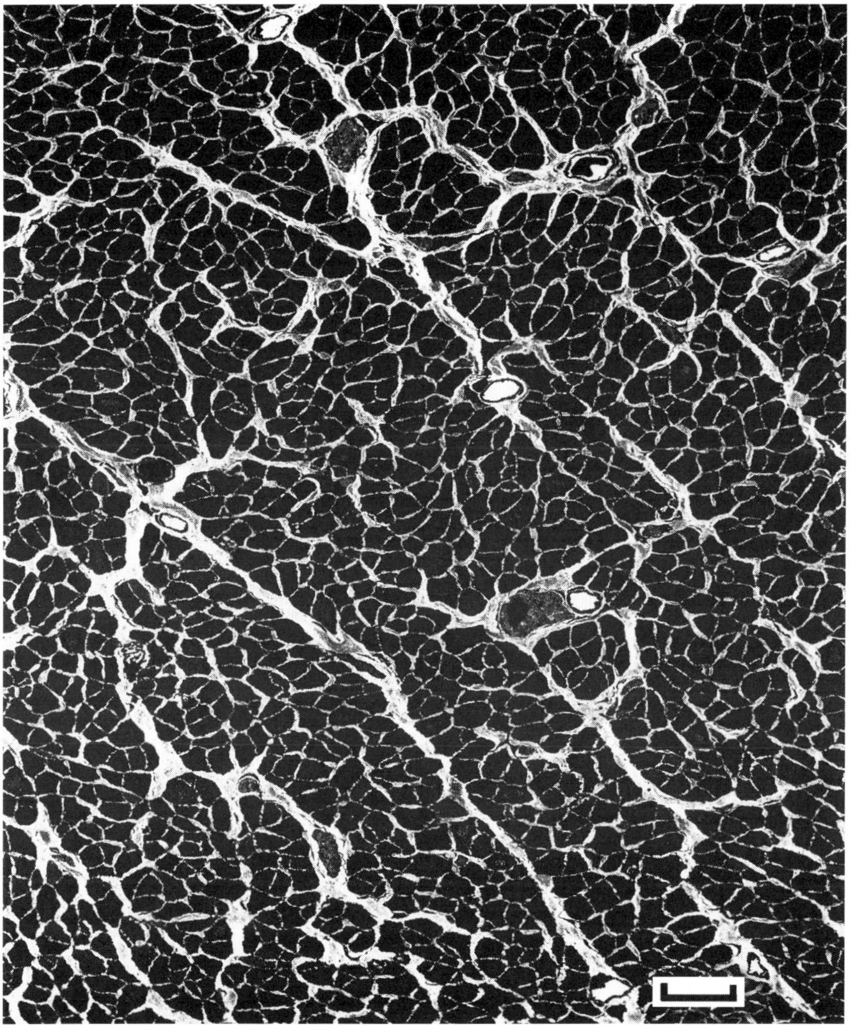

Fig. 7.2 Low-power electron micrograph of a guinea-pig taenia caeci in transverse section. The muscle cell profiles appear subdivided into groups by intramuscular septa, where blood vessels (capillaries) and nerve trunks can be seen. Scale bar: 10 μm. Micrograph kindly supplied by G. Gabella.

of the cell, between the dense bands (see below). The caveolae are characteristically associated with the superficial elements of the sarcoplasmic reticulum, and at present their functional significance is not known. However, it has been proposed that they may be involved in calcium homeostasis, as they are often surrounded by superficial elements of the sarcoplasmic reticulum (Fig. 7.3).

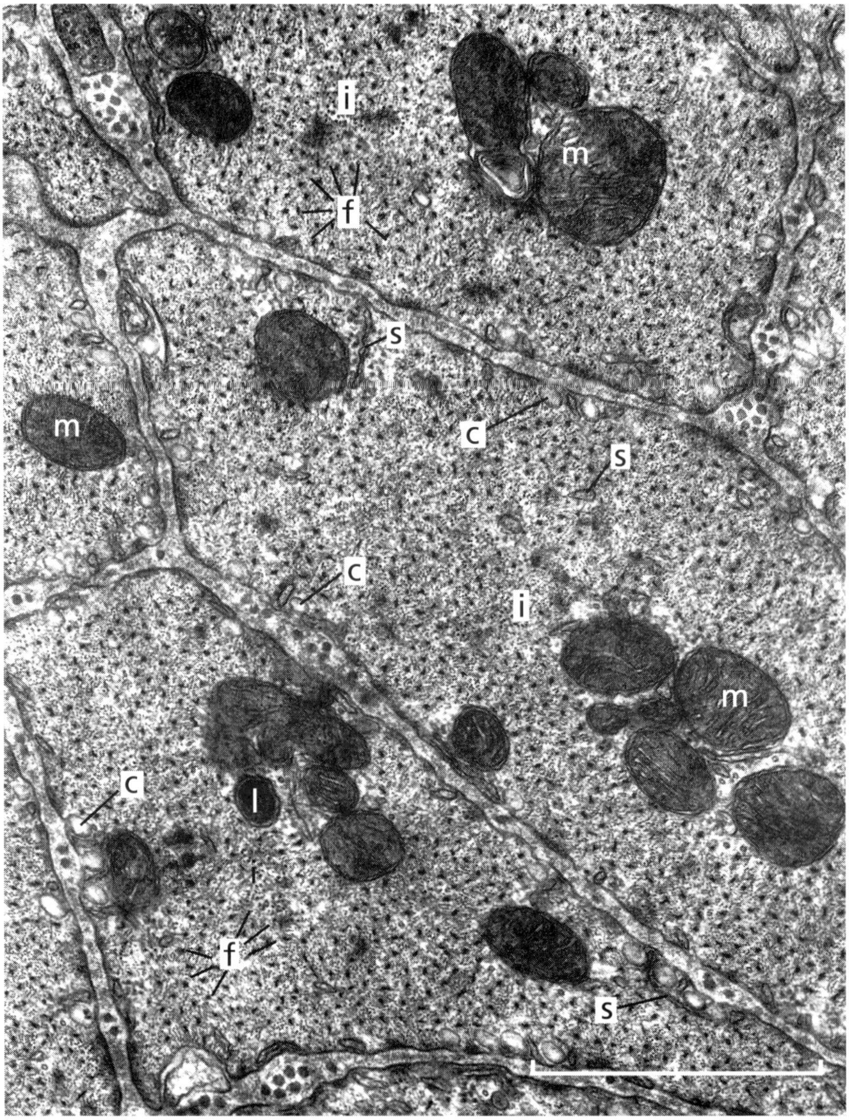

Fig. 7.3 Visceral muscle cells in transverse section in the electron microscope. In the narrow space between the cells some collagen fibrils are visible. Several organelles are found inside the cells: mitochondria (m), lysosome (l), sarcoplasmic reticulum (s), caveolae (c), myosin filaments (f) (the small dots between them are actin filaments), intermediate filaments (i). Scale bar: 1 μm. Micrograph kindly supplied by G. Gabella.

Most of the sarcoplasm is packed full of the contractile elements, and in high-powered electron micrographs such as that shown in Fig. 7.4, three filament types can be seen – thick, thin and intermediate – in proportions that are characteristic for each type of smooth muscle. Also seen are patches of densely staining material interspersed with the filaments (dense bodies),

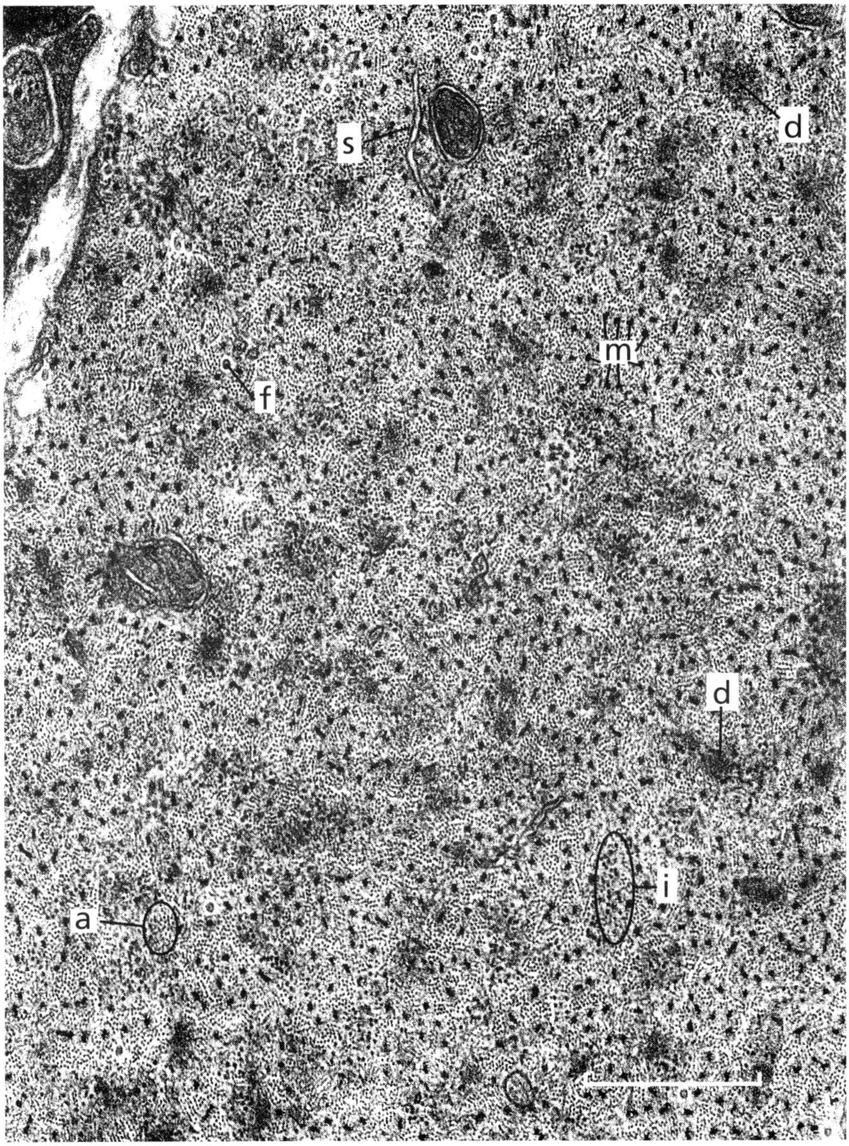

Fig. 7.4 Part of a smooth muscle cell profile, a small portion of its cell membrane visible to the top left. The cell is almost entirely made up of the contractile apparatus: dense bodies (d), myosin filaments (f), actin filaments (a), intermediate filaments (i), interspersed with a few mitochondria (m) and sacs of sarcoplasmic reticulum (s). Scale bar: 0.5 μm. Micrograph kindly supplied by G. Gabella.

or associated with the cell membrane (dense bands). Mitochondria are present, although these are less common than in striated muscles. Some are scattered through the sarcoplasm, often associated with elements of sarcoplasmic reticulum, and others are at the poles of the nucleus, where there are also elements of Golgi apparatus.

Muscle bundles and cell–cell connections

The arrangement of the smooth muscle cells within the tissue is of great importance, and in the larger smooth muscles they are arranged in anatomically discrete bundles of similarly oriented cells. Within a bundle, individual cells are interconnected by low-resistance electrical pathways. This means that current flowing through one cell membrane will spread to neighbouring cells, and this ensures that a group of cells acts in a coordinated manner. Gap junctions are known to be structures that provide low-resistance pathways between cells, but although they are found in

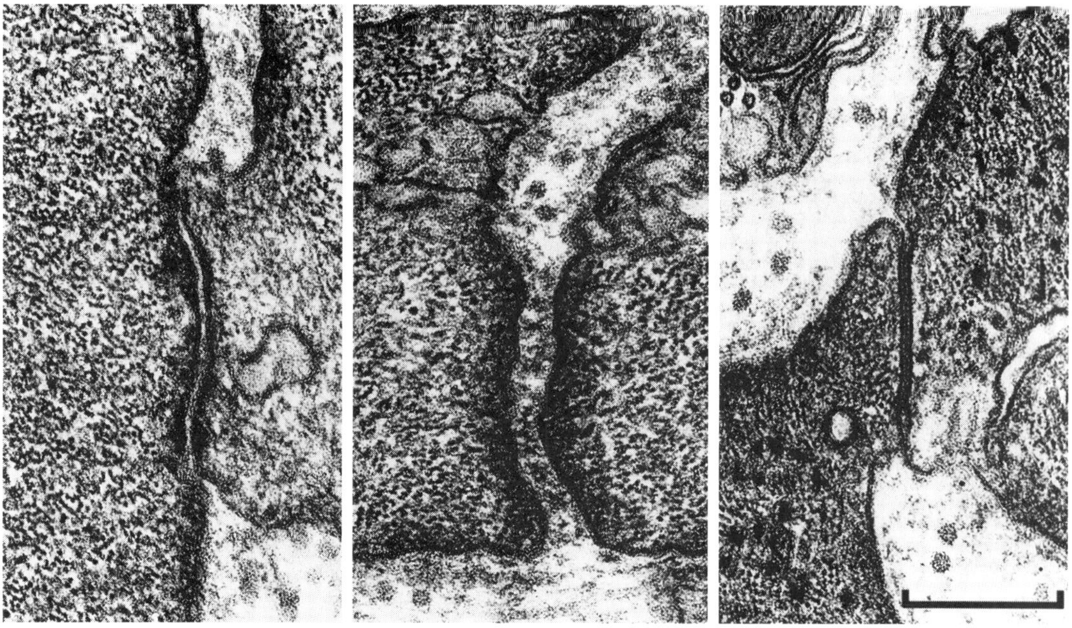

Fig. 7.5 Three common junctions between smooth muscle cells. In the centre is a junction of the adherens type which provides mechanical coupling between the cells: the paired membranes bear a band of dense material which is associated with intermediate filaments of the cytoskeleton and with bundles of actin filaments of the contractile apparatus; the membranes are separated by a wide gap occupied by electron-dense material. To the right is a gap junction or nexus, which provides electrical and ionic coupling between the cells: the paired membranes are very close to each other, separated by a barely visible gap of 2 nm, and are not associated with electron-dense material. To the left is a third type of junction which probably produces additional adhesion between the cells. Scale bar: 0.2 μm. Micrograph kindly supplied by G. Gabella.

some smooth muscles (for instance, circular intestinal smooth muscle and uterine smooth muscle at the time of parturition), not all smooth muscles have been shown to possess them. However, electron microscopy demonstrates many types of intimate contact between cells (Fig. 7.5), and it is possible that pores can form transiently linking cells even if stable gap junctions do not exist.

The arrangement of the muscle bundles again varies from tissue to tissue. In some cases, the bundles tend to branch and interdigitate, mainly in two dimensions, to form the longitudinal or circular layer surrounding many hollow organs, for instance (Fig. 7.6). In other cases, for instance the urinary bladder, the branching is more three-dimensional, and it is difficult to distinguish precise layers. Cell coupling has been found in *all* smooth muscles, even in arterioles, where only a single layer of smooth muscle cells surrounds the vessel. However, even in the larger organs, the extent of the spread of electrical activity along a bundle or from one bundle to another varies markedly, presumably reflecting the need for synchronisation of

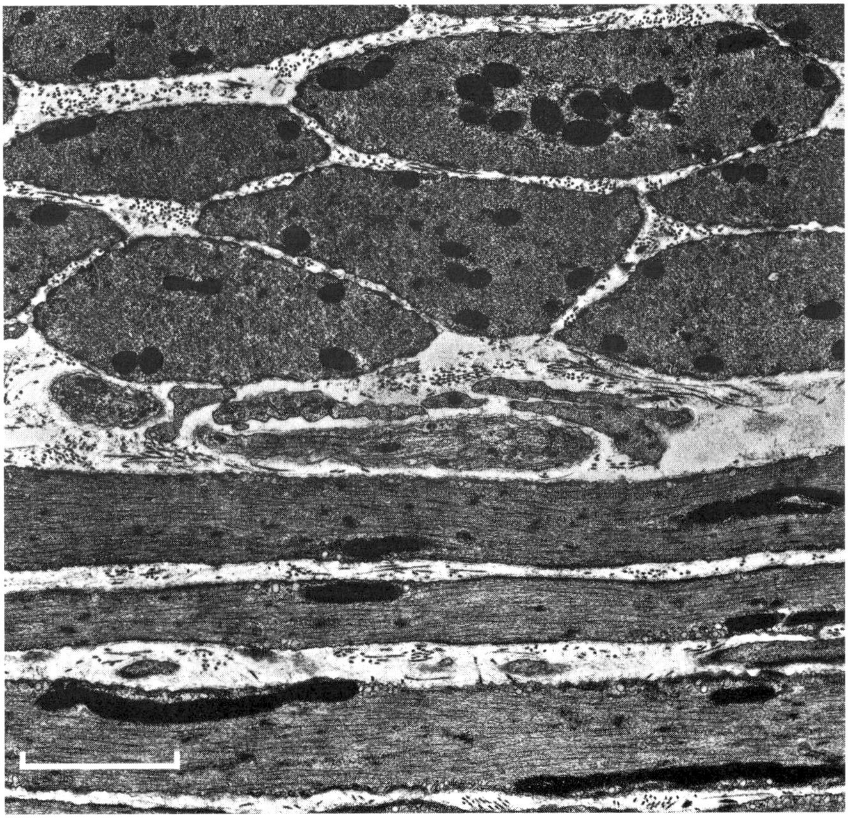

Fig. 7.6 Section through the muscle coat of the small intestine, in the electron microscope, showing distinct arrangement into two layers. Smooth musculature appears in transverse section (top) and in longitudinal section (bottom). A small nerve bundle lies between the two components. Scale bar: 2 μm. Micrograph kindly supplied by G. Gabella.

activity. It is notable that in tissues in which synchronous activity is largely initiated by nerve impulses (such as the urinary bladder or vas deferens), the electrical coupling between bundles may be less well developed than in organs that have spontaneous patterns of co-ordinated activity (such as the intestines, ureter and uterus).

7.1.3 Smooth muscle contraction

Structure of the contractile machinery

Smooth muscles, by definition, do not show striations, yet they possess thick and thin filaments, and evidence suggests that the sliding filament theory of contraction also applies to smooth muscles. The main structural differences between striated and smooth muscles are the lack of Z lines and clearly organised sarcomeres in smooth muscle, and the variable ratio of thick to thin filaments (in cross-sections 1 : 2 in striated muscles, but ranging from 1 : 5–1 : 20 or more in different smooth muscles). The dense bands and dense bodies in smooth muscle seem to be analogous to the Z lines, in that they are the sites for insertion of the thin filaments. Smooth muscles also have a network of non-contractile intermediate fibres (10 nm in diameter) linking the dense bodies, and probably playing a cytoskeletal role.

Thin filaments are mainly composed of actin and tropomyosin, and are about 7 nm in diameter and much longer than the myosin filaments (possibly up to five times their length). Thick filaments are myosin, 14 nm in diameter and 2.2 μm long – somewhat longer than in striated muscles (1.6–1.7 μm). The myosin molecules are arranged differently in the thick filaments from those in striated muscle. In striated muscle, there is a central bare region containing no cross-bridges. This is due to the myosin filaments being arranged with a different polarity at each end of the filament (end polarization), leaving the central zone bare of the myosin heads (cross-bridges). It is thought that, in smooth muscle, the myosin filaments may be polarized in alternate rows along the whole of the thick filaments (side polarization), allowing the thin filaments to be pulled along the length of the thick filaments by cross-bridge activation in both directions simultaneously. Since most of the thin filaments are inserted onto dense bands on the plasma membrane, the muscle cells can shorten dramatically. This can be shown well in isolated cells, which can reduce their length to about 25% of the relaxed length (Fig. 7.7). This is associated with the dense bands being pulled inward, and the areas where the caveolae are, bulging outward. Remarkably, these isolated cells will spontaneously lengthen – probably due to the elasticity of the cytoskeletal elements (such as the 10 nm filaments). In contrast, the shortening of single isolated striated muscle fibres is limited structurally and functionally by the sarcomeric structure, and lengthening requires force to extend the fibres. The extent of shortening of

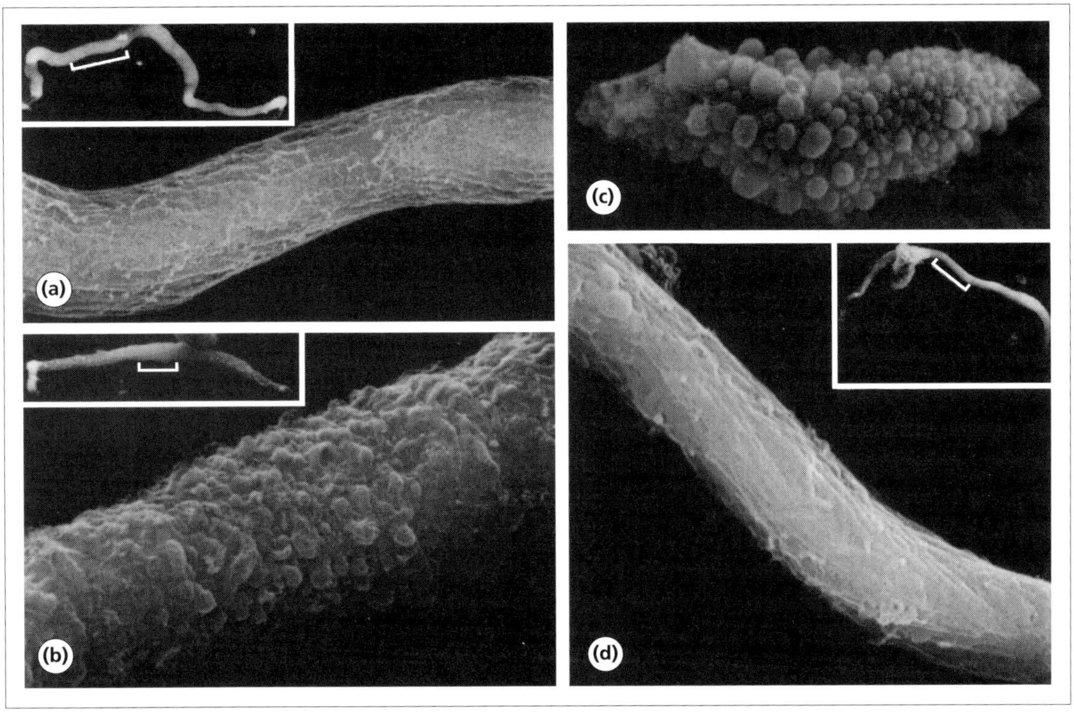

Fig. 7.7 Scanning electron microscope pictures showing shortening and re-extension of isolated smooth muscle cells fixed at various times after activation by electrical stimulation. Insets show the whole muscle cell indicating the region displayed at higher magnification below. Note the relatively smooth outline of the relaxed cell in (a), the appearance of small evaginations after half-maximal shortening in (b), which develop into nearly spherical bulbous projections attached to the main cell by thinner stalks in (c). The cell in (d) has relaxed and re-extended spontaneously. Scale bar ≏ 20 μm. Reproduced from Fay *et al.* (1976), with permission from the publisher, Lippincott-Raven.

smooth muscle cells *in situ* may be limited by their arrangement in the whole organ.

Activation of the contractile machinery

Ca^{2+} ions trigger contraction in all muscles, including smooth muscles. The relationship between free Ca^{2+} concentration and force is similar in all muscles, although the sensitivity may vary between muscles. However, in smooth muscles, the mechanism by which a rise in free Ca^{2+} leads to activation of the cross-bridges is quite different from that seen in vertebrate striated muscles.

It is instructive here to consider cross-bridge cycling in more detail (Box 7.1).

Box 7.1 The cross-bridge cycle

In all muscles, the cross-bridges are the double heads of the myosin molecules, which both possess adenosine triphosphatase (ATPase) activity and can also interact with a specific site on each of the actin monomers that make up the thin filaments. After attaching, first binding weakly, and then attaching more strongly, the myosin heads undergo a change in shape to generate the power stroke, pulling the actin filaments

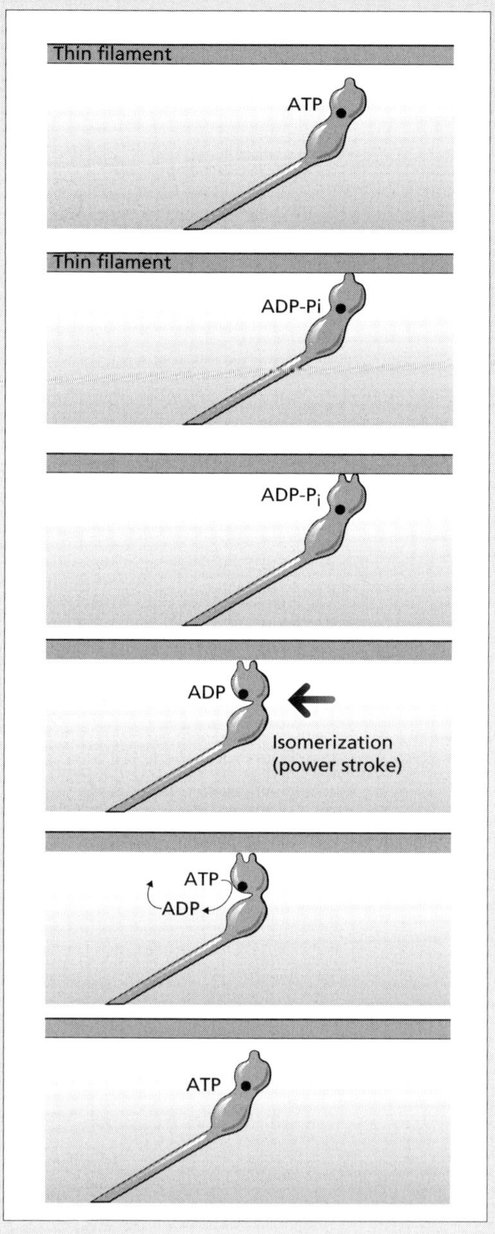

Fig. B7.1.1 Cross bridge cycle. The cross bridges are the myosin heads that project from the thick filament, and attach to the actin monomers of the thin filament. In the sequence of events shown from the top down, binding of ATP to the myosin head causes detachment of the cross bridge. The ATPase of the myosin head results in break-down of the ATP into ADP and inorganic phosphate (Pi), thus activating the cross bridge, and allowing weak attachment to the thin filament. In the activated state, conversion of this weak attachment to a strong attachment occurs, followed by loss of Pi and an alteration in the configuration of the head (isomerization) which is the power stroke. This results in tension production under isometric conditions, or shortening by sliding the thick and thin filaments past each other under isotonic conditions. After the power stroke, the affinity of the head for ADP decreases, it is replaced by ATP, which causes detachment and recovery of the resting configuration.

Continued

Box 7.1 *Continued*

one notch along the thick filament. This allows a release of adenosine diphosphate (ADP) and inorganic phosphate from the myosin heads, and adenosine triphosphate (ATP) can then bind to the enzymatic site, leading to detachment of the cross-bridge from the actin. On breakdown of ATP, the myosin head is energised, and it can bind again to the actin and repeat the cycle. This cycle is probably quite similar in all muscles.

In striated muscle, the regulation of cross-bridge cycling occurs at the level of the thin filament attachment site. In the resting state, attachment of cross-bridges in the strongly binding configuration is sterically prevented by tropomyosin, which lies in the helical groove of the actin filament. The position of the tropomyosin is controlled by the protein troponin – when Ca^{2+} is bound to troponin, the tropomyosin moves and allows weakly bound cross-bridges to enter the strongly bound state, and the cross-bridge cycle can start. Thus, in striated muscles, a preparation of pure actin and pure myosin shows Ca-independent ATPase activity, and the Ca^{2+} dependence only returns if the tropomyosin–troponin system is added back. Smooth muscles do not possess the complete tropomyosin–troponin–Ca^{2+} disinhibitory system of striated muscles. Instead, activation of the system is at the level of the myosin head itself. The myosin heads in all muscles each have two short protein chains as part of their structure, the light chains (Fig. 7.8). In smooth muscle, one of these chains in the resting state is thought to inhibit the ATPase activity of the myosin head, possibly either sterically, or by inhibiting product release. Thus, a preparation of pure actin and smooth muscle myosin has very little ATPase activity in the presence or absence of Ca. The light chain, however, possesses a phosphorylation site, and when phosphorylated, the myosin ATPase is activated and cross-bridge cycling can occur. The Ca^{2+} sensitivity of the system resides in the enzyme responsible for phosphorylating the myosin light chains – myosin light chain kinase (MLCK). The initial steps of smooth muscle activation by Ca^{2+} ions are illustrated in Fig. 7.9 and are as follows: Ca^{2+} binds to a Ca^{2+} binding protein, calmodulin. The Ca^{2+} calmodulin then binds to and activates MLCK. This enzyme then uses ATP to phosphorylate the myosin light chains, and cross-bridge cycling begins. When the free Ca^{2+} levels decline, a Ca-independent phosphatase dephosphorylates the light chains, and the ATPase activity is switched off.

This is not the whole story, however, since there is evidence that other regulatory systems can occur in smooth muscles. In particular, some smooth muscles can enter what is called the 'latch state', a condition in which they can generate tension for long periods of time with relatively little cross-bridge cycling, and thus only a small amount of energy consumption. In the latch state, free Ca^{2+} levels decline, and some cross-bridges are dephosphorylated but remain attached to the thin filaments (Fig. 7.10).

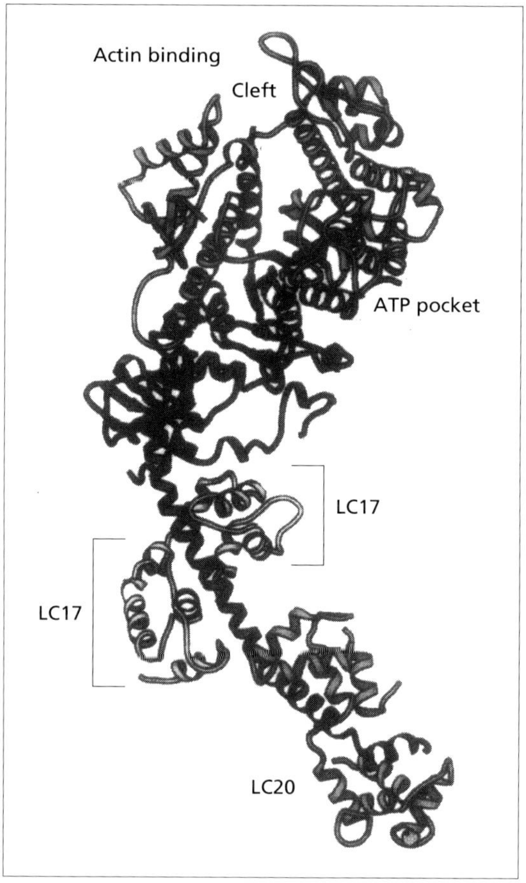

Fig. 7.8 Structure of the myosin head. The two light chains (LC17 and LC20) are on the stem area which leads into the main body of the thick filament. The ATP pocket is where the ATP binds and is hydrolysed. The actin binding site is on the side opposite the ATP pocket. Modified from the figure of I. Raymant in Adelstein & Sellers (1996).

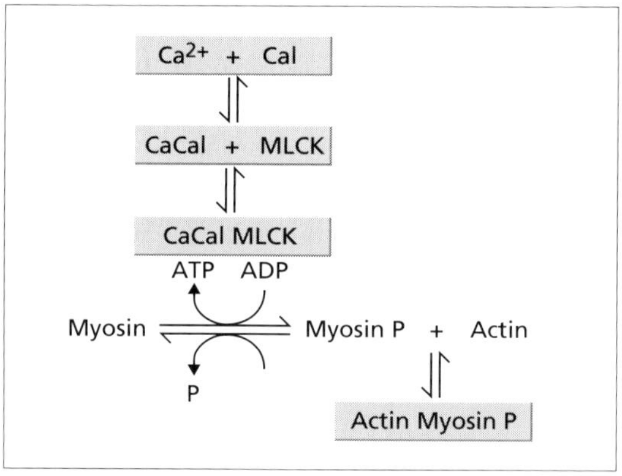

Fig. 7.9 Smooth muscle activation by Ca^{2+}. Ca^{2+} interacts with calmodulin (Cal) and the CaCal complex binds to and activates myosin light chain kinase (MLCK). This in turn phosphorylates the regulatory light chain on the myosin and allows cross-bridge cycling to proceed.

A further drop in free Ca^{2+} allows cross-bridge detachment and relaxation. This may be regulated at the level of the thin filaments. It is known that there are other proteins associated with the thin filaments in smooth muscles, such as calponin and caldesmon. These are Ca^{2+}-binding proteins with properties that can be altered by phosphorylation, and which can also

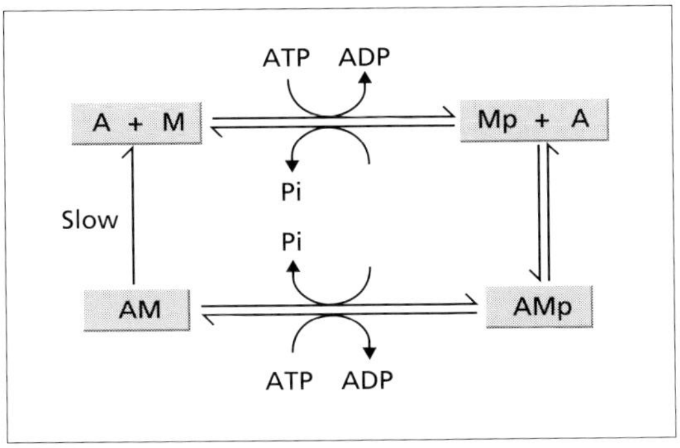

Fig. 7.10 Smooth muscle cross-bridge cycle. After the elevation of Ca^{2+} triggers phosphorylation of the myosin light chains, interaction between actin (A) and phosphorylated myosin (Mp) occurs (AMp), allowing cross-bridge cycling. Dephosphorylation is produced by myosin phosphorylase. If the rate of phosphorylation is reduced (for instance by a small decrease in [Ca^{2+}]), this can result in accumulation of attached dephosphorylated myosin heads (AM), which only slowly dissociate, thus becoming 'latch' bridges.

interact with actin. *In vitro*, the unphosphorylated form of these proteins can interfere with actin–myosin interactions. The precise role of these proteins *in vivo* remains to be elucidated.

7.1.4 Membrane properties

Ionic distribution

As in all cells, the membrane provides a relatively impermeable barrier to most ions and all but the smallest solutes. The resistance per unit area of smooth muscle membranes is higher than in many larger cells, reflecting the low passive permeability to ions. The ionic distribution between the extracellular and intracellular solutions follows a pattern similar to that found in most mammalian excitable cells. Table 7.1 gives examples typical of smooth muscles, showing the ionic activity and equilibrium potentials (calculated from the Nernst equation) for the main ions.

Smooth muscle membranes, in common with most excitable tissues, are more permeable to K^+ than to the other ions, and thus the resting membrane potential is determined most by the K^+ equilibrium potential. A large number of different types of K^+ channel have been identified, several of which may contribute to the 'resting' permeability, while others open in response to many extracellular or intracellular signals. An outline of the various types is given in Box 7.2.

One notable difference between smooth and skeletal muscle is the Cl^- equilibrium potential, which in all smooth muscles so far studied is positive to the membrane potential. Although the resting Cl^- permeability in smooth muscles is low, it may be responsible for the less negative resting potentials

Table 7.1 Typical values for intracellular ionic concentrations and Nernst potentials for ions in smooth muscle cells. Note that in this example the bathing medium is an artificial saline solution, and differs somewhat from normal tissue fluid.

	Intracellular	Extracellular	Nernst potential
Na^+	9 mM	137 mM	+68 mV
K^+	165 mM	5.9 mM	−88 mV
Ca^{2+}	100 mM	2.5 mM	+134 mV
Mg^{2+}	0.35 mM	1.2 mM	+16 mV
pH	7.06	7.4	−20 mV
HCO_3^-	7.3 mM	15.5 mM	−20 mV
Cl^-	54 mM	134 mM	−24 mV

Box 7.2 Ion channels in smooth muscles

Calcium channels. Voltage-sensitive calcium channels carry inward current during action potential generation in electrically excitable smooth muscles. Normally, the channels are L-type calcium channels, characterised by their sensitivity to blockade with calcium antagonists such as the dihydropyridines, and their activation at relatively positive potentials. L-type calcium channels inactivate relatively slowly and continuous activity may occur at the resting potential and be responsible for the resting tone generated in many sphincteric smooth muscles. Their opening probability can be modulated by activation of several types of receptor. Some smooth muscles (e.g. coronary artery) possess T-type calcium channels which activate at more negative potentials, and inactivate completely and rapidly.

Potassium channels. Many types of potassium channel are present in smooth muscles; they play an important role in determining whether or not a smooth muscle is excitable, and in excitable cells, the shape of the action potential. There are several types of potassium channel that are activated primarily by depolarization, including the delayed rectifier (analogous to that in nerves and striated muscle, these channels show little inactivation) and the A-type channels (which inactivate rapidly). Inwardly rectifying potassium channels are present in some smooth muscles (such as small blood vessels); they are activated by hyperpolarizing the membrane, and their voltage sensitivity is affected by alterations in extracellular potassium concentrations, allowing vasodilation in response to increased extracellular potassium. At least two types of calcium-activated potassium channels exist in smooth muscles, one large conductance (maxi-K channels) and one small

Continued

Box 7.2 *Continued*

conductance. Both are activated by a rise in intracellular calcium concentration, and are additionally voltage sensitive, being activated by depolarization. Also present are glibenclamide-sensitive potassium channels which are activated in response to changes in the metabolic state of the muscle, and can help prevent depolarization during ischaemia. These channels are activated when intracellular ATP levels fall, and induce membrane hyperpolarization.

Chloride channels. Calcium-activated chloride channels are present in some smooth muscles, and since the membrane potential is normally more negative than the chloride equilibrium potential, these channels serve to depolarize the cells, and may be involved in mediating the depolarizing responses to some transmitters (e.g. the response of some blood vessels to noradrenaline).

Receptor-activated channels. Receptor activation may lead to production of second messengers that can modulate the function of many ion channels. There are also several channels that are specifically receptor-activated, such as the non-selective cation channel activated by ATP (which is a directly coupled channel) and the non-selective cation channel which probably requires interaction with a G-protein to activate it, and is involved in the response to many depolarizing transmitters such as acetylcholine.

of some smooth muscles, and many smooth muscles have Cl^- channels that can be opened by various stimuli, and will result in membrane depolarization. Membrane potentials vary widely from one smooth muscle to another, and range from about –70 mV to –80 mV in relatively quiescent tissues, such as vas deferens, to –40 mV to –50 mV in more active tissues, such as longitudinal gut muscle. A study of the ionic distributions in Table 7.1, however, shows that, even with this wide range of membrane potentials, all of the ionic equilibrium potentials lie outside this range, and thus none of the ions is passively distributed. Recent experiments have demonstrated that smooth muscles have a large number of ion transport processes in their membranes, as shown in Fig. 7.11, including the sodium pump (Na^+,K^+-ATPase) and the Ca^{2+} pump, which both use ATP to pump ions against their electrochemical gradients – the former being responsible for the low Na^+ and high K^+ concentration in the cells, and the latter for the low intracellular Ca^{2+} concentration. The other ion transport mechanisms are co-transport and counter-transport mechanisms, which couple the movement of one ion down its electrochemical gradient with the movement of another ion against its electrochemical gradient, and are responsible for the relatively high intracellular Cl^- concentration and the lower than expected intracellular acidity. Examples are Na–Ca exchange, Na–Mg exchange, Cl–HCO_3

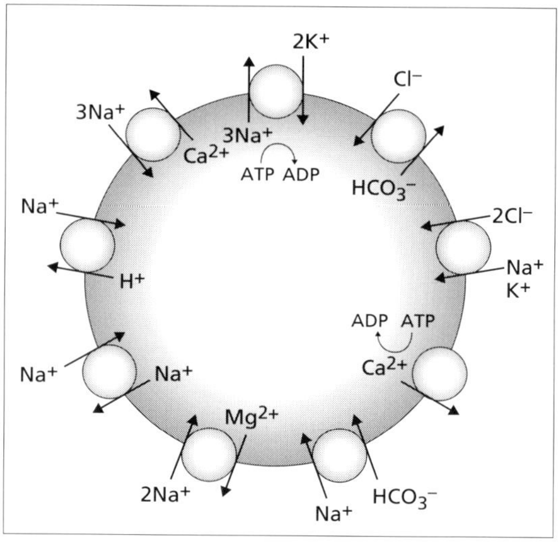

Fig. 7.11 Diagram of the various ion translocating mechanisms that have been shown in smooth muscle membranes. Two primary active transport mechanisms are present (the Na^+ and Ca^{2+} ATPases), both of which are probably electrogenic, three neutral cation exchange processes (Na^+/H^+, Na^+/Na^+, $2Na^+/Mg^{2+}$), one electrogenic cation exchange (Na^+/Ca^{2+} exchange), one neutral anion exchange (Cl^-/HCO_3^-) and two probably neutral co-transport processes (Na^+-HCO_3^-, Na^+-K^+-$2Cl^-$). Other transport mechanisms (not shown) link Na movement down its gradient with the uptake of metabolites such as glucose and amino acids.

exchange, Na–H exchange, Na,HCO_3 co-transport and Na,K,Cl co-transport. The relative proportions of the transport processes again vary between smooth muscles. The main determinant of the resting membrane potential is almost certainly the K^+ permeability, those cells with the highest P_K having the most negative resting potentials.

Electrical activity

The concept of a resting potential is valid in those smooth muscles that show no spontaneous electrical activity, but in spontaneously active tissues it is somewhat unreal, and usually refers to the most negative value recorded between action potentials. This is another area in which smooth muscles show remarkable variability. Not only are many smooth muscles quiescent, but many of them are in fact electrically inexcitable – in other words, even if they are artificially depolarized, they do not generate action potentials. Electrically inexcitable smooth muscles include those in many arteries, and tracheal and bronchial smooth muscles. Quiescent muscles that can generate spikes when stimulated include vas deferens, arteriolar smooth muscles and the smooth muscles of the eye. Most gut muscles, the smooth muscles of the lower urinary tract and the myometrium generate spontaneous electrical activity.

In electrically excitable smooth muscles, the action potentials are generated by the opening and closing of various ion channels. The depolarizing phase of the action potential requires inward current, and thus opening of channels permeant to ions that have an inwardly directed electrochemical gradient. In nerves and skeletal muscle, Na^+ ions and voltage-sensitive Na^+ channels are responsible for the upstroke of the action potential, and the channels are selectively blocked by tetrodotoxin (see Chapter 3). In smooth muscle, this type of channel is very rarely seen, and the predominant inward current mechanism uses voltage-sensitive Ca^{2+} channels and inward Ca^{2+} current. Inspection of Table 7.1 shows that there is an even greater inward driving force for Ca^{2+} than for Na^+. However, the very much lower extracellular Ca^{2+} concentration and the properties of the channels result in a much smaller current density when the channels are opened, and thus a slower rate of membrane depolarization (this results from the necessity of discharging the membrane capacity, which can only be achieved rapidly with large currents). The action potentials in smooth muscle thus have a rate of rise some 10-fold slower than in nerves and skeletal muscle, and are not blocked by lowering extracellular Na^+ or by tetrodotoxin. Instead, the spikes are sensitive to lowering extracellular Ca^{2+}, to Ca^{2+} channel-blocking drugs such as the dihydropyridines, and to many divalent and trivalent cations, such as Mn^{2+} and La^{3+}. The spike shape again varies dramatically from one smooth muscle to another, and examples are given in Fig. 7.12. Some smooth muscles have spikes with a long plateau phase and slow repolarization, some repolarize faster than they depolarize, and some show large negative after-potentials. Underlying these shapes are a great variety of channels, which are discussed in more detail in Box 7.2.

The spike frequency can be determined by different mechanisms in different smooth muscles. In the taenia from the guinea-pig caecum (a much studied smooth muscle) and the rat portal vein, the frequency varies with the membrane potential, and seems to depend on a voltage-sensitive pacemaker mechanism (Fig. 7.13). In many of the other gut muscles, action potentials are triggered on the top of slow rhythmic depolarizations or slow waves. The mechanisms underlying these are poorly understood, but their frequency is relatively independent of the level of membrane potential, and they may be generated by some electrogenic ion transport in specialised cells. In some tissues such as the uterus, slow depolarizations trigger trains of spikes, whose frequency depends on the level of potential reached in the underlying depolarization. These slow waves and slow potentials are often modulated by peptide hormones, such as gastrin in the stomach and oxytocin in the uterus – both increasing the frequency of the waves. The behaviour of individual smooth muscles is discussed more fully in Chapters 8–10.

Tissues that are electrically inexcitable also possess voltage-sensitive ion channels, but cannot normally produce regenerative action potentials. Action potentials are positive feedback mechanisms in which a net inward

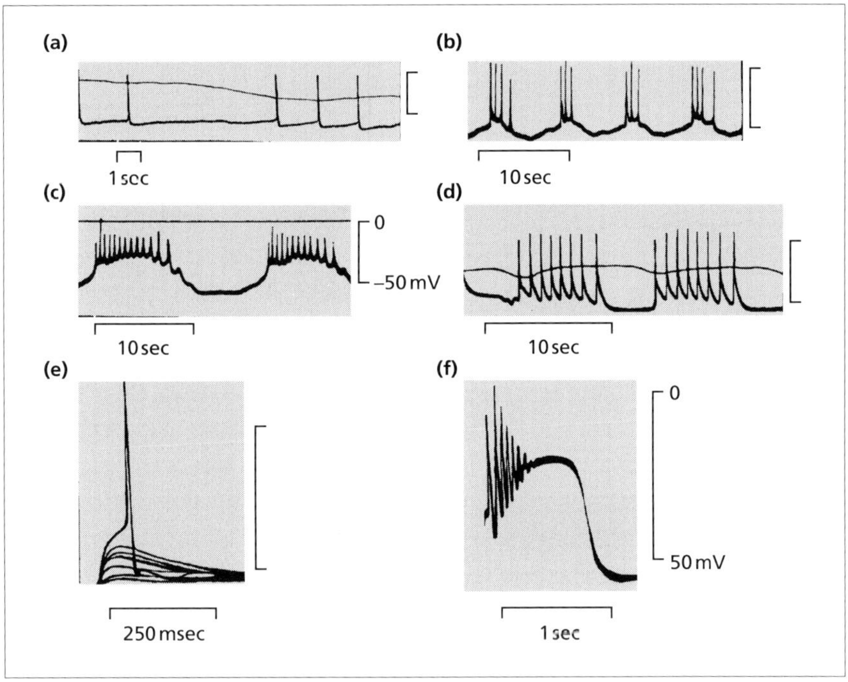

Fig. 7.12 Examples of different patterns of electrical activity seen in guinea-pig smooth muscles. (a) From taenia caeci, (b) jejunum, (c) stomach, (d) uterus, (e) vas deferens, (f) ureter. Note simple spontaneous spikes with negative after-potential in the taenia and the underlying slow wave activity with superimposed spikes in the stomach, jejunum and uterus. The vas deferens shows no spontaneous activity and simple action potentials arise from excitatory junction potentials. The ureter has action potentials that arise spontaneously from a pacemaker region in the kidney, and have this very complex form.

current occurs, which depolarizes the tissue and opens more channels, resulting in an increase in inward current. This process continues until halted by a spontaneous inactivation of the inward current or the opening of sufficient outward current channels to counteract the inward current. In the inexcitable smooth muscles, the K^+ channels seem particularly well developed, and in response to depolarization they open rapidly, and their outward current overlaps the inward Ca^{2+} current that is also generated. Thus, no net inward current occurs, and no spikes, although Ca^{2+} ions may enter the cells in considerable numbers. Many of these inexcitable cells can be made to fire action potentials if some of the K^+ channels are blocked pharmacologically. Agents blocking K^+ channels include tetraethylammonium (TEA) ions, 4-aminopyridine (4AP) and procaine (Fig. 7.14). Electrically inexcitable smooth muscles are often found surrounding small tubes such as blood vessels and airways, where their role is to control the diameter of the tube. In this case, phasic activity triggered by spike potentials may be less appropriate than the ability to respond to the local environment with smooth changes in tone.

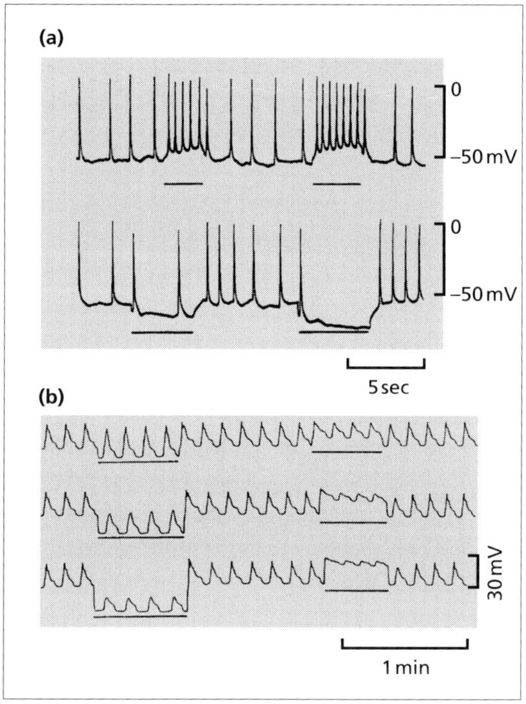

Fig. 7.13 The effects of depolarizing and hyperpolarizing the membrane on the electrical activity of the guinea-pig taenia caeci (a) and stomach (b). Note that the spike frequency in the taenia is markedly affected by the membrane potential, suggesting that voltage-sensitive pacemaker mechanisms are involved, whereas the frequency of the slow waves in the stomach is hardly affected by membrane potential changes. Figures kindly provided by T. Tomita.

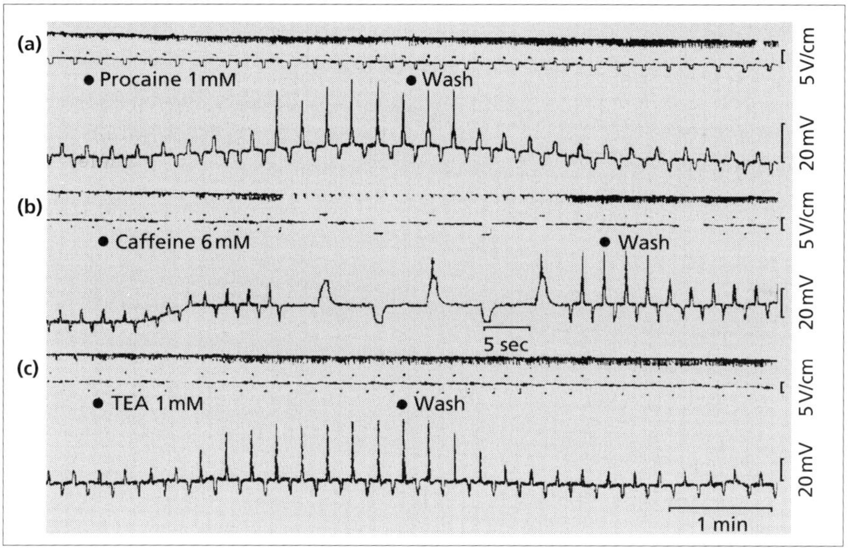

Fig. 7.14 The effects of agents blocking K^+ channels on the response of arterial smooth muscle to depolarizing and hyperpolarizing current pulses. On the right of the traces the depolarizing current injection did not elicit an action potential, since this smooth muscle is normally electrically inexcitable. Addition of TEA, 4AP or procaine caused an initial increase in the size of the voltage responses, indicating a decrease in the membrane conductance, and the depolarizing pulses then began to elicit action potentials. These drugs probably have several different mechanisms of action on the cells, but all result in a decrease in K^+ permeability, which allows the inward current through the voltage-sensitive Ca^{2+} channels to become regenerative. Reproduced from Itoh *et al.* (1981).

7.1.5 Sources of calcium for activation of contraction

An elevation of the free intracellular calcium concentration from a value of about 100 nM in relaxed smooth muscle is the normal trigger for contraction. The relationship between free calcium and force is shown in Fig. 7.15. The position of the curve may vary in different smooth muscles, but a level of 10^{-4} M Ca^{2+} will achieve maximal contraction. The total Ca^{2+} content of most smooth muscle cells is much higher than this, but Ca^{2+} ions are buffered in the cells, either by sequestration in the sarcoplasmic reticulum or binding to various cell proteins. As mentioned above, Ca^{2+} ions enter the cell during the action potential, and in small specimens of spontaneously firing tissues, a good correlation between phasic contractions and spikes is commonly seen (Fig. 7.16). The amount of Ca^{2+} entering the cell with each spike can be calculated, and if this calcium were unbuffered, it could probably elevate the free calcium into the range that could initiate contraction. Experiments indicate, however, that the rapid buffering of the Ca^{2+} entering will probably prevent a sufficient increase occurring, and the current view is that Ca^{2+} entering, at least in the shorter action potentials, may trigger further release of Ca^{2+} from the intracellular stores by a Ca-dependent Ca release mechanism.

The voltage-sensitive Ca^{2+} channels in different smooth muscles may vary in property. Most are L-type Ca channels, which inactivate relatively rapidly with large depolarizations and are responsible for the upstroke of the spikes in electrically excitable smooth muscles. With these spikes, relatively little Ca enters the cell. However, in many tissues, these channels can

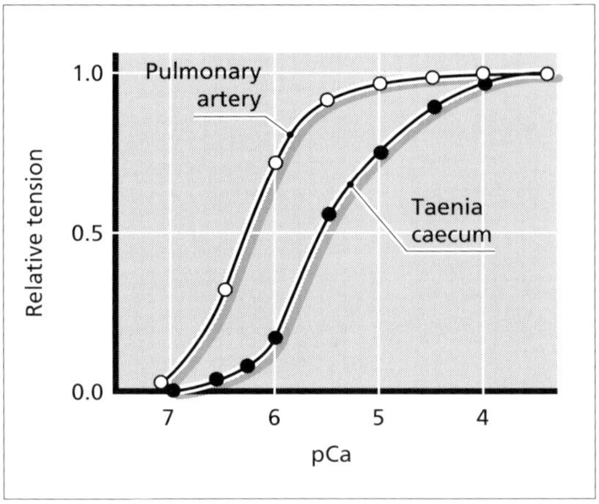

Fig. 7.15 The relationship between pCa (negative log of the concentration of Ca^{2+}) and tension in strips of smooth muscle chemically skinned by exposure to saponin. This type of experiment allows the sensitivity of the contractile apparatus to calcium to be examined. Note that the arterial muscle shows greater sensitivity than the smooth muscle from the caecum. Both tissues are maximally activated at 10^{-4} M Ca^{2+}. Adapted from Endo *et al.* (1977).

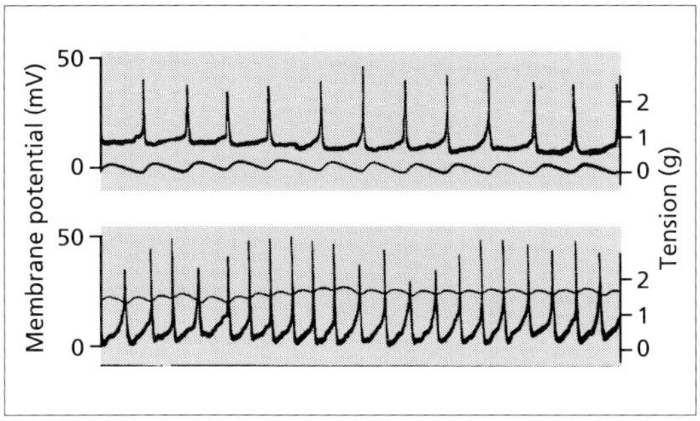

Fig. 7.16 Correlation between spike activity recorded with an intracellular microelectrode from one cell in a strip of guinea-pig taenia caeci and the contractile response of the whole strip. The upper traces were obtained in a strip that had little applied stretch, and the lower traces when the tissue had been stretched slightly. Note that each action potential correlates with a small phasic contraction of the whole strip. The cells are well coupled electrically, allowing synchronous electrical activity. In the upper trace each phasic contraction relaxes to baseline between spikes. Stretch depolarises the cells and increases the spike frequency, allowing the phasic contractions to generate fused tetanic activity. Adapted from Bülbring & Kuriyama (1963).

remain open during prolonged depolarization to less positive values, and can thus allow much larger amounts of Ca^{2+} to enter the cell – certainly enough to activate the contractile machinery. Any external stimulus that results in the depolarization of the cell membrane (e.g. the action of excitatory neurotransmitters, or an increase in extracellular K^{+}) will thus allow Ca^{2+} entry. These contractions are blocked by removing extracellular Ca^{2+}, and by the organic Ca^{2+} channel antagonists such as the dihydropyridines, to which L-type Ca^{2+} channels are very sensitive. However, it is frequently apparent that, even when Ca^{2+} entry through these voltage-sensitive channels is excluded, many agonist drugs can still induce contraction of the tissue. It is possible that drug–receptor interactions can trigger Ca^{2+} entry through some potential-independent mechanism, but even in Ca-free solutions, it can be shown that such interactions can lead to the release of intracellular Ca^{2+} from the sarcoplasmic reticulum through second-messenger systems. The most important of these is inositol trisphosphate, a water-soluble breakdown product of a naturally occurring membrane lipid, phosphatidylinositol-4,5-bisphosphate (see Section 6.2.3). Drug–receptor interaction may result in activation of the enzyme phospholipase C, which catalyses this break-down. Such a mechanism is called 'pharmacomechanical coupling', since it may occur under conditions in which there is no change in membrane potential.

7.1.6 Regulation of activity

Smooth muscle activity is regulated by nerves, hormones, autacoids and changes in the local environment of the cells. More details are given in the discussion of the control of the various organ systems. Here, we will give an overview of the types of smooth muscle and how they are regulated.

Smooth muscles range from those that will only contract under normal conditions in response to nervous activity, through those with myogenic activity that is regulated by their innervation, to those whose activity is almost entirely independent of nerves. The density of the innervation varies in proportion to the amount of neurogenic control. Tissues such as the vas deferens, arterioles and the smooth muscles of the iris are very densely innervated, with the terminal varicose portions of nerves penetrating between the cells, with close contacts between naked varicosities and most, if not all, of the smooth muscle cells. Lower urinary tract smooth muscles are also densely innervated. In contrast, in intestinal smooth muscles, the innervation is more diffuse, and only a small proportion of the individual cells have contact with a naked varicosity. The innervation of the trachea is also very sparse, with little penetration of varicose nerve terminals into the muscle bundles. In many arteries, the innervation is confined to the adventitia, and the inner layers of smooth muscle receive no innervation.

Classification of smooth muscles

An early classification of smooth muscle was proposed by Emil Bozler in 1948. He divided smooth muscles into 'multi-unit' and 'single-unit' types, in the mistaken belief that in some smooth muscles the individual cells were as independent of their neighbours as in skeletal muscles – hence the term 'multi-unit' smooth muscles. Tissues with synchronous spontaneous activity with clearly coupled smooth muscles were called 'single-unit'. Since we now know that all smooth muscles are coupled to some extent, it seems a less appropriate division. Another useful classification is in terms of the mechanisms responsible for regulating contractile activity in smooth muscles.

Neurogenic smooth muscles. The first class of muscles includes those showing no myogenic activity, whose contraction is initiated entirely through nervous activity. Examples include smooth muscles of the iris, in which the radial smooth muscles are under control of the sympathetic nerves and the circular ones under control of the parasympathetic nerves; the ciliary muscles of the lens again being controlled by parasympathetic nerves; the arterioles, which are under the control of the sympathetic nerves; and the vas deferens, under sympathetic nervous control. These are the densely innervated smooth muscles described above, and characteristically the predominant innervation is excitatory in nature, and of one division only. If there are other nerves, these are of minor importance. The muscle tone is governed almost entirely by the frequency of the nerve impulses. A single action potential propagating through the nerve network will release quanta of transmitter from some of the varicosities (low probability of release), and

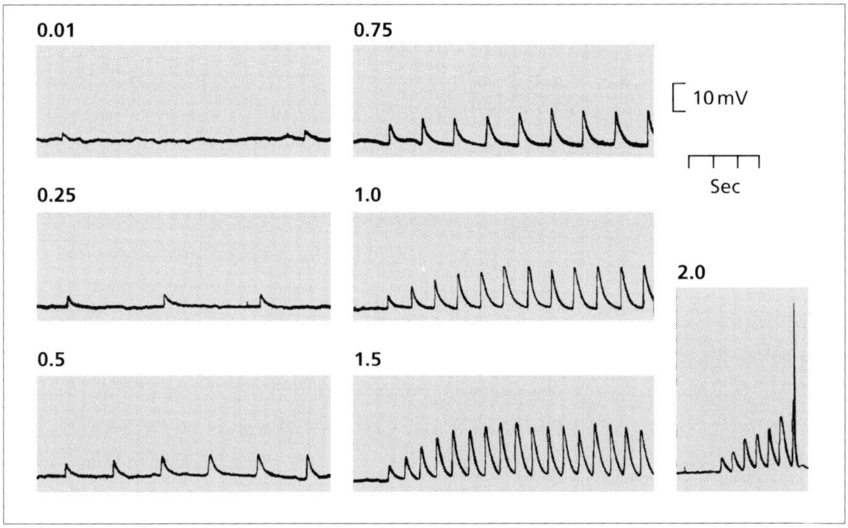

Fig. 7.17 Facilitation of excitatory junction potentials (EJPs) in the guinea-pig vas deferens. Nerve stimulation was applied at increasing frequencies and the EJPs recorded with an intracellular microelectrode. The stimulation frequency is indicated in stimulations/s. At 2/s, the EJPs facilitate sufficiently to reach threshold for initiation of an action potential. Adapted from Burnstock *et al.* (1964).

intracellular recording from a cell will show the summed effect of activity in all the neighbours as a transient junction potential similar to, but much smaller than, the end-plate potential in striated muscle. This is described in some detail in Chapter 4. Excitatory junction potentials (EJPs) are caused by net inward current flowing through channels opened as a result of the transmitter interaction at the postjunctional membrane. They are usually not large enough to reach the threshold for firing an action potential in the smooth muscle cell, and it may require repetitive activity in the nerves with summation of the EJPs to reach the threshold (Fig. 7.17). This type of smooth muscle does have more in common with skeletal muscle than the other types, except that the cells are electrically interconnected, there are no well-defined postsynaptic end plates, and the amount of transmitter released per smooth muscle cell is far less. The excitatory nerves are usually cholinergic or adrenergic (adrenergic in vas deferens), but ATP is often co-released with noradrenaline or acetylcholine, and may play a major role in the excitation.

Myogenic smooth muscles. The second class is a large one, and would include all those smooth muscles which generate spontaneous contractions. It can be divided into two subclasses, those that generate spontaneous electrical activity, and those that are electrically inexcitable, but nevertheless generate myogenic tone.

The smooth muscles whose contractile activity is myogenic and related to the electrical activity of the membrane include those of the gut, the ureter, bladder and urethra, the uterus, and a few blood vessels, such as the portal veins. In these, smooth muscle myogenic activity continues in the presence of tetrodotoxin to block all conducted nerve activity, but the tone can be modulated by activation of both excitatory and inhibitory nerves. This is normally achieved by the transmitters altering the excitability of the membrane by opening or closing ion channels. Discrete inhibitory synaptic potentials are often seen in response to single stimuli of inhibitory nerves, but excitatory synaptic potentials are less often seen, although slow changes in membrane potential may occur with repetitive stimulation. Action potentials may be generated by slow depolarizations (pacemaker potentials) or slow waves. Pacemaker potentials have voltage-sensitive properties, so that the action potential frequency increases as the membrane is depolarized, often leading to a fused or partially fused tetanus (Fig. 7.18). Slow waves are particularly pronounced in the gut. Their frequency is usually relatively insensitive to membrane potential changes, although it can be altered by locally produced substances (autacoids), and in particular peptides (Fig. 7.19). Changes in membrane potential can, however, alter the size or frequency of the spikes triggered by the slow wave, and thus affect the contractile response. The innervation of these tissues is often very complex, with excitatory, inhibitory and modulatory innervation. They may have both parasympathetic (cholinergic) and sympathetic (usually adrenergic) innervation, and in addition there may be several other classes of nerves, often called non-adrenergic, non-cholinergic (NANC) nerves because no-one is really sure what the transmitters are. Recently, it is becoming clear that many inhibitory neurones use NO as a transmitter, and these have been called nitrergic neurones. Other potential inhibitory transmitters include amino acids, purines and peptides.

The other subclass of the myogenic smooth muscles contains those that

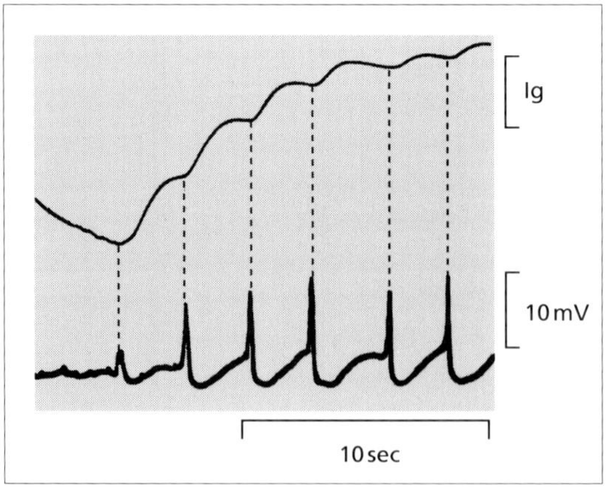

Fig. 7.18 Electrical and mechanical activity from the guinea-pig taenia caeci. A burst of spontaneous action potentials leads to a fused tetanic contraction. This is one of the earliest published records of action potentials and contraction in a smooth muscle, and does not record the full size of the action potential. Adapted from Bülbring (1957).

are normally electrically inexcitable, but can nevertheless generate spontaneous tone. Many of the blood vessels fall into this class, both arteries and the smaller blood vessels responsible for regulating local blood flow to meet the metabolic need of the tissues, and also the smooth muscles round the airways. Although these muscles are often innervated (and, again, the innervation can be quite complex), they characteristically respond most readily to alterations of the environment (such as changes in $P\mathrm{O}_2$, $P\mathrm{CO}_2$, pH and the availability of metabolites) and are affected by autacoids (locally produced substances such as kinins, prostanoids, histamine, serotonin, endothelium-derived factors, etc.). In many instances, when the smooth muscles are causing fine adjustments in the diameter of small tubes, it may be sensible for them not to have regenerative spikes that would result in phasic tension changes in the muscle, but rather to respond to the changes in their environment with smooth, graded responses. It is likely that all these stimuli cause changes in the movement of Ca^{2+} ions into and out of the cells, or can alter the release from and uptake of Ca^{2+} into intracellular stores, or alter the sensitivity of the contractile apparatus to Ca^{2+}.

The enormously diverse properties of different smooth muscles seem to be determined by which of the large number of basic pieces of cellular machinery available to them they express. These mechanisms include the different receptors, ion channels, transport mechanisms, G proteins and intracellular enzymes, many of which are described more fully in Chapter 6.

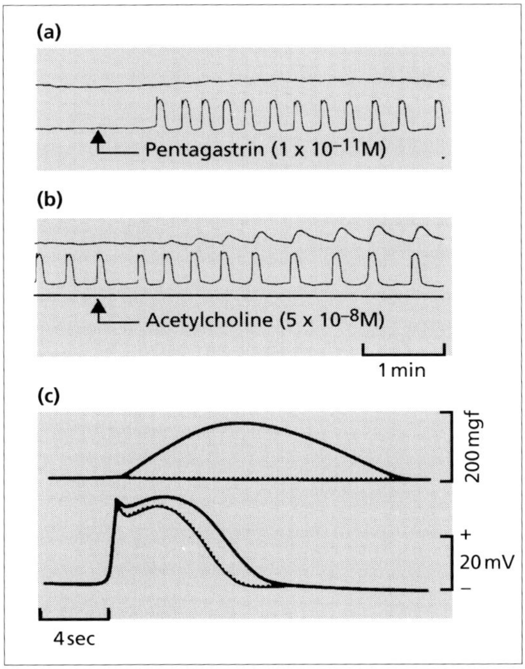

Fig. 7.19 Effect of pentagastrin and acetylcholine on the smooth muscle of the stomach. In each pair of traces the upper trace is tension, and the lower trace membrane potential. Pentagastrin (a) increases the frequency of the electrical slow waves without generating any contractile responses. Acetylcholine (b) results in an enlargement of the slow depolarizations, so that they now reach threshold for activation of the contractile activity. Figure provided by J. Szurszewski.

It seems that these mechanisms may be combined in a variety of ways to ensure that the cell produces an appropriate response to a stimulus. It might be thought that smooth muscles in organs with the same function in different species would use identical mechanisms, but this does not always seem to be the case – the same responses often being produced by different sets of mechanisms. This has to be borne in mind when developing drugs for modulating smooth muscle behaviour in the treatment of human pathological conditions.

7.2 Cardiac muscle

The contractile activity of the heart is myogenic, and the heart can beat and vary its contractile strength to match input and output within its chambers in the complete absence of any innervation. The autonomic nervous system, however, plays an important role in regulating the heart in response to the demands of the body. The frequency of the heartbeat is under the control of both the parasympathetic and the sympathetic nervous systems, and the contractile strength of the muscles is regulated by the sympathetic nervous system. It is a combination of the intrinsic properties of the cardiac muscles and their autonomic innervation that results in the amazing efficiency of the heart, which performs its function economically and unceasingly throughout our lives.

7.2.1 Function of cardiac muscles

It is worth spending time thinking precisely what the functions of the cardiac muscles are before looking in detail at their properties. There are several distinctly different classes of cardiac muscles. These are: the pacemaking cells (the primary pacemaker is the sino-atrial (SA) node and the secondary pacemaker the atrioventricular (AV) node), the atrial muscle, the conducting tissues (bundle of His and Purkinje fibres) and the main working muscle of the ventricles.

Pacemaking cells

These cells are responsible for initiating the beat of the heart, and their contractile properties are unimportant. The SA node is the normal pacemaker, but if for some reason this cannot function, the AV node will take over. These cells must be able to respond to autonomic innervation and circulating hormones by altering the frequency of their action potentials, and the SA node must be connected electrically to the atrial cells, and the AV node to the conducting tissues of the ventricle. The conduction through the AV node is slow, to allow the atria to contract before the ventricles. The conduction velocity is under autonomic control and can be altered to accommodate different rates of heartbeat.

Atrial muscle

The atria receive the blood returning to the heart and conduct the cardiac impulse from the SA node to the AV node. When the ventricles are contracting, the atria act as a low-pressure reservoir. During diastole, the blood flows through them into the ventricles, and early in systole, the atrial muscles contract and complete the filling of the ventricles, supplying about 15–20% of the input. The contractile strength of the muscle fibres does not need to be great.

Conducting tissues

These muscle fibres are specialised for rapid conduction of the impulse to the ventricular muscle. Their contractile properties are unimportant, but they can act as a tertiary pacemaker if there is a block of conduction from the AV node (complete heart block).

Ventricular muscle

This is the most important cardiac muscle, being responsible for the work of the heart. When the heart muscle is relaxed (during diastole), filling of the heart occurs, blood flowing from the vena cava and pulmonary vein through the atria into the ventricles. The filling pressure from the vena cava is very low, and there may only be an average pressure gradient during filling of 2 mmHg. This means that the ventricular muscles must be very easily stretched. When the heart beats (systole), blood is expelled from the ventricles into the aorta and pulmonary artery. The pressure at the end of diastole in the aorta is likely to be between 60 and 90 mmHg (depending on age) and in the pulmonary artery between 4 and 12 mmHg. Thus, to expel blood, the pressure in the ventricles has to rise significantly above these pressures. In order to achieve this, the muscle fibres must be arranged so that, if they shorten, they will reduce the volume of the ventricles. Since the muscle is so easily extensible, pressure will only rise in the ventricles if all the fibres are contracting simultaneously, and there has to be an efficient method of synchronising the beat. This is achieved by electrical coupling between the myocytes and by the specialised conducting tissues. On average, each beat must expel the amount of blood that is entering the heart during the cardiac cycle. The muscle has therefore to contract for long enough and with enough strength to achieve this, and must vary these parameters depending on the amount of blood that has entered the heart (end-diastolic volume). This is achieved intrinsically through the length–tension relationship of the muscle fibres (they contract harder when stretched further), and extrinsically through the action of the sympathetic nerves and circulating adrenaline, which can alter the position of the length–tension curve so that force can be increased without stretching the fibres. The ventricular muscles have to relax completely between beats for long enough to ensure adequate filling. They must not be re-excited rapidly by any stray impulse, and this is achieved by the electrical properties of the membrane. The action potential has a plateau that is nearly as long as the contraction it initiates, and there is thus a long absolute refractory period (during which it is impossible to fire another action potential), and also a long relative refractory period, during which a larger than normal stimulus is needed to excite the muscle. The ventricular muscle must always have enough oxygen and a sufficient source of energy, however hard it is working. It is therefore heavily vascularised. Since the heart has to work harder when the other muscles of the body are also working harder (thus depleting the blood of glucose), the cardiac muscles must be able to use other sources of energy, such as lactate, pyruvate, lipids and ketone bodies.

7.2.2 Properties of cardiac muscle

Size, shape and structure of the cells

Cardiac muscles, unlike the fused muscle fibres of skeletal muscle, are composed of individual myocytes, between 35 and 130 μm long and 10–15 μm wide, depending on their location. The cells are linked together by various junctional complexes to form a functional syncytium, which allows passage of current between the cells, and also tension transmission in the working myocytes. The junctions are particularly well developed between ventricular myocytes at the intercalated discs. These have areas of gap junction providing electrical continuity, and desmosomes and fasciae adherens providing mechanical continuity (Fig. 7.20). All the myocytes have visible striations, although they are poorly developed in the pacemaking and conducting muscles.

7.2.3 Cardiac muscle contraction

Structure of contractile machinery

The contractile machinery in cardiac muscles is very similar to that found in skeletal muscles. The thick and thin filaments are arranged in myofibrils consisting of sarcomeres separated by Z lines. The thin filaments insert on the Z lines. At the end of the myofibril, the thin filaments insert onto the cell membrane at the intercalated disc, which replaces the last Z line. There are twice as many thin filaments as thick filaments, and they are arranged to form a hexagonal interdigitising pattern in cross-section (Figs. 7.21 & 7.22). As in skeletal muscle, thin filaments are composed of globular actin units, arranged in a double helix, and have the long filamentous tropomyosin molecules lying in the groove of the helix. The thin filaments also possess the complete globular troponin complex, with troponin T, C

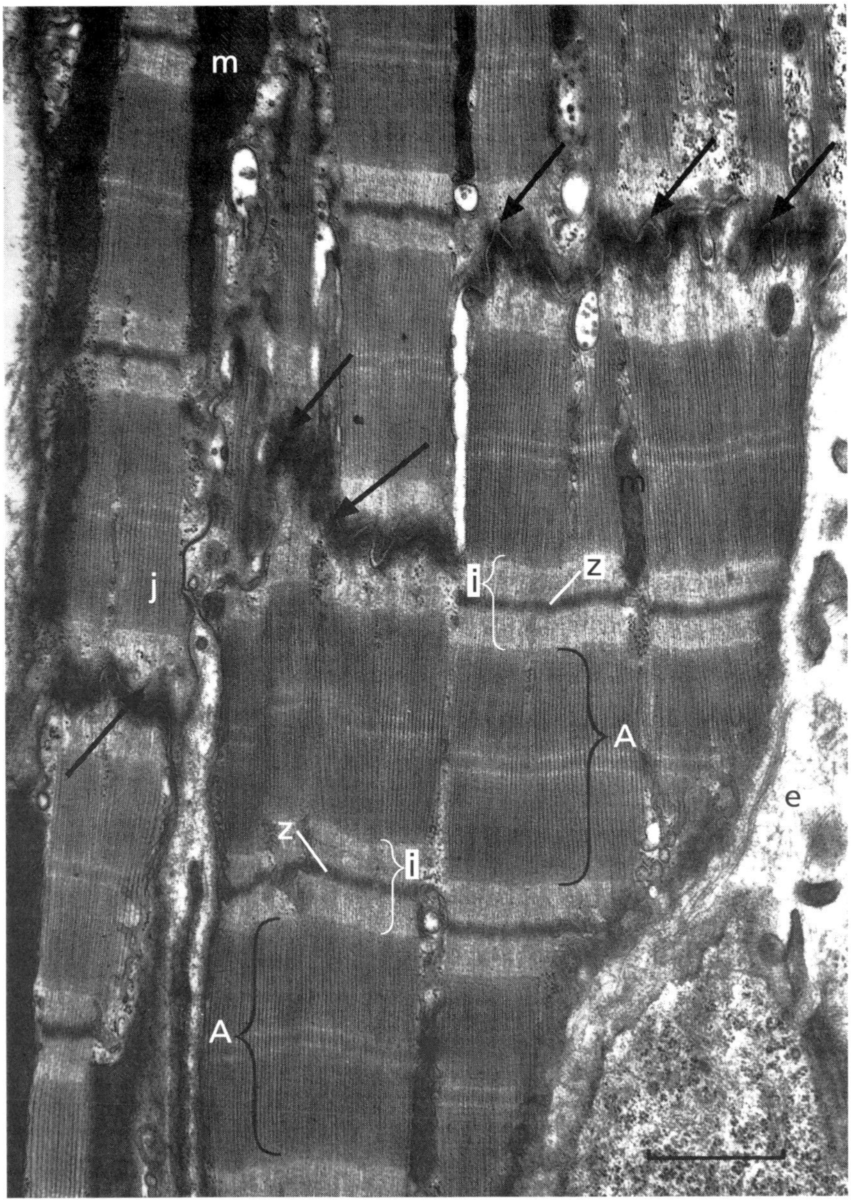

Fig. 7.20 Longitudinal section of cardiac muscle. The sarcomeres are well outlined, with Z lines (z), I bands (i) and A bands (A). An intercalated disc (arrows) separates the sarcomeres of adjacent cells, while providing mechanical and electrical continuity between them. (m) Mitochondria, (e) extracellular space, (j) gap junction. Scale bar: 1 μm. Micrograph kindly supplied by G. Gabella.

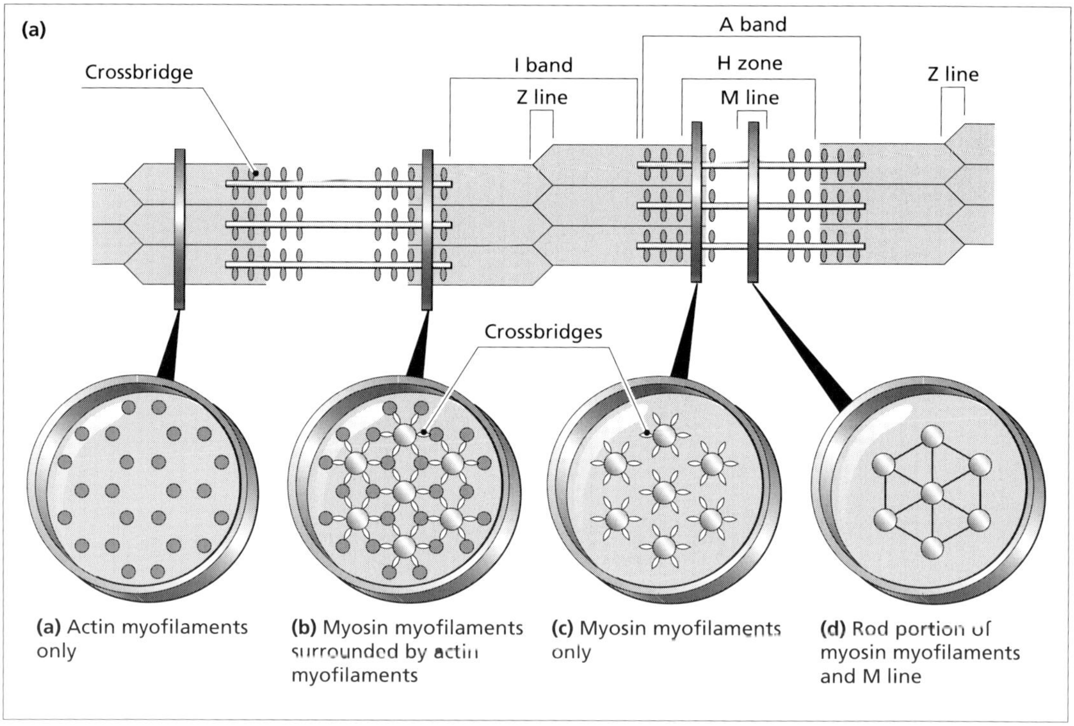

Fig. 7.21 Structure of sarcomeres in a myofibril taken from cardiac muscle. (a) Diagram of the arrangement of filaments in the sarcomere, with cross-sections taken at the positions indicated. (b) High-powered electron micrograph of cardiac muscle in cross-section. Several myofibrils are intersected by the plane of the section at different levels of the sarcomere. (Z) Z-line, (I) I band, (A) A band, (M) middle of the A band or M line. There are numerous mitochondria (m) near the edges, a lipid vacuole (L), tubules and cisternae of sarcoplasmic reticulum (s) and T-tubules (T). Scale bar: 0.5 μm. Micrograph kindly supplied by G. Gabella. *Continued opposite.*

and I, each tropomyosin molecule having one troponin complex bound to it through the T unit (Fig. 7.23). Thick filaments are again similar to those of skeletal muscle. The myosin molecules point in different directions at each end of the filament (end-polarized), leaving a central zone free of cross-bridges. Shortening occurs in the normal sliding filament manner, with cross-bridges pulling the thin filaments between the thick filaments. As mentioned above, the myofibrils are less well developed in the pacemaking tissues of the heart.

Activation of contractile machinery

Cross-bridge cycling is switched on by an increase in free intracellular Ca^{2+} as in all muscles (see Box 7.1 and p. 195). The sensitivity of the contractile machinery to Ca^{2+} can be altered by cyclic adenosine monophosphate

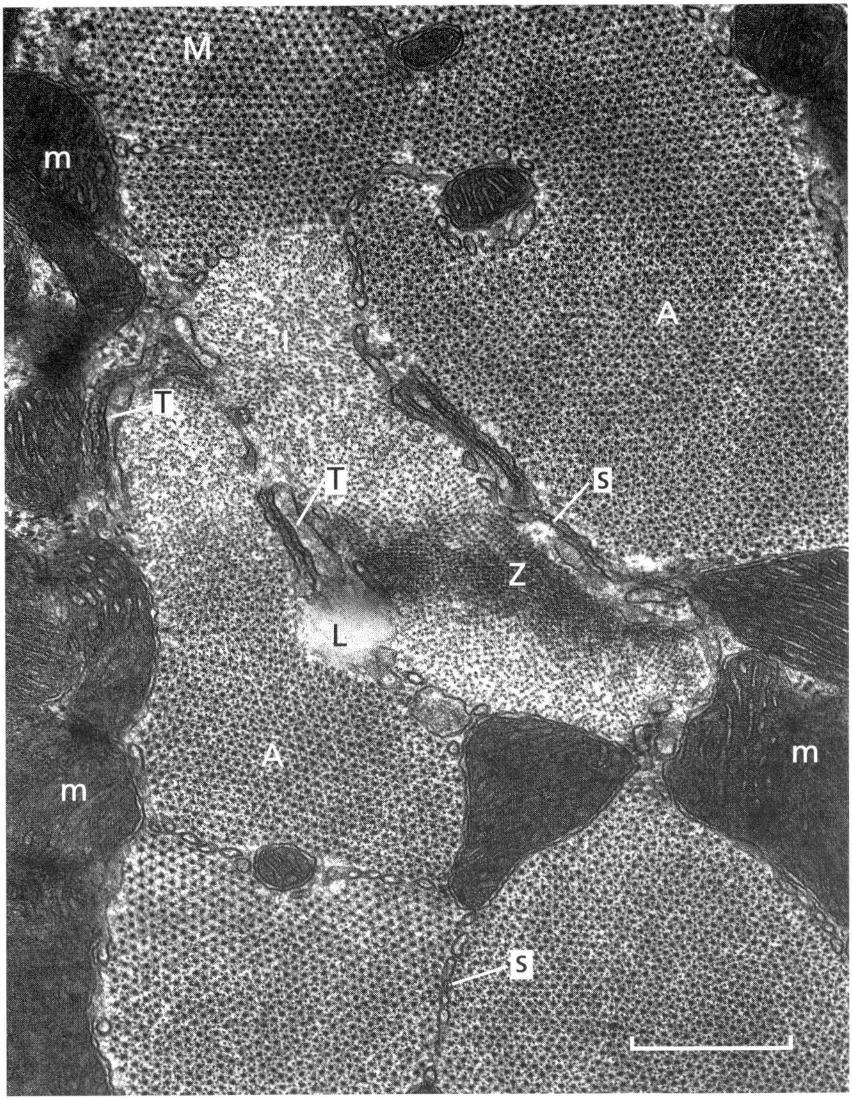

(b)

Fig. 7.21 *Continued.*

(cAMP)-dependent phosphorylation of the troponin molecule, which reduces its affinity for calcium ions.

7.2.4 Membrane properties

Ionic distribution

Cardiac muscles have fairly typical intracellular ionic concentrations. The intracellular Na^+ is low and the K^+ is high. The intracellular Cl^- is higher than would be predicted by a passive distribution. As in smooth muscle,

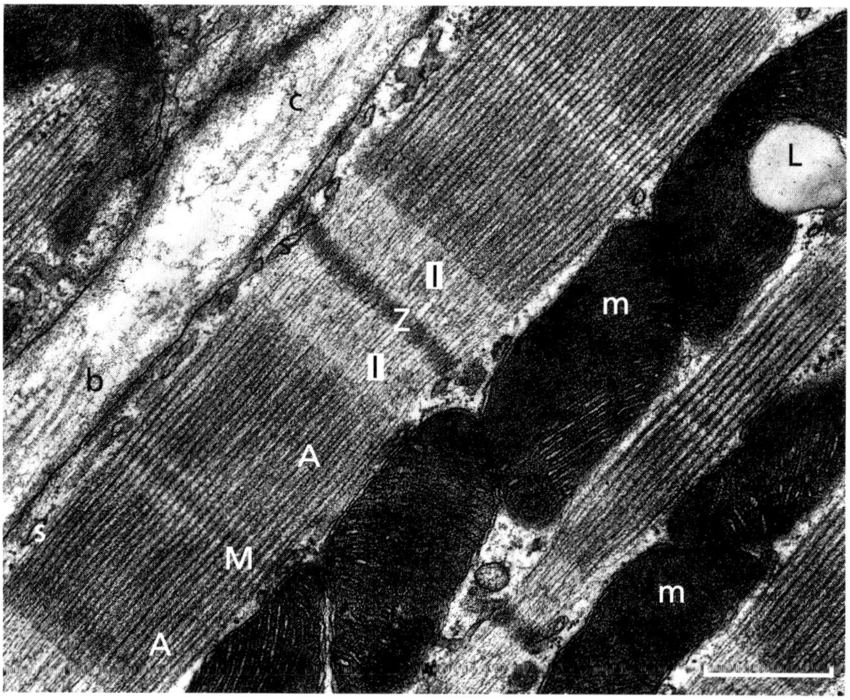

Fig. 7.22 Longitudinal section of the edge of a cardiac muscle cell, showing well-developed sub-plasmalemmal sarcoplasmic reticulum (s). The arrangement of the myofilaments in the sarcomeres is well illustrated. (Z) Z line; (I) I band; (A) A band; (M) M line. Note closely packed mitochondria (m), lipid vacuole (L), basal lamina (b) and collagen in the extracellular space (c). Scale bar: 0.5 μm. Micrograph kindly supplied by G. Gabella.

few if any of the ions are passively distributed, and the membranes possess a large number of membrane transport processes. Particularly important are those controlling intracellular Ca^{2+} and intracellular pH, since these may have effects on the contractile strength of the muscle. In comparison to most smooth muscles, in cardiac muscle Ca^{2+} entering the cell is extruded by a powerful plasma membrane Na–Ca^{2+} exchange, and the ATP-driven Ca^{2+} pump, although present, is less important. Ca^{2+} is also taken up by intracellular Ca^{2+} stores. Intracellular pH is regulated by Na–H exchange, Na,HCO_3 co-transport and by Cl–HCO_3 exchange. This latter exchange also helps determine the intracellular Cl^- level. Because of the spontaneous activity, it is difficult to define a true resting potential of the cells, but the most negative potential reached during the cycle (maximum diastolic potential) varies between the different types of cardiac muscle. Typical values are: ventricle –80 mV; Purkinje fibres –80 mV; atria –75 mV; SA node –65 mV; AV node –65 mV. The pacemaker cells tend to be less polarized than the working and conducting tissues.

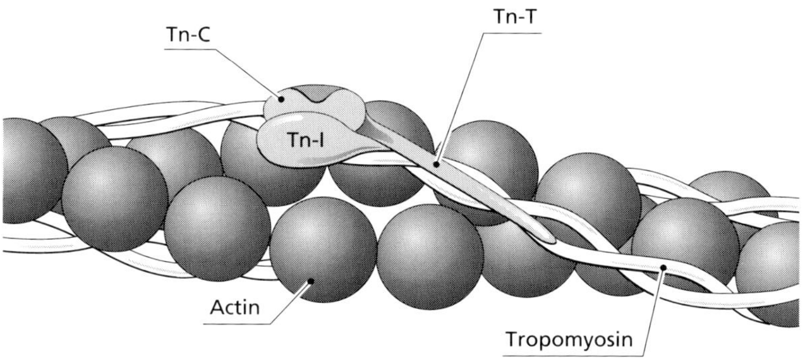

Fig. 7.23 Thin filament in striated muscles. The globular actin monomers combine to form a double helix which is the main component of the thin filament. Lying in the groove is the double helical strand of the filamentous tropomyosin. Each molecule overlaps seven actin monomers. At the end of each tropomyosin molecule is a troponin complex, consisting of a long troponin T (Tn-T) which interacts with the tropomyosin, and troponin I (Tn-I) which interacts with Tn-T and the third component, troponin C (Tn-C). Tn-C binds to calcium, and mediates a change in conformation of the troponin complex, causing a movement in the tropomyosin which allows the strong binding of the myosin head to occur, and cross-bridge cycling.

Action potential shapes

The heart beats spontaneously in the absence of any nervous input, and thus the action potentials are myogenic. The shape of the action potential is characteristic of the cardiac muscle type. Figure 7.24 shows typical action potentials from the SA node, atrium, AV node, Purkinje fibre and ventricle.

One obvious difference is the rate of the depolarization during the upstroke of the action potential. In the nodal tissues, this is clearly much slower than in the other tissues. This is associated with the less negative maximum diastolic potential, and also with a slow conduction velocity (about 5 cm/s in the nodes). The conduction velocity is determined by the rate at which current can spread from one cell to another. This depends on the time taken to change the charge on the membrane. The greater the current flow, the faster the membrane can depolarize and the faster the action potential can propagate. Rapid upstrokes are thus associated with rapid conduction, and this is necessary in the atria, conducting and working tissues of the heart. The conduction velocity is about 200 cm/s in Purkinje fibres.

Another difference is the pacemaker depolarization that is characteristic of the nodal cells and the Purkinje fibres. This is the slow depolarization that occurs during diastole. The pacemaker potential is steepest in the SA node, and this tissue thus reaches the threshold for action potential production most frequently, and acts as the primary pacemaker in the heart. As explained earlier, the AV node and the Purkinje fibres can also act as

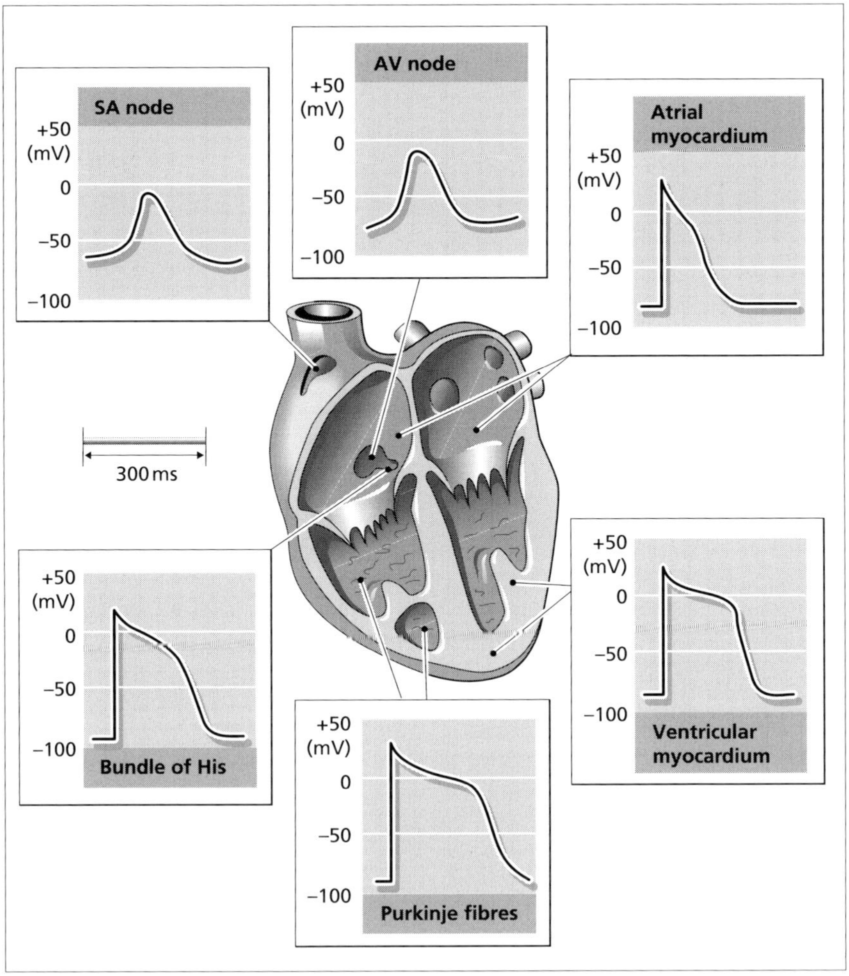

Fig. 7.24 Diagram of the heart, showing the shape of action potentials recorded with microelectrodes from muscle cells of each part.

secondary or tertiary pacemakers. The diastolic potential in the atria and ventricles is constant, and these tissues will not generate spontaneous action potentials, but rely for their activation on the spread of current from adjacent tissues.

The third characteristic difference is the presence of the plateau in the tissues of the ventricles. This is essential firstly to allow sufficient time for propagation of the potential to all regions of the ventricle so that synchronous contraction can occur, and secondly for preventing tetani, by ensuring that the refractory periods are long.

7.2.5 Action potential mechanisms

The mechanisms underlying the action potential have been most intensely studied in Purkinje fibres, as these are easily removed from the heart. If you open the ventricles in a mammalian heart, the Purkinje fibres can be seen looping out of the ventricular muscle and looking like short, thin strands of cotton. It is a comparatively easy matter to dissect one of these strands off without damaging the cells. The action potential is determined by many different mechanisms.

Fast inward current

The rapid upstroke of the action potential is triggered by depolarization, and due to Na^+ ions flowing through voltage-sensitive channels with similar properties to the Na^+ channels in nerves and striated muscle. This is called the fast inward current, and the threshold for generating an all-or-none action potential is about –70 mV. The current is tetrodotoxin-sensitive, and inactivates rapidly if the membrane is held slightly depolarized. This current plays little part in the upstroke of the nodal cells, since the diastolic membrane potential seldom, if ever, reaches a level at which sufficient of these channels are reactivated. In the Purkinje fibre, there is a partial repolarization phase that can often be seen before the plateau – it is probably due to inactivation of the Na^+ channels, and also to activation of a transient outward current.

Slow inward current

When the membrane potential is depolarized sufficiently, another inward current, the slow inward current, is switched on. This is a Ca^{2+} current, and may have several different components. The major and most rapid component is due to voltage-sensitive Ca^{2+} channels, which are activated more slowly and at less negative membrane potentials than the Na^+ channels. These channels also inactivate, but comparatively slowly. This component plays a part in the end of the upstroke and the beginning of the plateau in the Purkinje fibres and ventricles, but is also entirely responsible for the upstroke of the action potential in the nodal tissues. Slower components of inward Ca^{2+} current are responsible for maintaining a net inward current during the plateau in the Purkinje and ventricular fibres.

Potassium currents

The cardiac cells also possess voltage-sensitive K^+ channels, which on opening will tend to repolarize the membrane. Again, there is more than one type. The transient outward current mentioned above is present in some myocytes, and is activated and rapidly inactivated by depolarization. The delayed rectifier current is only slowly activated by depolarization, and becomes important towards the end of the plateau, helping repolarization. Some potassium channels are present that are open at all potentials, but have the interesting property that, although they are open, their conductance to the outward flow of K^+ ions gets smaller as the membrane is depolarized (inward rectifier K^+ channels). This means that, during the plateau, the outward current through these channels will be small, and only a relatively small inward current is needed to keep the membrane depolarized. As the inward current declines and the membrane begins to repolarize, these channels increase their conductance and aid the rapid repolarization of the action potential.

Plateau currents

The components of the slow inward current that operate during the plateau, particularly in the ventricular muscle, may be partially triggered by the rise in free intracellular calcium that will occur during contraction. It is known that this can trigger Na–Ca^{2+} exchange. This mechanism is electrogenic, since at least three Na^+ ions enter the cell in exchange for each Ca^{2+} ion extruded, and thus a net inward current is generated. The membrane may also have non-selective cation channels that are activated by intracellular Ca^{2+} and could generate inward current. The plateau is terminated by the decline in the inward current (either as a result of the drop in intracellular Ca, or the slow inactivation of voltage-sensitive Ca^{2+} channels), which causes an initially slow repolarization, but as the K^+ channels start to increase their conductance, a rapid repolarization develops.

Pacemaker currents

In the Purkinje fibre, the main pacemaker current is called I_f (f was originally for 'funny'). This current is carried by relatively non-selective cation channels that are switched on by hyperpolarization, and switched off by depolarization. When the repolarization after the plateau reaches a sufficient level, these channels are switched on, and because of the large inwardly directed electrochemical gradient for Na^+ ions, a net inward current flows through them. This begins the depolarization, which represents the pacemaker potential. I_f is a self-limiting current, since the depolarization switches the channels off. In the absence of an invading action potential, I_f can reach the threshold for activating the upstroke. This pacemaker current may play a lesser role in the nodal tissues, since the diastolic potential never normally reaches a sufficiently negative potential to activate it fully. Two other mechanisms also probably contribute to the pacemaker potential, and are more important in the nodes than in the Purkinje fibres. The first is the delayed rectifier potassium current, which is activated during the depolarization of the action potential and only switches off slowly after repolarization; and the second is the slow inward calcium current. I_f and the switching off of the K^+ current are probably responsible for the initial phase of the nodal pacemaker potential. In these cells, the leak

Na^+ current (passive sodium permeability) may be relatively high, so that reducing the K^+ outward current can result in a net inward current and contribute to the pacemaker depolarization. The depolarization is continued by the slow inward Ca^{2+} current, which will begin to be activated towards the end of the pacemaker potential, and will take it to threshold.

7.2.6 Sources of calcium for activation of the contractile machinery

The working cardiac muscle uses both intracellular and extracellular calcium for activation of the contractile machinery. The sarcoplasmic reticulum in the ventricular muscle is well developed, but not quite to the same extent as in skeletal muscle. T tubules exist, but the connections with the sarcoplasmic reticulum form diads rather than triads with the T tubules. Elements of the sarcoplasmic reticulum, as well as wrapping round the myofibrils, also approach the plasma membrane and make foot-like contacts with it as well as with the T tubules. There is significant entry of calcium into the heart during each action potential, and calcium is also released from the sarcoplasmic reticulum at each beat as a result of both a depolarization-dependent mechanism (excitation–contraction coupling through the diads) and also by a calcium-activated calcium release mechanism. Figure 7.25 shows the well-developed sub-sarcolemmal sarcoplasmic reticulum. The calcium entering from the outside has to be returned to the extracellular space, and the main mechanism for this is Na–Ca^{2+} exchange, Na^+ entering down its electrochemical gradient being used to expel Ca^{2+} against its electrochemical gradient. The Na^+ is then expelled through the Na^+ pump. There is also an ATP-dependent Ca^{2+} pump in the plasma membrane, and another type in the sarcoplasmic reticulum membrane.

7.2.7 Length-dependent changes in contractile force

The ventricular muscle generates increased force when it is stretched over a certain range which includes its normal range *in situ*. Further stretching will result in reduced force production similar to that seen in skeletal muscle, when the length of the sarcomeres is increased to a point where the overlap between thick and thin filaments is reduced. In the intact heart this can result in heart failure. In the range where stretch increases the force production, improved alignment of the thick and thin filaments probably plays little role in generating the increased force. Evidence suggests that the initial responses to rapid increases in length are due to an increased sensitivity of troponin to calcium. Slower responses involve increases in the calcium released from the sarcoplasmic reticulum. The mechanisms involved in these changes are not well understood, but the changes are important physiologically, resulting in the well-known 'Starling's law of the heart' enabling the contractility of the ventricles to change in response to their filling, and thus to match the inflow and outflow of blood. In people with

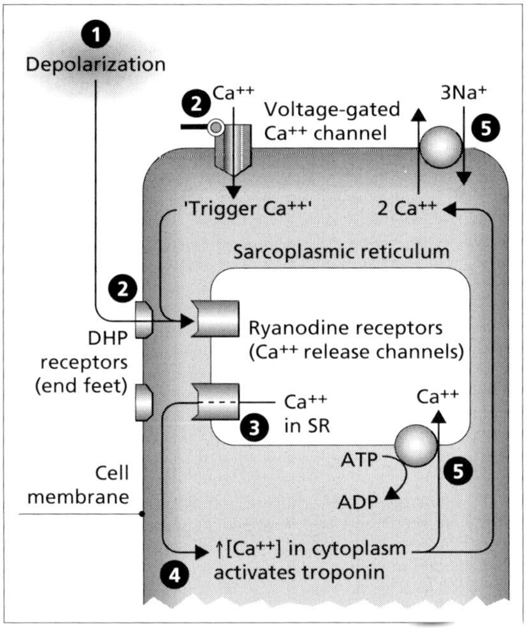

Fig. 7.25 Excitation–contraction coupling in myocardial cells. Depolarization of the membrane (1) can act both by opening voltage-gated Ca^{2+} channels in the plasma membrane and by activating the dihydropyridine (DHP) receptors in the T tubules (2). Through Ca^{2+}-activated Ca^{2+} release and mechanical coupling with the DHP receptors, Ca^{2+} is released from the sarcoplasmic reticulum (3). Ca^{2+} can then bind to troponin C and initiate cross-bridge cycling and contraction (4). Ca^{2+} is removed from the cytoplasm by re-uptake into the sarcoplasmic reticulum and extrusion from the cell via Na-Ca exchange (5).

heart transplants and no autonomic innervation to the heart, this is the main mechanism available for altering cardiac output.

7.3 Transporting epithelia and glands

7.3.1 Introduction

The autonomic nervous system plays a major role in stimulating secretion from exocrine glands, such as sweat glands, salivary glands, pancreatic acinar cells, lachrymal glands, nasopharyngeal glands and bronchial glands. It plays a secondary role in stimulating or inhibiting secretion from several endocrine glands, such as pancreatic islet cells, juxtaglomerular cells of the kidney and the pineal gland. The enteric division of the autonomic nervous system, with extrinsic input from the parasympathetic and sympathetic systems, plays an important role in the control of secretion from the various glands in the wall of the gastrointestinal tract, and in determining the rates of secretion and reabsorption of ions and water. In this section, some of the basic mechanisms involved in the secretion and reabsorption of ions, and in, release of hormones and enzymes, will be outlined, and the mechanisms by which the autonomic nervous system can influence these functions will then be discussed.

In view of the common embryological origin of many glands and epithelia, it is not surprising to find that secretion of ions and water in exocrine glands and secreting epithelia, and their reabsorption in the ducts of exocrine glands and in reabsorbing epithelia, have many molecular mechanisms in common. Although much of the basic molecular machinery is shared, the distribution and relative contribution of the different ion channels, transporters and pumps vary from tissue to tissue, and will determine the directionality of the transport and which ions undergo net movements.

The exocytotic mechanisms involved in the secretion of enzymes and hormones in different glands again have many elements in common, although it is likely that only in transmitter release from nerve terminals has exocytosis evolved to become the extremely rapid process seen in the nervous system.

7.3.2 Epithelial transport

Epithelial transport regulated by the autonomic nervous system occurs in the gut, the ducts of exocrine cells, and probably also in the kidney tubule. Similar mechanisms also occur in acinar cells in exocrine glands, which are modified epithelia.

Transporting epithelia are columnar epithelia. The cells consist of an apical membrane facing the lumen of the organ, and a basolateral membrane facing the serosa. The two membrane domains are separated anatomically by junctions between the cells, usually near the luminal membrane, which may be of several types (Fig. 7.26). Desmosomes and adherens junctions hold epithelial cells together, gap junctions may exist which allow communication from cell to cell, and tight junctions can limit the movement of ions and water between the cells.

Structural modifications may be seen, depending on the amounts of ions and fluids transported and on whether or not the epithelium builds up ionic or osmotic concentration gradients. In epithelia that transport large amounts of fluids, with little build-up of gradients, expansion of the membrane surfaces is provided by microvilli on the apical membranes and infoldings of the basolateral membranes, often with numerous mitochondria in association (Fig. 7.27). In these epithelia, the junctions between the cells are leaky, and allow paracellular movements of ions and water. Epithelia that build up large concentration gradients, on the other hand, have smaller surface areas, and have tight junctions between the cells preventing back-diffusion of ions and water.

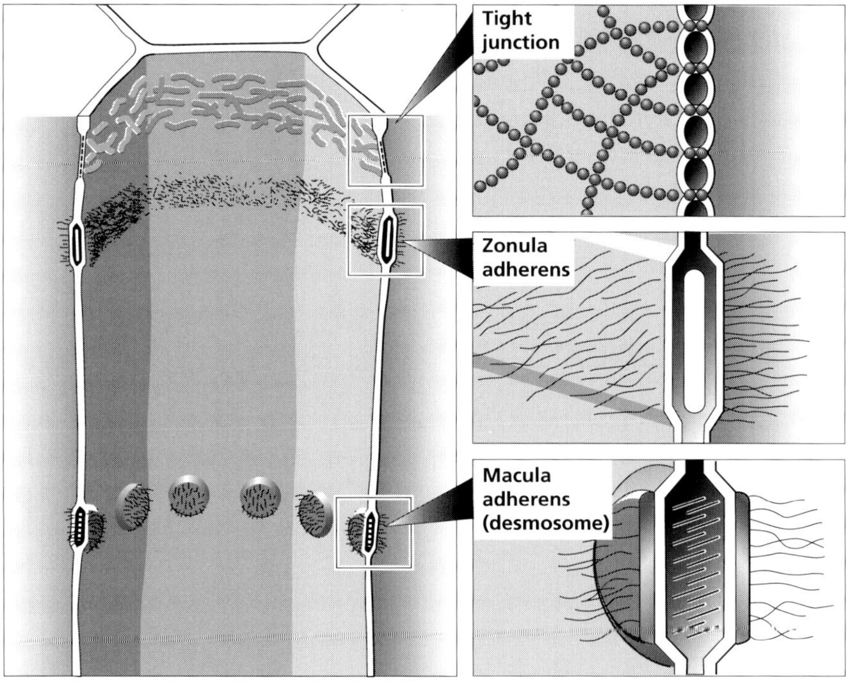

Fig. 7.26 Diagram of junctions between columnar epithelial cells. On the left is a three-dimensional view showing the inner surface of the membrane, and the specialized junctions are shown at higher magnification on the right. The tight junction can limit the paracellular movement of solutes and water, and the adherens junctions strengthen the luminal surface and prevent disaggregation of the cells. Gap functions between the cells may also be present.

Basic principles

When considering ion transport, there are several basic principles that should be borne in mind.

1 The movement of water across an epithelium is always secondary to the movement of solutes, and is thus driven by osmotic (and occasionally hydrostatic) gradients.

2 Net movement of ions across an epithelium can only occur if equal numbers of positive and negative charges move.

3 The passive movement of ions can only occur down their electrochemical gradient, which is determined both by their concentration gradient across a barrier and the electrical potential difference across the barrier. This applies both when considering movement across the cell membrane, and movement across the whole epithelium. An exception to this is solute drag, when net fluid movement down osmotic or hydrostatic gradients can drag solutes with the flow.

4 The driving force for solute movement is always an ATP-driven ion pump, which is usually referred to as the primary active transport mechanism.

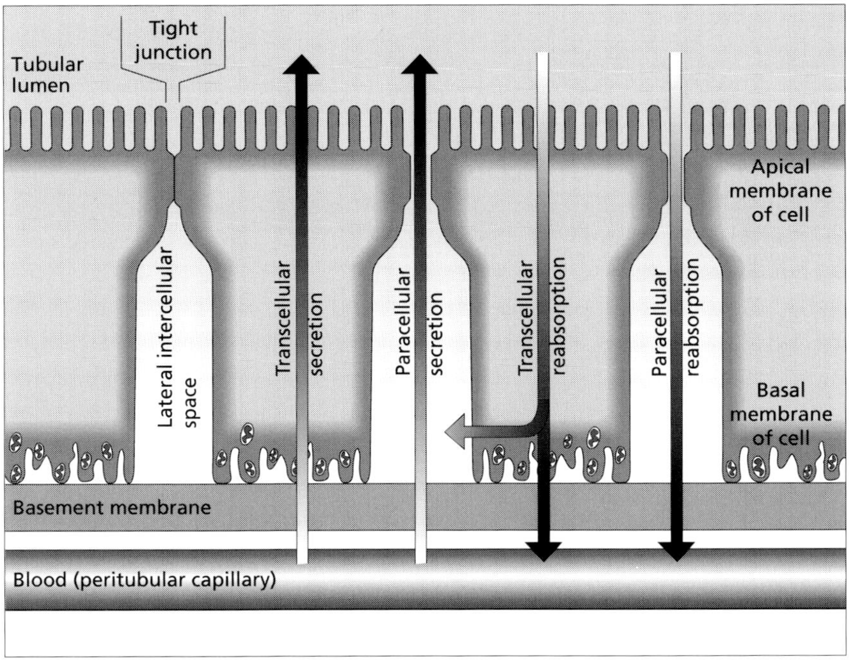

Fig. 7.27 Diagram of pathways for transepithelial secretion or reabsorption. Depending on the permeability of the tight junctions between the cells, ion and solute movement may occur through transcellular or paracellular pathways. Epithelia with leaky 'tight' junctions can transport large quantities of salts and fluids, but cannot build up large transepithelial gradients. In epithelia with impermeable tight junctions, transport is mainly transcellular, and limited in amount, although large gradients can be established.

5 The primary transport generates potential energy for the movement of other ions or solvents.

The sequence of events is where the energy-dependent primary transporter sets up an electrochemical gradient for the transported ions across the cell membrane. This gradient can then be used to allow passive movement of ions down their electrochemical gradients into or out of the cells, if the correct channels or translocating molecules are present and switched on. It can also provide the energy for movement of ions or solutes up their electrochemical or concentration gradient by co-transport or counter-transport mechanisms, which couple the downhill movement of the primary ion to secondary transport of ions or solutes. This process is often referred to as secondary active transport. If the transport processes result in the generation of a potential difference across the epithelium or an increase in osmolarity – for instance, in the restricted spaces between the cells – this can also provide an energy source for paracellular movement of permeant ions or water. Whether or not reabsorption or secretion is the final result, and what is reabsorbed or secreted, depend entirely on the transport mechanisms present and switched on, and their distribution between the apical and basolateral membranes (Fig. 7.27).

Primary active transport

There are three primary ion pumps involved in ion transport in mammalian cells: Na^+,K^+-ATPase, H^+,K^+-ATPase and Ca^{2+}-ATPase.

Na^+ pump. By far the most important primary transporter is Na^+,K^+-ATPase, usually called the Na^+ pump. All mammalian cells possess this pump. It is an electrogenic ion pump, using the energy derived from one molecule of ATP to extrude three Na^+ ions out of the cell in exchange for the uptake of two K^+ ions. In this process, one positive charge is moved out of the cell. The activity of this pump ensures a low intracellular Na^+ concentration and a high intracellular K^+ concentration. Since the majority of cell membranes have a much lower permeability to Na^+ than to K^+, the K^+ distribution generates an inside negative membrane potential close to the K^+ equilibrium potential. There is thus a very large electrochemical gradient available for Na^+ entry into the cells. In transporting epithelia, the pump is asymmetrically distributed in the cell membrane, and occurs almost exclusively in the basolateral membrane, whether or not the cell is secreting or absorbing ions. The rate-limiting step for Na^+ pump activity is the intracellular concentration of Na, since this is normally well below the equilibrium constant for binding of Na^+ to the pump sites. The pump will thus extrude towards the serosa any Na^+ entering the cell through whatever pathway, although it should be borne in mind that significant amounts of net Na^+ can move only if exchanged for another cation or accompanied by an anion. The Na^+ pump is specifically blocked by ouabain and the cardiac glycosides.

H^+ pump. H^+,K^+-ATPase is responsible for active proton secretion. In the parietal cell in the stomach, Cl^- accompanying protons in the secretion of HCl is carried on a K^+-Cl symporter, the K^+ being reabsorbed on the proton pump. This pump is blocked by omeprazole.

Ca^{2+} pump. Ca-ATPase is present in most cells. It is probably not primarily involved in generating fluid transport, but may play a role in the trans-epithelial transport of Ca^{2+} ions.

Ion channels

The term 'ion channels' refers to conductive channels that allow ions to flow through them down an electrochemical gradient as a current. In transporting epithelia, several specific ion channels have been identified, which can be switched on and off and may be responsible for triggering or modulating epithelial transport. Examples are an amiloride-sensitive Na^+ channel, and Ca^{2+}-activated K^+ and Cl channels.

Table 7.2 Epithelial transporters and blockers.

Co-transport
Na^+-glucose, electrogenic, blocked by phlorizin
Na^+-neutral amino acid, electrogenic
Na^+-HCO_3^-, electrogenic ($1Na^+:3HCO_3^-$)
Na^+-HCO_3^-, electroneutral
Na^+-Cl^-, electroneutral
K^+-Cl^-, electroneutral
Na^+-K^+-$2Cl^-$, electroneutral, blocked by loop diuretics (bumetanide)
There are probably also Na^+-PO_4^- and Na^+-SO_4^- co-transport mechanisms.

Counter-transport
Na^+/H^+ exchange, blocked by amiloride
Na^+/Ca^{2+} exchange, electrogenic ($3Na^+/1Ca^{2+}$ or possibly $4Na^+/1K^+$, $1Ca^{2+}$), blocked by dichloribenzamil and bepredil
Na^+/Mg^{2+} exchange
Cl^-/HCO_3^- exchange, blocked by SITS and DIDS

Secondary transport systems

These can be subdivided into co-transport systems (symport), in which the ion or solute moves in the same direction as the primary ion, and counter-transport systems (antiport), in which the movement is in the opposite direction. The mechanisms may be neutral if no net charge is moved, or electrogenic if there is net charge movement. In the latter case, a current is generated during operation of the transporter.

Many different transport systems have been proposed, but the absolute identification of a system may be difficult, and really requires that a selective blocker of the transport is available. Table 7.2 lists some of the more important transporters found in epithelia, with an example of a blocker for each where available.

Absorption

Absorption of ions and water depends largely on entry of Na^+ into the cell through the apical membrane, and its active extrusion through the basolateral membrane (Fig. 7.28). Continuous activation of the Na^+ pump requires there to be K^+ channels in the basolateral membrane, to allow the K^+ entering on the pump to diffuse back down its electrochemical gradient. In epithelia such as the gut, where solute absorption is important, much of the Na^+ entry will be on the Na^+-glucose or Na^+-amino acid co-transport. Thus, Na^+ absorption will generate a net luminal–serosal current, and in systems specialised for mass fluid reabsorption with leaky junctions, Cl^- ions will flow through the paracellular pathway. Water will follow through either pathway. In tight epithelia, Na^+ and Cl^- may both enter through the apical membrane, using the Na^+-K^+-$2Cl^-$ co-transport, or by the combined actions of Na^+–H^+ exchange taking Na^+ into the cell, and Cl^-–HCO_3^- exchange taking chloride in. In the latter case, the cell will have to generate H^+ ions and HCO_3^- ions from water and CO_2. Na^+ entry may also occur through the amiloride-sensitive Na^+ channels.

Secretion

Secretion of ions and water depends largely on Cl^- entering the cells through the basolateral membrane using Na^+-K^+-$2Cl^-$ co-transport (Fig. 7.28). Na^+ is then pumped out again through the same membrane, and the K^+ taken up in this process leaks out down its electrochemical gradient through K^+ channels. Cl^- moves out of the cells across the apical membrane down its electrochemical gradient through Cl^- channels, making the lumen negative and Na^+ ions flow through the paracellular pathway. Water

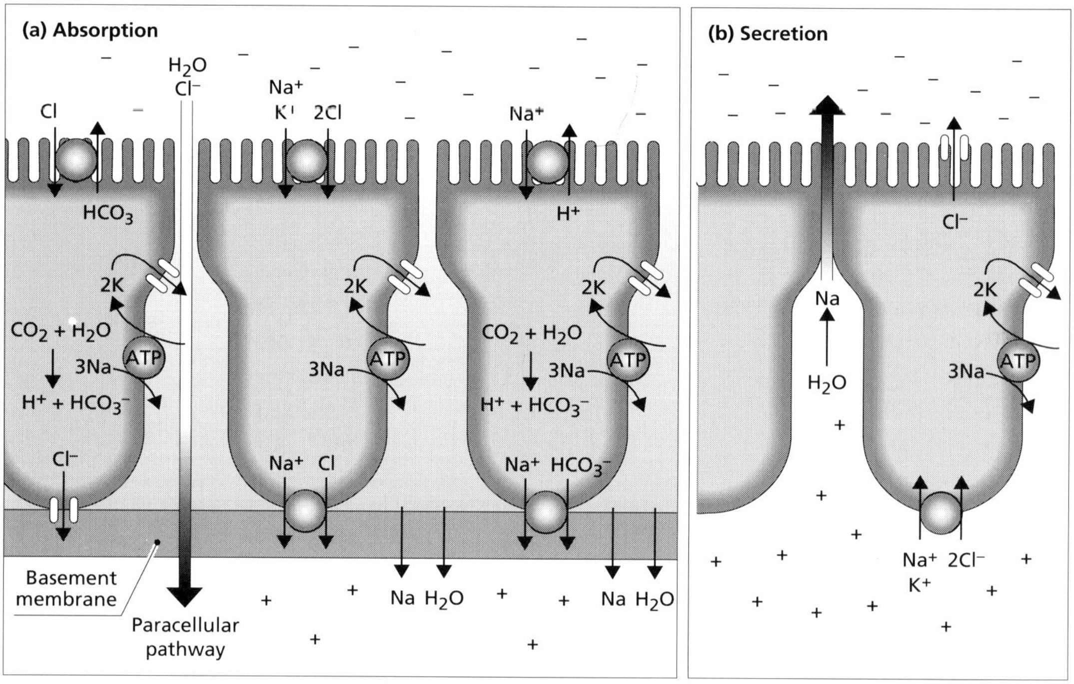

Fig. 7.28 Diagram of transepithelial absorption and secretion. (a) Absorption. Na^+ enters the epithelial cells through the apical membranes via co- or counter-transport processes, down its electrochemical gradient. The Na^+ pump extrudes Na^+ through the basolateral membranes, and the K^+ entering the cell during the pumping leaves through K^+ channels to allow continuous activation of the pump. This generates a driving force for the movement of anions from the cells through basolateral co-transport exchanges and Cl^- channels or through the paracellular pathway. Water follows isosmotically. (b) Secretion. The Na^+ pump generates the driving force for Cl^- entry into the cells via Na^+-linked co-transport mechanisms, and the Cl^- ions leave the cells through apical Cl^- channels, generating a potential gradient which allows paracellular Na^+ and fluid movement.

follows. It is interesting to note that, in many of the exocrine glands, after the primary secretory event from the acinar cells, the composition of the fluid secreted (initially iso-osmotic and predominantly NaCl) can be modified both in ionic composition and osmolarity by further secretion or reabsorption from the epithelial cells of the ducts. A similar effect is seen in the gut, where secretion from the crypt cells may be modified by the actions of the epithelium of the villi.

Mechanisms for regulation of ion transport

Secretion and reabsorption of ions and water can be regulated through alterations in the activity of the various ion transport mechanisms. This can occur either by regulation of the activity of the ion transport mechanisms already in the membrane, or by stimulating their insertion into the membrane. Two ion channels that are frequently regulated to control ion transport are the Cl^- channels and the K^+ channels. Evidence suggests that the number of Cl^- channels can be increased by elevation of cAMP levels in the cell, suggesting that phosphorylation of the channel protein by a cAMP-dependent protein kinase may be involved. Cl^- and K^+ channels can also be opened by an increase in intracellular Ca^{2+} ions. Transmitters can induce elevation of cAMP through the receptor G protein–adenylyl cyclase pathway, and can elevate intracellular Ca^{2+} by activating the phosphoinositide pathway, with IP_3 inducing Ca^{2+} release from intracellular stores. It is interesting that, in cystic fibrosis, a disease caused by a single genetic defect, the symptoms are due to a reduced Cl^- permeability of epithelial cells, and the defect is apparently in the regulation of Cl^- channel activity. Insertion of ion transporters may occur through fusion with the plasma membrane of preformed membrane vesicles containing the mechanism. This may be triggered by the same pathways as responsible for exocytosis outlined below. Recently, it has been suggested that the permeability of the junctional complex between the epithelial cells may also be modified by the action of transmitters.

7.3.3 Secretion of hormones and enzymes by exocytosis

In the majority of cases, exocytosis can be triggered by one of two pathways, one resulting in elevation of intracellular Ca^{2+}, and the other resulting in elevation of intracellular cAMP (Fig. 7.29). Artificially elevating either will also trigger exocytosis. There are, however, a few exceptions. Increasing intracellular Ca^{2+} will inhibit secretion in parathyroid cells and the juxtaglomerular cells in the kidney, and in these cells exocytosis is associated with a lowering of free intracellular Ca^{2+}. Raising intracellular cAMP will inhibit exocytosis by mast cells and platelets.

The initial steps in the processes elevating intracellular Ca^{2+} and cAMP are separate, and may be triggered by activation of different receptors.

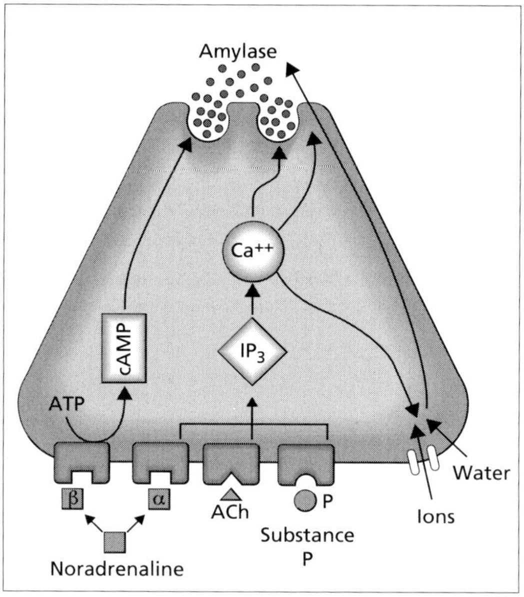

Fig. 7.29 Mechanisms involved in the secretion of saliva. Receptors in the basolateral membrane are coupled via G-proteins to either the production of cAMP or IP_3. cAMP can activate protein kinase A and phosphorylate some step in the pathway that can trigger exocytosis. IP_3 releases Ca^{2+} from internal stores, and can result in activation of protein kinase C, which may be involved in triggering exocytosis. The mechanisms involved in the secretion of ions and water are also activated by a rise in intracellular Ca^{2+}, probably by activating Cl^- or K^+ channels.

Elevation of intracellular Ca^{2+} is triggered through the phosphoinositide pathway, with IP_3 triggering release of Ca^{2+} from intracellular stores. The simultaneous production of diacylglycerol and activation of protein kinase C may also be important in some cases. Elevation of cAMP is through G protein activation of adenylyl cyclase. It is thought that, in either case, the final trigger to exocytosis is the phosphorylation, by a cAMP-dependent or Ca-dependent protein kinase, of some protein that can then initiate membrane fusion of the secretory vesicle and the plasma membrane. In glands, the process is too slow for direct binding of Ca^{2+} to be the trigger for exocytosis, although this probably occurs in exocytotic transmitter release from nerve terminals.

7.4 Brown fat

The function of brown fat (also known as brown adipose tissue or BAT) is to generate metabolic heat. It has been described as an internal heating jacket that overlies parts of the systemic vasculature, which when switched on becomes an active metabolic heater applied directly to the flowing blood stream as it passes to and from the cooler periphery. It is particularly important in neonatal mammals and hibernators. Its potential for generating heat is enormous, with a thermogenic capacity of some 500 W/kg. The interesting things to consider are its structure and distribution, the mechanisms involved in heat generation, how these mechanisms are switched on both acutely and chronically, and their importance in the life of the animal.

7.4.1 Structure and distribution

The tissue is composed of the fat-containing cells, or adipocytes, and is richly supplied with blood vessels and sympathetic nerves. The individual adipocytes are smaller and the tissue contains only about half the lipid content of white fat. The fat is present in numerous small lipid vacuoles (multilocular), in contrast to the single large vacuole (unilocular) of white adipocytes (Fig. 7.30). The cells also contain large numbers of mitochondria, and it is a combination of the high levels of mitochondrial cytochrome and flavin compounds and the capillary networks that gives brown fat its characteristic colour.

In the human infant, brown fat may account for between 2% and 6% of the total body weight. It is found in a thin, diamond-shaped sheet between the shoulder-blades, and in small masses around the muscle and blood vessels of the neck, extending under the collar-bone and into the armpits (Fig. 7.31). In the thorax, it is present around the great vessels, also extending along many of the intercostal and mammary vessels, and discrete masses are present between the oesophagus and trachea. In the abdomen, discrete masses occur along the aorta, and in association with the pancreas, autonomic ganglia and chromaffin tissue, with a large abdominal mass enveloping the kidneys and adrenals. During ageing, much of the brown fat becomes very similar to normal white adipose tissue, but significant amounts of true brown fat remain, particularly around the kidneys.

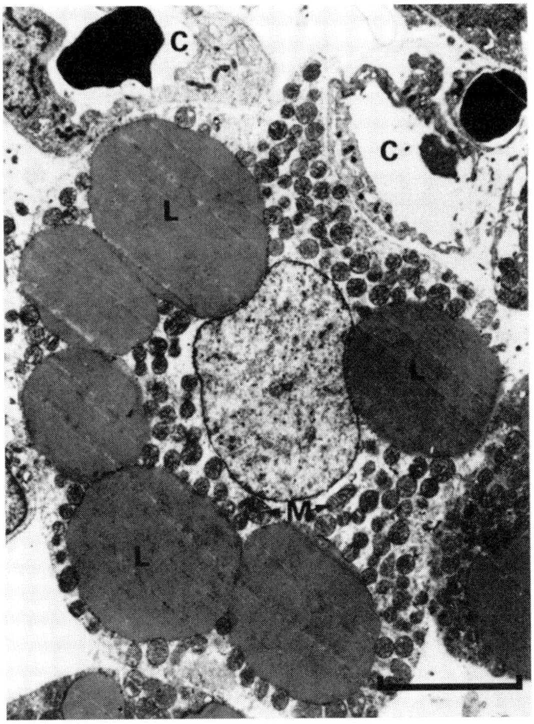

Fig. 7.30 Brown adipose tissue is composed of lobules divided by fibrous septa which carry blood vessels and sympathetic nerves to the fat cells. The cells are interspersed with a rich network of capillaries. They have exocentric nuclei, and the lipid is stored in multiple droplets. The cytoplasm is packed with mitochondria which give the tissue its brown colour. Scale bar: 5 μm. From Burkett *et al.* (1993), with permission from the publisher, Churchill Livingstone.

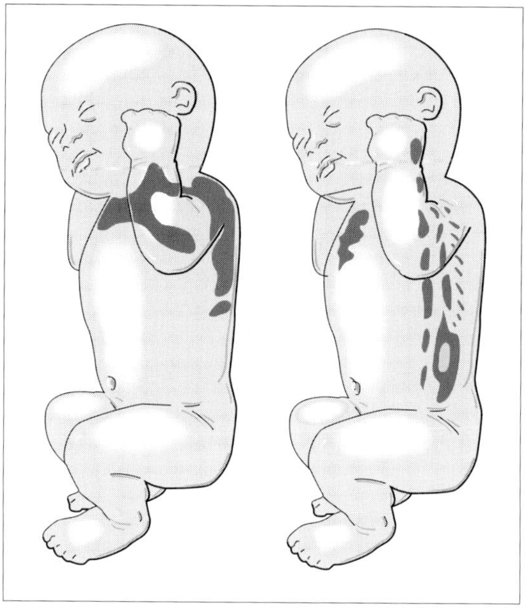

Fig. 7.31 Location of brown adipose tissue (shaded areas) in the new-born baby.

7.4.2 Mechanisms of thermogenesis

The brown adipocytes can both synthesise and metabolise lipids. Thermogenesis requires lipid metabolism. This occurs through a series of steps: lipases release fatty acids from the lipid droplets; fatty acids are oxidised by the fatty acid oxidation cycle in the cytosol to produce acetyl coenzyme A (CoA); acetyl-CoA is oxidised by the Krebs cycle, which generates the energy-rich compounds, reduced nicotinamide adenine dinucleotide (NADH) and reduced flavin adenine dinucleotide ($FADH_2$). The energy of these is recovered by oxidation in the mitochondria through the respiratory chain.

In normal mitochondria, the energy of oxidation liberated through the electron transport chain is directly harnessed for the synthesis of ATP. The sequence of events is as follows: electrons from NADH and $FADH_2$ pass through a series of asymmetrically arranged carriers (the electron transport chain) in the inner mitochondrial membrane, while at the same time hydrogen ions are moved in the opposite direction, creating a proton gradient across the membrane. ATP is synthesised using the proton gradient as an energy source, by coupling the leaking back of protons down their gradient through a channel that is associated with an ATP-synthesising coupled ATP synthase. It is therefore the proton gradient across the inner mitochondrial membrane that allows oxidation of NADH and $FADH_2$ to be coupled with ATP synthesis. In normal mitochondria, this proton gradient is maintained by the impermeability of the inner mitochondrial membrane to protons. In the mitochondria in brown fat, during thermogenesis, mitochondrial respi-

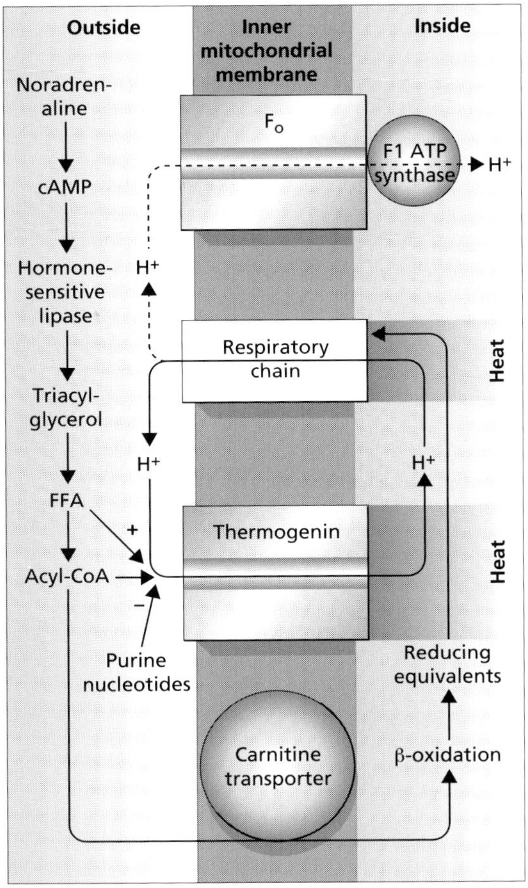

Fig. 7.32 Thermogenesis in brown adipose tissue. Thermogenin is normally switched off by purine nucleotides such as ATP. The H^+ ion gradient generated by the respiratory chain across the inner mitochondrial membrane is then coupled to the synthesis of ATP. Noradrenaline through the cAMP pathway activates a lipase and liberates free fatty acids and acetyl-CoA which both remove the inhibition on thermogenin. This molecule then allows H^+ ions to flow down their concentration gradient generating heat.

ration is partially uncoupled from ATP synthesis, and the energy of oxidation is dissipated as heat. This is achieved by the use of a leak pathway for protons. Experimentally used uncouplers of mitochondrial respiration, such as carbonyl cyanide *m*-chlorophenyl hydrazone (CCCP), can make the inner mitochondrial membrane permeable to protons, resulting in dissipation of the gradient, thus preventing synthesis of ATP and allowing the energy of oxidation to be liberated as heat. In brown fat mitochondria, a naturally occurring uncoupling protein (also called thermogenin) is present in the inner membrane. The molecule is a dimer, with a monomeric weight of 33 kDa. It is a member of a family of solute transporters with a high percentage of apolar residues that allow it to span the membrane, but is unique because it is the only known transporter that carries protons alone. Thermogenin can make up as much as 16% of the total inner mitochondrial membrane protein in brown fat, and allows it to generate heat instead of ATP (Fig. 7.32). The function and amount of this protein can be regulated.

Acute regulation

The proton translocating properties of thermogenin can be acutely switched on and off. Each dimer of the protein has a nucleotide binding site on the cytosolic face, which under physiological conditions normally will bind to ATP. This switches off translocation. However, in the presence of fatty acids, the relationship between ATP and thermogenin is altered in such a way that higher levels of cytosolic ATP are required to inactivate the protein. The normal signal for inducing thermogenesis is via the sympathetic nervous system, and the effects of noradrenaline. A possible sequence of events is as follows. Noradrenaline activates both β- and α-adrenoceptors on the adipocyte membrane (activation of both seems necessary). Through the normal G protein–adenylyl cyclase interaction initiated by β-adrenoceptor activation, a rise in cAMP occurs, leading to activation of a protein kinase, phosphorylation and thus activation of lipase and liberation of fatty acids from the fat globules. Accumulation of free fatty acids reverses the ATP inhibition of thermogenin, and leads to an increase in proton permeability of the inner mitochondrial membrane and uncoupling. Other agents that may also play a role in activating the thermogenin are thyroid hormones, steroids, insulin, glucagon, endorphins and melatonin.

Long-term regulation

The amount of thermogenin and also of lipase can be regulated through gene expression. Cold stress and circulating noradrenaline can both lead to an increase in thermogenin mRNA, particularly in the presence of normal levels of thyroid hormones. These conditions can also lead to an increase in the number of mitochondria. There is also evidence that, under such conditions, the neonatal brown fat that has reverted in the adult to behaving like normal adipose tissue can be reactivated. Clinically, it is interesting that, in humans with phaeochromocytomas (catecholamine-secreting tumours), brown fat levels are increased, and the patients suffer from weight loss, which may be very rapid in some cases.

7.4.3 Role of thermogenesis

Three types of thermogenesis are important: non-shivering thermogenesis, diet-induced thermogenesis, and thermogenesis in recovery from hibernation, this last having no importance in humans.

Non-shivering thermogenesis

This is particularly important in the human infant, since the shivering response does not develop until some time after birth. Ability to withstand cold relies almost entirely on this mechanism. There have been suggestions that abnormalities in this system may be implicated in 'cot deaths'. Non-shivering thermogenesis can also be induced in some animals in response to cold adaptation, as described above.

Diet-induced thermogenesis

This has been studied largely in rats. These animals, when fed on a 'cafeteria' diet of varied and palatable food, may increase their energy intake by 80%, while only showing a weight gain of 27% in comparison to that of control rats. There is a concomitant increase in both resting oxygen consumption and its sensitivity to noradrenaline, and a significant increase in the weight of brown fat, suggesting that diet-induced thermogenesis may be a significant mechanism for weight regulation. It has been suggested that deficiencies in brown fat thermogenesis may predispose to obesity in humans. Reduced effectiveness of the sympathetic innervation could be involved.

Further reading

Smooth muscle

Bárány, M. (ed) (1996) *Biochemistry of Smooth Muscle Contraction.* Academic Press, San Diego.

Bülbring, E., Brading, A.F., Jones, A.W. & Tomita T. (eds) (1970) *Smooth Muscle.* Edward Arnold, London.

Bülbring, E., Brading, A.F., Jones, A.W. & Tomita T. (eds) (1981) *Smooth Muscle: An Assessment of Current Knowledge.* Edward Arnold, London.

Horowitz, A., Menice, C.B., Laporte, R. & Morgan, K.G. (1996) Mechanisms of smooth muscle contraction. *Physiol. Rev.* **76**, 967–1003.

Heart

Di Francesco, D. (1993) Pacemaker mechanisms in cardiac tissue. *Ann. Rev. Physiol.* **55**, 455–72.

Levick, J.R. (1991) *An Introduction to Cardiovascular Physiology.* Butterworths, London.

Noble, D. (1979) *The Initiation of the Heartbeat.* Clarendon Press, Oxford.

Epithelia

Spring, K.R. (1998). Routes and mechanisms of fluid transport by epithelia. *Ann. Rev. Physiol.* **60**, 105–19.

Brown fat

Lafontan, M. & Berlan, M. (1993) Fat cell adrenergic receptors and the control of white and brown fat cell function. *J. Lipid. Res.* **34**, 1057–91.

References

Adelstein, R.S. & Sellers, J.R. (1996) Myosin structure and function. In: *Biochemistry of Smooth Muscle* (ed M. Bárány) pp. 3–19. Academic Press, San Diego.

Bülbring, E. (1957) Changes in configuration of spontaneously discharged spike potentials from smooth muscle of the guinea-pig's taenia coli. The effects of electronic currents and of adrenaline, acetylcholine and histamine. *J. Physiol.* **135**, 412–25.

Bülbring, E. & Kuriyama, H. (1963) The effects of adrenaline on the smooth muscle of the guinea-pig's taenia coli in relation to the degree of stretch. *J. Physiol.* **169**, 198–212.

Burkett, H.G., Young, B., Heath, J.W., Wheater, P.R. & Deakin, P.J. (1993) *Wheater's Functional Histology.* Churchill Livingstone, Edinburgh.

Burnstock, G., Holman, M. & Kuriyama, H. (1964) Facilitation of transmission from autonomic nerve to smooth muscle of guinea-pig vas deferens. *J. Physiol.* **172**, 31–49.

Endo, M., Kitazawa, T., Uagi, S., Iino, M. & Kabuta, Y. (1977) Some properties of chemically skinned smooth muscle fibres. In: *Excitation–Contraction Coupling in Smooth Muscle* (eds R. Casteels, T. Godfriand & J.C. Ruegg) pp. 199–209. Elsevier, Holland.

Fay, F.S., Cooke, P.H. & Canaday, P.G. (1976) Contractile properties of isolated smooth muscle cells. In: *Physiology of Smooth Muscle* (eds E. Bülbring & M. Shuba) pp. 249–64. Raven Press, New York.

Itoh, T., Kuriyama, H. & Suzuki, H. (1981) Excitation–contraction coupling in smooth muscles of the guinea-pig mesenteric artery. *J. Physiol.* **321**, 513–35.

8 : Cardiovascular and Respiratory Systems

CHAPTER 8
Cardiovascular and Respiratory Systems

In this chapter, we will consider the heart, blood vessels, lymphatics and lungs, outlining their innervation, the transmitters involved in their control and some relevant pharmacology for the treatment of dysfunction.

8.1 The heart

8.1.1 Neuroanatomy

There are two cardiac plexuses associated with the heart – the superficial plexus, lying in the concavity of the aorta, and the deep plexus, lying between the tracheal bifurcation and the aortic arch. As in other autonomic plexuses, elements of both autonomic systems converge, and there is also input from sensory neurones. Preganglionic parasympathetic fibres from the cardiac branches of the vagus run into the plexuses and synapse with ganglion cells in the cardiac ganglia, which are embedded in the plexuses. Some of these fibres run through the plexuses and synapse with ganglion cells in the walls of the atria, especially close to the two nodes. The plexuses also receive postganglionic sympathetic fibres from the three cervical cardiac nerves, and through branches of the first four thoracic sympathetic ganglia. Nerves leaving the plexuses run to the heart along the main arterial and venous trunks. A simplified diagram of the origin of the autonomic input is shown in Fig. 8.1.

8.1.2 Parasympathetic nervous system

The postganglionic neurones of the parasympathetic nervous system innervate the sino-atrial (SA) and atrioventricular (AV) nodes, the atria and the ventricular conducting system (Purkinje fibres), but not the ventricles. Parasympathetic activation results in slowing of the heart rate, a reduction in the force of contraction in the atria and a reduction in the conduction velocity through the AV node. Evidence strongly suggests that the transmitter responsible for these effects is acetylcholine, acting on muscarinic receptors, predominantly of the M_2 subtype. Exogenous acetylcholine will also reduce the force of contraction of the ventricles.

The majority of the experiments designed to elucidate the mechanisms involved in these actions have been carried out using bath-applied muscarinic agonists such as acetylcholine and carbachol. Some care needs to be taken in interpreting such experiments, because it is clear that muscarinic receptors exist on cardiac muscle that is not directly innervated by the parasympathetic neurones. It is known, for example, that ventricular muscle is supplied with these receptors, although it is likely that in life it is never normally activated by acetylcholine.

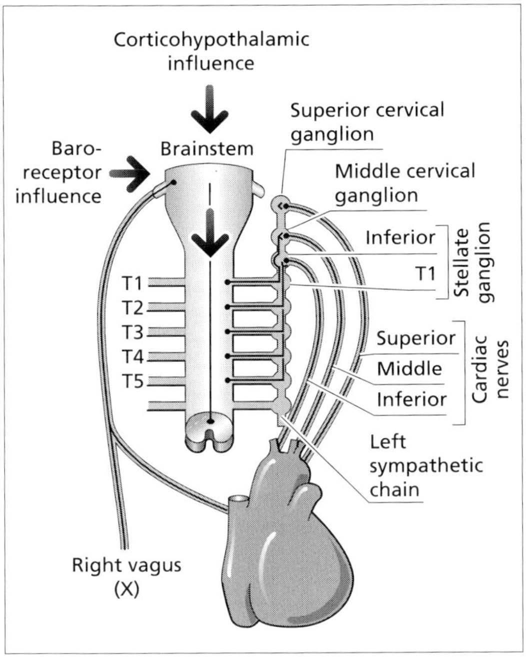

Fig. 8.1 Simplified diagram of the innervation of the heart through the autonomic nervous system. The innervation is symmetrical, but the parasympathetic system is shown on the left and the sympathetic on the right for clarity. Preganglionic parasympathetic neurones lie in the brainstem, and innervate the nodes, atria and Purkinje fibres through local ganglia in the cardiac plexus via the vagus nerve. Preganglionic sympathetic nerves arise in segments T1–T5 of the spinal cord and activate ganglia in the superior cervical and stellate ganglia. Postganglionic neurones enter the heart via the cardiac nerves, and innervate all the tissues.

Mechanisms involved in slowing heart rate (negative chronotropy)

Figure 8.2 shows classic examples of the effects of stimulation of the vagus on the membrane potential of the sinus venosus of the frog and sino-atrial SA node of the kilten. In the frog, there is a clear hyperpolarization that is triggered by vagal stimulation, and during recovery, a reduced slope of the pacemaker potential, whereas in the pacemaker cells of the rabbit node, the main effect is slowing of the pacemaker potential, with little effect on the membrane potential. Any factors hyperpolarizing the cells, increasing the threshold or reducing the slope of the pacemaker will result in a slower heartbeat (Fig. 8.3). A small reduction in the height of the action potential in the nodes and atria is also seen, and a shortening of their action potential duration.

Recent evidence has shown that those tissues that are innervated by the parasympathetic system may respond differently to acetylcholine released from the nerve terminals at physiological rates of stimulation (causing predominantly slowing of the pacemaker potential), and acetylcholine applied

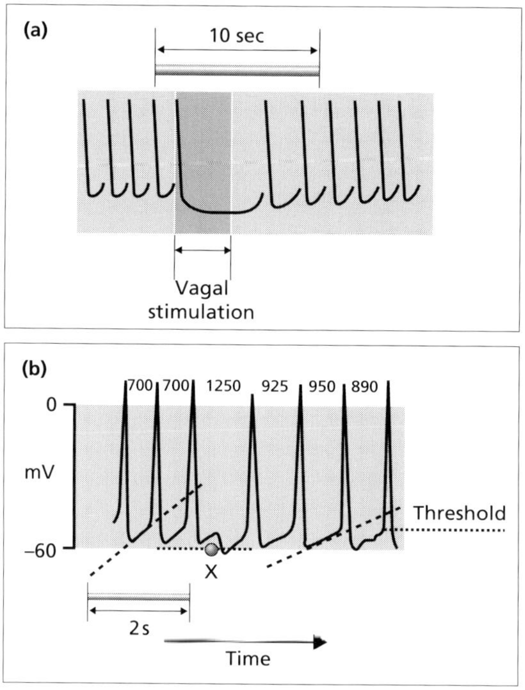

Fig. 8.2 Effect of vagal stimulation on the heart. (a) The effect of vagal stimulation on the spontaneously beating frog sinus venosus. The pacemaker potential is abolished during the nerve stimulation, and the membrane hyperpolarized, temporarily stopping the heart. The first few beats after the stimulation have slowed pacemaker potentials. (b) The effect of brief vagal stimulation (at X) on the sino-atrial node of a kitten. Note brisk transient hyperpolarization, followed by a reduced slope of the pacemaker potential. The numbers at the top of the trace are the time between beats in ms. (a) from Hutter (1961), (b) from Jalife & Moe (1979).

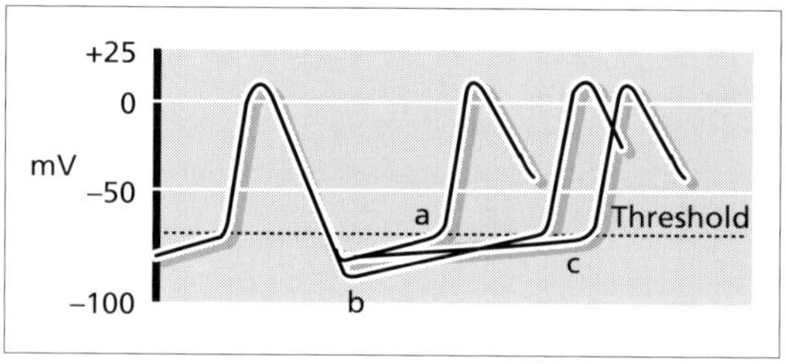

Fig. 8.3 Possible methods of slowing the heart rate. Under resting conditions, the next beat comes at (a). Hyperpolarization of the membrane without a change in the pacemaker slope will result in trace (b) and reducing the pacemaker slope will result in trace (c). Elevating the threshold without altering the pacemaker will also slow the heartbeat.

in the bathing solution (causing predominantly hyperpolarization), suggesting that individual myocytes may have junctional and extrajunctional receptors that may be coupled to different cellular processes.

Hyperpolarization. This is caused by the opening of specific acetylcholine-activated K^+ channels, which results in the membrane potential moving towards the potassium equilibrium potential. Muscarinic receptor stimulation activates G proteins in the membrane, one of which (G_k) is somehow linked to the K^+ channels. The activated G protein exchanges guanosine diphosphate (GDP) for guanosine triphosphate (GTP) and splits into α and βγ subunits. Evidence suggests that one of these (probably the βγ subunit)

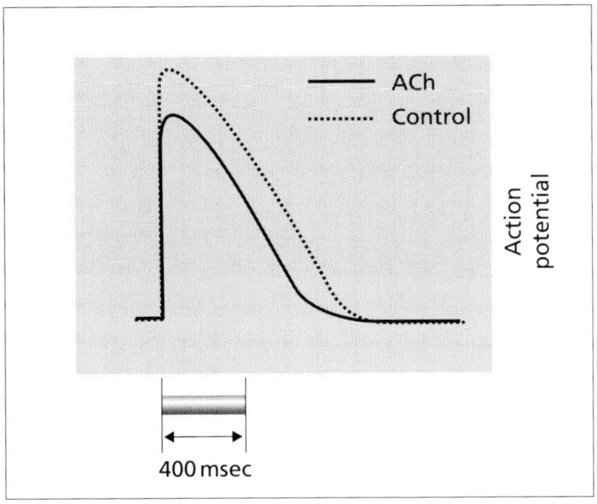

Fig. 8.4 Acetylcholine shortens the action potential in frog atrium. From Giles & Noble (1976).

can directly activate K^+ channels without the involvement of other second-messenger systems. The activation of the potassium channels could also account for the action potential shortening seen (Fig. 8.4).

Reduction of pacemaker slope. There is now evidence that the inward Ca^{2+} current and the non-selective hyperpolarization-activated cation current (I_f), both of which are involved in pacemaker activity, can be reduced as a result of muscarinic receptor activation (see Section 7.2.1). In both cases, the suppression of the current seems to be caused by a reduction in intracellular cyclic adenosine monophosphate (cAMP). cAMP concentrations are regulated through G proteins, which can activate (G_s) or inhibit (G_i) adenylyl cyclase. This enzyme catalyses the synthesis of cAMP from adenosine triphosphate (ATP). Muscarinic receptors, on activation, interact with G_i, inhibit adenylyl cyclase and reduce cAMP levels.

The slow inward Ca^{2+} current is regulated by phosphorylation through protein kinase A (a cAMP-dependent protein kinase). Phosphorylation increases the number of channels that can be opened at any potential without altering the voltage sensitivity of the activation process. In the pacemaker cells, there seems to be a high resting level of cAMP present, probably important to ensure a large Ca^{2+} current for generating the upstroke of the action potential in these tissues. Muscarinic receptor activation can reduce this current by lowering the cAMP levels and, in turn, the degree of phosphorylation of the Ca^{2+} channels. Thus, there is reduced involvement of Ca^{2+} inward current at the end of the pacemaker potential, a decreased slope of depolarization and slowing of the heart rate. A reduced slow inward current could also account for the changes in action potential configuration seen (Fig. 8.4).

The mechanism by which I_f is affected by the levels of cAMP in the cell is somewhat different. Increased intracellular cAMP shifts the activation curve of the current to the right (towards more positive potentials), so that

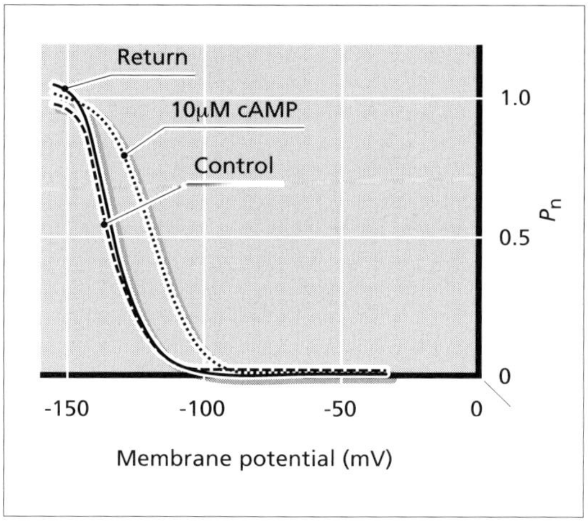

Fig. 8.5 The effect of cAMP on I_f. The graph shows the relationship between the open probability of the I_f channels and the membrane potential. Note this channel opens on hyperpolarization of the membrane. cAMP shifts the curve to the right, enabling the channel to open at less negative potentials, and thus increases the slope of the pacemaker potential. Adapted from Difrancesco & Mangoni (1994).

at any potential the inward current will be greater, and decreased levels of cAMP shift the curve to the left (towards more negative potentials), so that the inward current is reduced (Fig. 8.5). The effect of cAMP seems to be by direct interaction with the channel mechanism, and does not involve activation of adenylyl cyclase and phosphorylation. Muscarinic receptor activation, by reducing the cAMP levels in the cell, thus reduces the contribution of both the slow inward current and also I_f.

Mechanisms involved in reducing conduction velocity (negative dromotropy)

The rate of conduction of an impulse through the heart muscle depends on the speed with which the invading impulse can discharge the membrane capacity and thus depolarize the membrane (see Section 3.4.3). The larger the inward current, the faster this can be achieved. Increasing the resting K^+ conductance through activating the acetylcholine-dependent K^+ channels, and reducing the number of Ca^{2+} channels that can be opened, will both result in a reduction in the net inward current available to discharge the membrane conductance, and will thus slow the action potential propagation.

Mechanisms involved in reducing contractility (negative inotropy)

Contraction is determined largely by the amount by which intracellular free Ca^{2+} concentration rises as a result of the action potential, and also by the sensitivity of troponin to calcium. Ca^{2+} entering during the action potential may, in some cardiac tissues, raise intracellular Ca^{2+} enough to activate the contractile apparatus directly, but it may also stimulate Ca^{2+} release from intracellular stores (Fig. 8.6). The reduced entry of Ca^{2+} through the membrane during the action potential when the muscarinic receptors have been

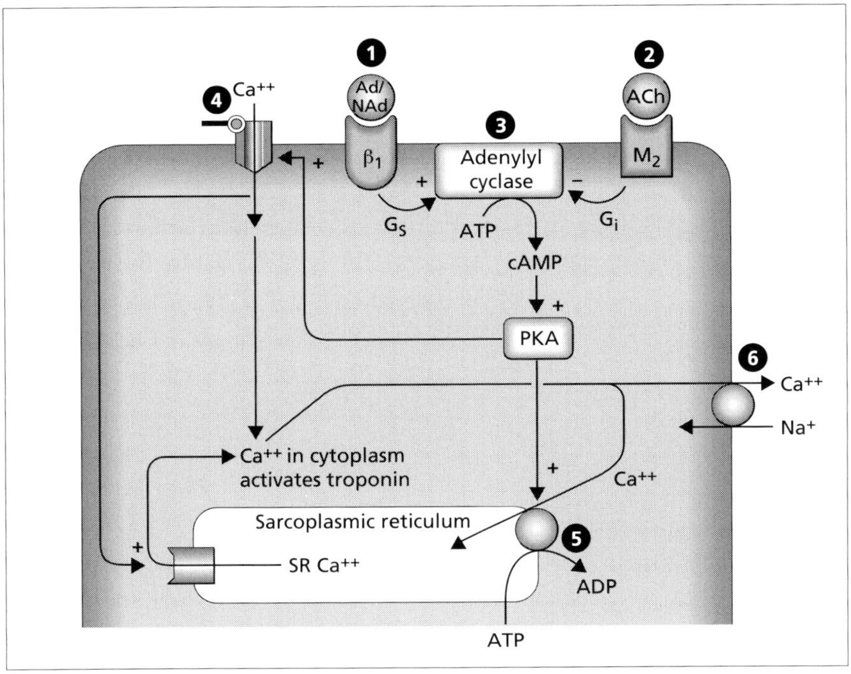

Fig. 8.6 Mechanisms involved in autonomic control of the strength of the heartbeat. Activation of β-adrenoceptors (1) and M_2 muscarinic receptors (2) leads to activation and inhibition of adenylyl cyclase activity (3) respectively, via the stimulatory and inhibitory G-proteins (G_s and G_i). Alterations in the level of cAMP modulate protein kinase A (PKA) activity. β-Adrenoceptors activation of PKA results in phosphorylation of the L-type Ca channels (4), allowing more channels to be opened by depolarization, and enhanced Ca entry. PKA also phosphorylates phospholamban, a protein that regulates the activity of the Ca^{2+}-ATPase (5) calcium can be extruded from the cell by sodium–calcium exchange (6), thus enhancing Ca^{2+} uptake into the stores. This both shortens the period of systole, and causes a larger release of Ca from the stores during the action potential, resulting in β-adrenoceptors positive inotropism. Muscarinic receptor activation, by reducing the level of activation of PKA, will have the reverse effects and cause negative inotropism.

activated will thus have a direct effect on contraction, and reduce Ca^{2+}-activated Ca^{2+} release. The amount of Ca^{2+} held in the sarcoplasmic reticulum will also fall, since there is less Ca^{2+} to be taken up, and there will be a progressive reduction in the amount of stored Ca^{2+} released at each beat. The sensitivity of troponin to Ca^{2+} can be reduced by phosphorylation through a cAMP-dependent kinase, and thus the ability of muscarinic receptor activation to lower cAMP may enhance the sensitivity of troponin and somewhat attenuate the negative inotropic effect of parasympathetic stimulation.

8.1.3 Sympathetic nervous system

The sympathetic neurones innervate all the tissues of the heart. Their activation results in an increased heart rate, force of contraction and conduction velocity through the AV node. The rate of relaxation is also increased, shortening systole, and there is a decrease in the efficiency of the heart (the oxygen consumption increases more than the work). Most of the effects of sympathetic stimulation are due to activation of β_1-adrenoceptors by noradrenaline released from the nerve terminals, and can be mimicked by application of adrenaline and noradrenaline. However, the situation is more complex than is the case for the parasympathetic system, since the nerve terminals also secrete other substances, such as ATP and peptides (e.g. calcitonin gene-related peptide (CGRP) and neuropeptide Y (NPY)), which may have their own effects on the heart, and the cardiac muscle also has β_2- and α_1-adrenoceptors that can be activated by the catecholamines. We will concentrate here on the β_1-adrenoceptor mechanisms, since they are best understood, and probably the most important.

The effects of β-adrenoceptor activation are due almost entirely to a rise in the intracellular concentration of cAMP. The G protein involved is G_s, which stimulates adenylyl cyclase. cAMP activates protein kinase A, which causes an increased phosphorylation of many substrate proteins (Fig. 8.6).

Mechanisms involved in increasing heart rate (positive chronotropy)

All three of the currents that may be involved in the pacemaker depolarization – the delayed rectifier K^+ channel, I_f and the slow inward Ca^{2+} current – can be enhanced by a rise in intracellular cAMP. The net result is a steepening of the pacemaker potential and an increase in the heart rate (Fig. 8.7). As described above, the number of Ca^{2+} channels opened by depolarization is increased without a change in the voltage sensitivity or kinetics of the channels, and the activation curve for I_f is shifted to more positive potentials. The mechanisms responsible for the increase in the delayed rectifier current are not well understood.

An increase in the rate of rise and size of the action potential is also seen in the nodal tissues, as would be expected from the enhanced slow inward current, but the effects of β-adrenoceptor stimulation on the shape and duration of the rest of the action potential are very variable – the increased

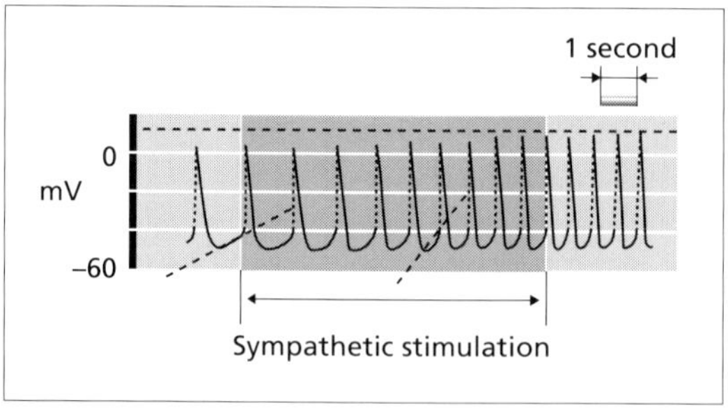

Fig. 8.7 The effect of sympathetic stimulation on the spontaneously beating frog sinus venosus. A progressive steepening of the pacemaker slope increases the frequency of the action potentials. From Hutter & Trautwein (1956).

slow inward current might also be expected to give rise to a more positive and prolonged plateau, whereas the enhancement of the delayed rectifier K^+ current would shorten the action potential. A more positive plateau potential is commonly seen, but the action potential duration may increase or decrease depending on the tissue studied.

An undesirable effect of β-adrenoceptor stimulation is the appearance of cardiac dysrhythmias. The effects on the pacemaker currents may result in the production of extrasystoles, which can contribute to this action.

Mechanisms involved in increasing conduction velocity (positive dromotropy)

The increase in conduction velocity is due to the increased slow inward Ca^{2+} current during the upstroke of the action potential, which allows faster discharge of the membrane capacity, and an increased rate of propagation of the impulse. This effect of β-adrenoceptor stimulation may also contribute to the production of ventricular arrhythmias, since the mechanism that increases conduction velocity will also shorten the refractory period and may allow extraneous action potentials in the atria (due, for example, to ectopic foci or re-entrant circuits) to invade the ventricles.

Mechanisms involved in increasing contractility (positive inotropy)

An increase in the slow inward Ca^{2+} current will increase direct activation of the contractile apparatus in some cardiac tissues, and will also enhance Ca^{2+}-activated Ca^{2+} release from intracellular stores. Increased filling of the sarcoplasmic reticulum with Ca^{2+} results both from the enhanced Ca^{2+} entry, and also from the cAMP-dependent phosphorylation of phospholamban, which stimulates the sarcoplasmic reticulum Ca^{2+} pump activity (Fig. 8.6). Increased Ca^{2+} pump activity is also one of the factors responsible for the enhanced rate of relaxation of contraction – an essential concomitant of the enhanced heart rate, since it will prevent the diastolic interval shortening enough to compromise ventricular filling (Fig. 8.8). Phosphorylation of troponin is known to reduce its affinity for Ca^{2+}, and this may result in more

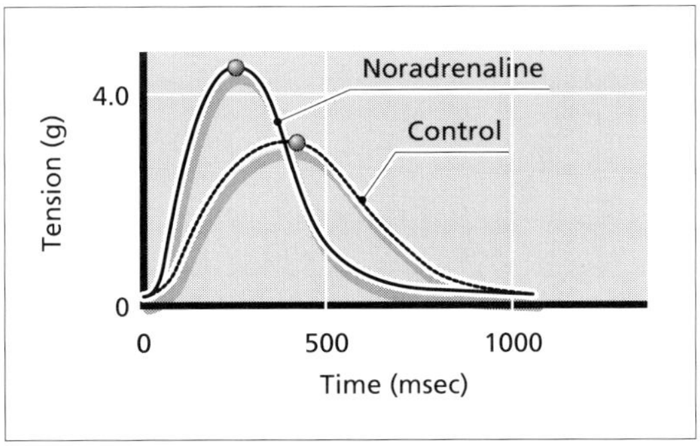

Fig. 8.8 A comparison of the magnitude and time course of the contraction of ventricular muscle in the absence (control) and presence of noradrenaline. Note the enhanced tension and shortened duration of the contraction produced by noradrenaline.

rapid dissociation of Ca^{2+} from the troponin complex and may also play a role in the enhanced relaxation rate. It will also attenuate the positive inotropic effects of β-adrenoceptor stimulation.

α_1-Adrenoceptor responses

Stimulation of these receptors results in a positive inotropic response of the heart, but does not cause any increase in the rate of relaxation of the contractions. There is evidence that the effect is in some way mediated through a G-protein activation of phospholipase C and the production of inositol triphosphate and diacylglycerol as second messengers.

8.1.4 Interactions between the parasympathetic and sympathetic systems

It is obvious from the above account that the parasympathetic and sympathetic systems interact at the level of the second messengers in the cell. β-adrenoceptor stimulation causes activation of adenylyl cyclase and a rise in intracellular cAMP, and muscarinic receptor activation inhibits the enzyme and lowers cAMP levels. The systems also interact in many other places. For instance, it seems that the terminal neurones of the two systems run close together, and that transmitters released from the nerves not only act on postjunctional receptors, but also on prejunctional receptors, both on the parent axon (autoreceptors) and on neighbouring axons. Thus, activation of muscarinic receptors on adrenergic neurones can lead to a diminished output of noradrenaline, and activation of adrenoceptors on cholinergic neurones can reduce the output of acetylcholine. There is also some evidence for interaction in the coeliac ganglion, where postganglionic sympathetic neurones may inhibit parasympathetic neurones. Reciprocal activation of one system and inhibition of the other is seen in response to increases or decreases in baroreceptor input to the medulla, and is probably organised at the level of the inputs from higher centres. Thus, although separate activation of both systems can occur, the overall design ensures that, when necessary, the appropriate one plays the predominant role.

8.1.5 Local control of cardiac output

In the section on cardiac muscle (Section 7.2), it was pointed out that the force of contraction of the ventricular muscle is increased with stretch. This is known as Starling's law of the heart, or the Frank–Starling mechanism, and allows the heart to adjust its output to changes in venous return without intervention of the autonomic nervous system. The relationship can be expressed as shown in Fig. 8.9, where the end-diastolic volume (and thus fibre length) is plotted against the resting pressure and the peak systolic pressure. The relationship can also be shown using ventricular func-

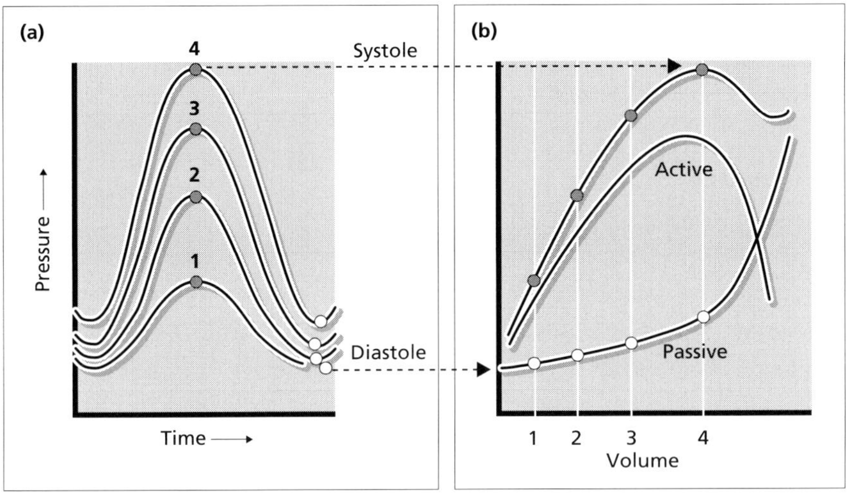

Fig. 8.9 The effect of increasing ventricular volume on the pressure generated during systole. In (a), the individual pressure traces are plotted with increasing volume. In (b), the pressure volume relationship is plotted (shaded circles) as the peak systolic pressure against the end-diastolic volume and also the passive force generated in the uncontracted ventricle is shown (open circles). The active force can be obtained by subtraction of the two curves. Adapted from Levick (1991).

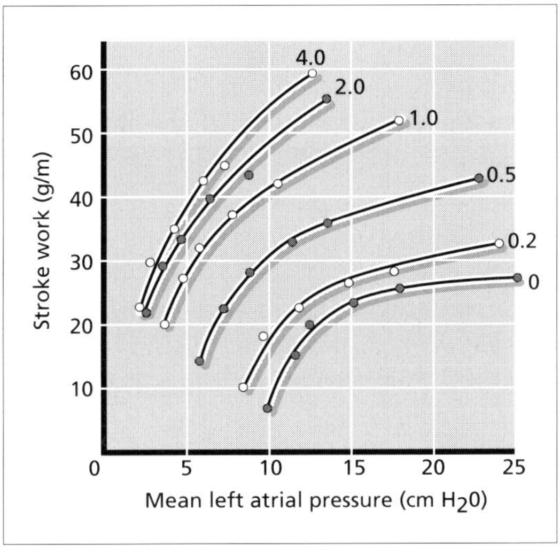

Fig. 8.10 Effect of sympathetic nerve stimulation on the ventricular function curves in an isolated dog heart–lung preparation. With increasing frequency of stimulation (numbers on the curves are frequency of stimulation in Hz), the curves are shifted upwards and to the left. Starling's law of the heart thus operates during sympathetic stimulation. Adapted from Sarnoff & Mitchell (1962).

tion curves, in which the end-diastolic pressure or the mean left atrial pressure (both of which can represent the diastolic volume) is plotted against left ventricular stroke work, computed from the mean pressure and mean flow (Fig. 8.10) .

In the denervated heart, Starling demonstrated the way in which alterations of the venous return (pre-load) or aortic pressure (after-load) could change the cardiac output. An increase in the venous return will increase the end-diastolic volume, and will increase the contractility of the muscle (see Section 7.2.7), allowing an increase in the amount of blood ejected per beat (stroke volume) at constant arterial pressure. An increase in the arterial pressure with a constant venous return will mean that the heart cannot expel as much blood in the next beat, thus leaving a larger residual volume. This will increase the end-diastolic volume for the following beat, and thus the stroke volume.

If the cardiac function curves are plotted in the absence and presence of increasing sympathetic stimulation, or after addition of increasing concentrations of catecholamines, the curves shift to the left and upwards, as shown in Fig. 8.10. There is therefore an increase in the work output of the heart at any given filling pressure, and the heart can increase its output without an increase in the end-diastolic volume.

Cardiac output is determined by the rate of the heartbeat and the stroke volume of the left ventricle. The heart rate is controlled by the autonomic system, but the stroke volume is determined by a complex interrelationship of different factors, including sympathetic tone, circulating catecholamines, and the pre-loads and after-loads that determine the end-diastolic volume of the heart.

8.1.6 Reflexes and central control

The autonomic nervous system is used as the efferent arm of many reflex systems that control cardiac output. The dual control via the parasympathetic and sympathetic systems, combined with the individual characteristics and distribution of the postganglionic neurones, ensures that the behaviour of the heart can be finely adjusted to suit the prevailing needs of the body. The autonomic output can be accessed through many reflex pathways, and also more directly from higher centres.

Reflex adjustment of the cardiac output includes the baroreceptor reflex. This is involved in maintaining a constant arterial blood pressure through alterations in cardiac output and peripheral resistance. Increase in the activity of baroreceptor nerves from the arterial baroreceptors in the aortic arch and carotid sinus triggers reduction in cardiac output, and vice versa. This is achieved by reciprocal alterations in the activity of the parasympathetic and sympathetic systems. Reflex adjustment also occurs in response to stretching of the great veins and atria caused by an increased venous return. This stimulates an increase in heart rate so that output matches inflow, but this occurs with little change in contractility, via sympathetic activity predominantly affecting the pacemakers. The heart is also controlled through various reflexes involved in breathing. Activation of stretch receptors in the lung, as occurs when there is an increase in tidal volume, leads to a reflex tachycardia, thus ensuring an increase in blood flow to match increased respiratory demand. Activation of the arterial chemoreceptors in the carotid and aortic bodies on its own will cause a bradycardia, but this is normally not seen due to the more dominant tachycardia from the lung receptors. However, the bradycardia will occur during asphyxia, when the pulmonary stretch receptors are not activated. Under these circumstances, a reduction in cardiac work can clearly increase the chances of survival.

Central control is seen, for instance, in the increase in heart rate that occurs when exercise is initiated, and also in response to emotional disturbances, such as fear and rage.

Figure 8.11 illustrates some of the pathways involved in the central and reflex control of the heart. Afferent information from the various receptors enters the medulla of the brain to synapse with cells in the nucleus of the solitary tract (NTS). The output from this nucleus goes to other areas of the medulla for the more direct reflex responses, and also ascends to the hypothalamus and cerebellum for co-ordination of activity. In the medulla, information passes to the nucleus ambiguus and the dorsal motor nucleus, which contain the cell bodies of the preganglionic neurones of the vagus, and thus excitation of these neurones provides a cardio-inhibitory parasympathetic outflow. Activity in the sympathetic preganglionic neurones of the spinal intermediolateral columns is normally tonically generated from cells in the rostral ventrolateral medulla, providing an excitatory drive to the heart and blood vessels. Another group of neurones in the caudal ventrolateral medulla provides inhibitory input, and these neurones are excited by the afferent input from the NTS. Thus, increased afferent input results in inhibition of the sympathetic outflow to the heart and blood vessels. This arrangement can mediate the reciprocal changes in the parasympathetic and sympathetic innervation seen in response, for instance, to alterations in the baroreceptor activity.

The hypothalamus is important in co-ordinating the overall cardiovascular responses. Of importance to the heart, it contains a depressor area in the dorsal part of the anterior hypothalamus which receives input from the NTS, and projects back to the medulla, initiating reciprocal activation and inhibition of the parasympathetic and sympathetic outflow to the heart. It also contains a defence area, which integrates input from the limbic system through the amygdala, and triggers the sympathetic and vagal responses to fear or rage (increased heart rate and blood pressure). It also inhibits the neurones in the NTS that are normally activated by baroreceptor input, thus preventing the reflex lowering of heart rate and blood pressure that would normally be activated.

The projection from the NTS to the cerebellum is involved in co-ordinating the cardiovascular responses to exercise. The cortex can influence the autonomic control of the cardiovascular system through input to the cerebellum and hypothalamus, and also via the brainstem raphe nucleus.

8.1.7 Relevant pharmacology

When considering the effects of drugs that interact in some way with the

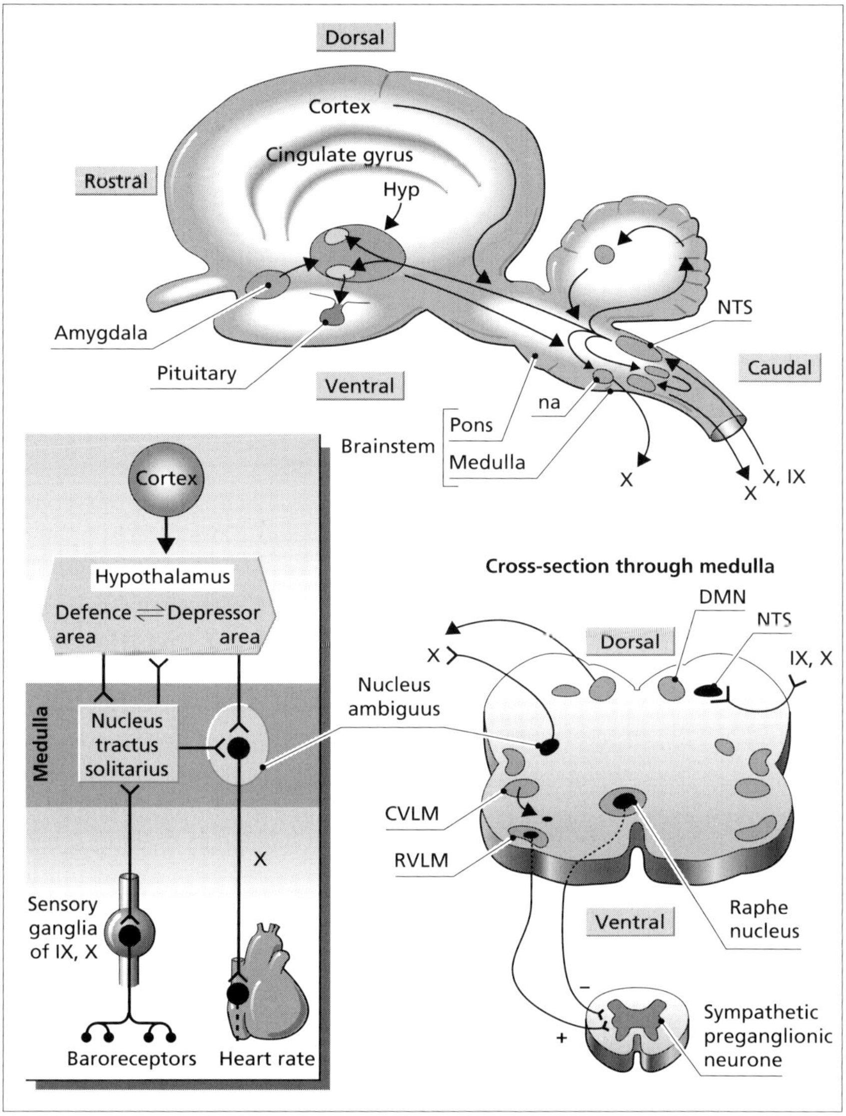

Fig. 8.11 Pathways involved in the central and reflex control of the heart. Afferent information from the various receptors enters the medulla of the brain to synapse with cells in the nucleus tractus solitarius (NTS). The output from this nucleus goes to other areas of the medulla for the more direct reflex responses, and also ascends to the hypothalamus (Hyp) and cerebellum for co-ordination of activity. In the medulla, information passes to the nucleus ambiguus (na) and the dorsal motor nucleus (DMN) which contain the cell bodies of the preganglionic neurones of the vagus (X), and thus excitation of these neurones provides a cardio-inhibitory parasympathetic outflow. Activity in the sympathetic preganglionic neurones of the spinal intermediolateral columns is normally tonically generated from cells in the rostral ventrolateral medulla (RVLM), providing an excitatory drive to the heart and blood vessels. Another group of neurones in the caudal ventro-lateral medulla (CVLM) provides inhibitory input, and these neurones are excited by the afferent input from the nucleus tractus solitarius.

autonomic control of the heart, it is essential to realise that, as well as their direct effects, the drugs are also likely to affect the vascular system. They can thus produce alterations in the pre-load and after-load on the heart, which will indirectly alter cardiac function and result in alterations of the baroreceptor activity, leading to reflex changes in cardiac function through the autonomic nervous system.

Parasympathetic pharmacology

Muscarinic antagonists. In the resting state, there is considerable vagal tone on the heart, although this tends to decline somewhat with age. Thus, muscarinic antagonists such as atropine and hyoscine will cause an increase in heart rate and conduction velocity by removing this vagal tone. Atropine is used clinically in the treatment of bradycardia and atrioventricular block.

Parasympathomimetics. Muscarinic agonists such as bethanechol and carbachol (the latter also with nicotinic actions) will have parasympathomimetic effects, slowing the heart rate and reducing the atrioventricular conduction velocity. They may also result in a reduced contractility of the ventricles. With excessive stimulation of muscarinic receptors, a drastic reduction in cardiac output can result, and it is quite easy to cause a cessation of the heartbeat. It is therefore very dangerous to administer muscarinic agonists intravenously. Cholinesterase inhibitors such as neostigmine and physostigmine will also have parasympathomimetic effects and slow the heart rate. Parasympathomimetics are not used in the treatment of cardiac disease, but as they are used for other conditions, their cardiac effects may be an important consideration, especially in cases in which the heart is already weak.

Cardiac glycosides. Another group of drugs of interest in this context is the cardiac glycosides such as digoxin, digitoxin and ouabain. These drugs are inhibitors of the Na–K pump in cell membranes, and are used because of their positive inotropic effects on the heart. They are prone to cause cardiac dysrhythmias, but are also used in cases of atrial tachycardia or atrial fibrillation, since they can restore a more normal heart rate. They do this by slowing conduction in the AV node and thus increasing the refractory period and reducing the number of impulses getting through to the ventricles – an effect due to their ability to activate the vagal input to the heart. It is thought that this activation is partly a central effect of the drugs, and partly due to decreasing the threshold for activation of the baroreceptors. In both cases, it is probably their ability to block the Na pump that underlies the action of the glycosides.

Sympathetic pharmacology

β-Adrenoceptor blockers. These are commonly used in the treatment of hypertension and angina, and for some types of cardiac arrhythmia. Non-selective β-blockers such as propranolol can block both β_1- and β_2-adrenoceptors, and have the clinical disadvantage that they prevent successful treatment of conditions such as asthma and anaphylactic reactions with β-agonists. Selective β_1-blockers such as atenolol are also in clinical use. The hypotensive actions of β-blockers are only partially due to their local reduction in the actions of the sympathetic nerves on the heart β-adrenoceptors. They also in some way reduce the amount of activity in the sympathetic nerves, and have long-term effects on the shape of the cardiac action potential. The anti-anginal effects of β-blockers can be accounted for by the decrease in the work output of the heart, which can relieve the oxygen deficit causing the angina. The antidysrhythmic actions of β-blockers are due to the antagonism of the arrhythmogenic actions of sympathetic activity.

Sympathomimetics. Catecholamines are used clinically for their cardiac effects. Adrenaline and noradrenaline are used as an emergency measure to try to reverse cardiac arrest, and isoprenaline to increase the heart rate. Isoprenaline is particularly effective at increasing the heart rate, because it also causes vasodilation, and through the baroreceptor reflex this will trigger a reduction in vagal tone. Noradrenaline, on the other hand, will constrict blood vessels, increase blood pressure and trigger a reflex increase in the activity of the vagus, which will reduce its positive chronotropic effects (Fig. 8.12). Dopamine is useful because it has positive inotropic actions, with

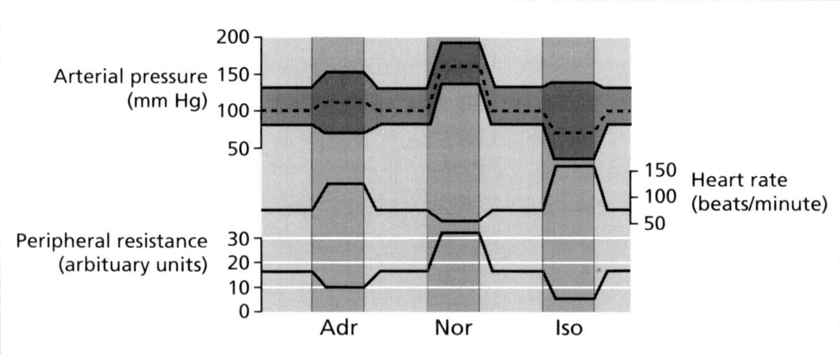

Fig. 8.12 Schematic diagram of the effects of intravenous infusion of adrenaline, noradrenaline and isoprenaline in humans. Noradrenaline causes vasoconstriction (through α-adrenoceptors), and increases systolic and diastolic pressures, resulting in a reflex slowing of the heart rate. Isoprenaline causes vasodilation, and also strongly increases force and rate of the heartbeat (through β-adrenoceptors), causing a drop in mean blood pressure with an increase in pulse pressure. Adrenaline, which has both actions, produces intermediate effects. Adapted from Rang *et al.* (1995).

little effect on the heart rate. It probably works on the α_1- and β-adrenoceptors in the heart, but because it causes little net change in blood pressure, it does not increase heart rate as much as isoprenaline. It is useful to provide inotropic support in cardiac surgery, infarction and cardiogenic shock. Dobutamine, a sympathomimetic agent, is also used in similar situations. It is a selective β_1-adrenoceptor agonist, and thus does not cause the vasodilation and reflex tachycardia of the non-selective β-agonists.

8.2 The vascular system

After describing the anatomy of the innervation of the vasculature, we will consider briefly here the importance of vascular smooth muscle in controlling the vascular system, and the factors important in regulating smooth muscle tone. We will then look at the overall properties of excitatory and inhibitory innervation, and finally examine in more detail the structure and innervation of the various types of blood vessel.

8.2.1 Neuroanatomy

The smooth muscles of the blood vessels are predominantly innervated by postganglionic sympathetic fibres, although some vascular beds also have a postganglionic parasympathetic supply. The cell bodies of the sympathetic fibres are in the paravertebral ganglia of the sympathetic trunks. The postganglionic fibres are distributed either with the spinal nerves (exiting the sympathetic trunks through the grey rami communicantes) that supply the blood vessels to the limbs, or via the arteries, where fibres emerging from paravertebral ganglia form plexuses around the arteries, and supply branches to the vascular smooth muscles (Fig. 8.13). Careful studies of the peptide contents of postganglionic fibres suggest that there may be several different classes of neurone, each of which may have a discrete distribution on blood vessels and secrete a unique combination of transmitters and peptide modulators. These neurones may be differentially activated in the various autonomic reflexes acting on the vasculature.

8.2.2 Haemodynamics

The autonomic nervous system plays a major role in controlling the blood pressure and the distribution of the blood flow to the various organs of the body. All the blood vessels, with the exception of the capillaries and some of the small veins, contain smooth muscle in their walls, and it is the contractile activity of these smooth muscles that can alter the dimensions of the vessels, and thus affect blood flow and blood pressure (Box 8.1).

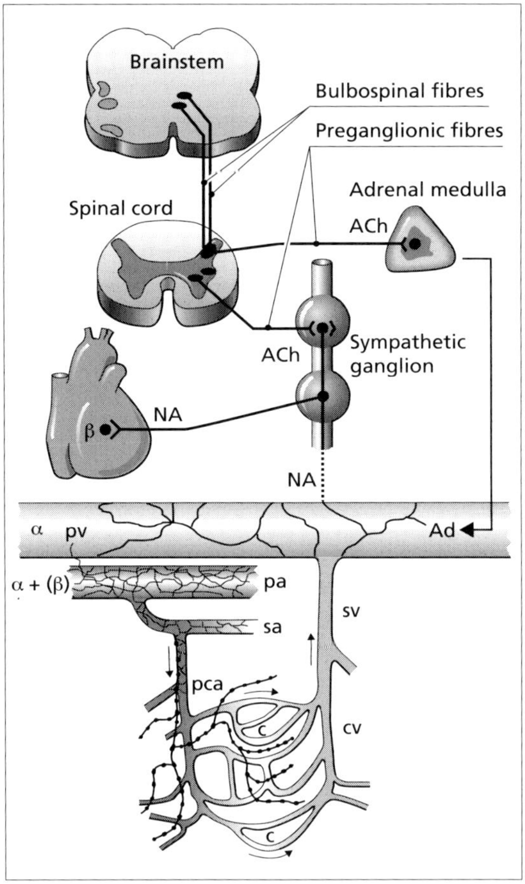

Fig. 8.13 Sympathetic innervation of the blood vessels. The cell bodies of the sympathetic fibres are in the paravertebral ganglia of the sympathetic trunks. The postganglionic nerves form plexuses around the arteries and branch to supply the vascular smooth muscles. α and β refer to the predominant adrenoceptor class on the end organ. NA, noradrenaline; Ad, adrenaline; ACh, acetylcholine; pa, pv, primary artery and vein to an organ; sa, sv, small artery and vein; pca, precapillary artery; c, capillary; cv, collecting venule. Adapted from Furness & Marshall (1974).

8.2.3 Factors controlling smooth muscle tone

The factors controlling the degree of activation of the vascular smooth muscles are many and various, and also depend on the type of blood vessel. The four main factors are as follows.

1 Intrinsic myogenic tone in the smooth muscle.

2 The effects of locally produced vasoactive substances.

3 The effects of substances circulating in the blood.

4 The degree of activation of the nerves innervating the smooth muscle.

Myogenic tone

In most blood vessels, blocking the action of excitatory nerves usually causes vasodilation, suggesting that under normal conditions part of the tone in blood vessels is neurogenic. However, in most blood vessels, significant tone persists in the absence of neural tone, and further dilation can be produced pharmacologically, for instance with calcium antagonists or activation of β-adrenoceptors. The degree of myogenic tone varies from vessel

Box 8.1 Haemodynamics

Theoretically, the relationship between blood flow and blood pressure depends on the resistance of the vessel to flow, in much the same way that current and voltage are related to electrical resistance in Ohm's law – flow = pressure difference/hydraulic resistance, or:

$$Q = (P_1 - P_2)/R$$

Considering the whole circulation, the flow will be equal to the cardiac output, the pressure gradient will be the difference between the mean arterial pressure and the central venous pressure, and the resistance will be equal to the total peripheral resistance.

The resistance to the flow of fluid in a tube depends on many factors, for instance the length of the tube, its diameter and the viscosity of the fluid. The relationship was established for steady laminar flow of a Newtonian fluid along a straight cylindrical tube by the French physician, J.L.M. Poiseuille, in 1840, and is:

$$R = 8\eta \times L/\pi r^4$$

where η is the viscosity of the fluid, L is the length of the vessel and r is the radius.

Combining these two equations gives Poiseuille's law:

$$Q = (P_1 - P_2) \times \pi r^4/8\eta \times L$$

From these equations, one can see how important the radius of the vessel is, since there is a fourth power relationship here. In the circulation as a whole, if the cardiac output remained constant, a very small decrease in the diameter of the resistance vessels (the arterioles) would result in a much larger increase in arterial blood pressure. For an individual circulation, a 16% reduction in the arteriolar diameter at constant arterial blood pressure would theoretically halve the blood flow through the organ concerned.

The viscosity is an important term in the equation, and will vary depending on the haematocrit (the percentage of red blood corpuscles). In practice, the blood does not actually behave like a Newtonian fluid, and in blood vessels less than 1 mm in diameter, the apparent viscosity decreases as the diameter decreases. This minimises the pressure needed to perfuse the microcirculation. The reason for the apparent drop in viscosity is that there are changes in the flow patterns of the red blood cells in narrow tubes.

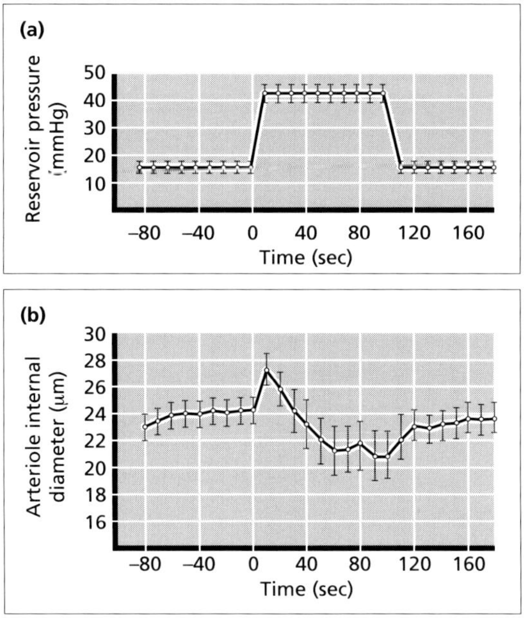

Fig. 8.14 Effect of increased intravascular pressure on the diameter of an arteriole in the mesentery of a cat. A step change in perfusing pressure leads to an initial increase of the arteriole diameter, followed by a reduction to less than the original diameter, caused by an active myogenic response of the smooth muscle. Adapted from Johnson & Intaglietta (1976).

to vessel; it is particularly well developed in vessels in the skin, for instance. In some of the smaller arteries and arterioles, this myogenic tone is affected by the intraluminal pressure. Increase in pressure can actually cause an increase in tone and a vasoconstriction, and vice versa (Fig. 8.14). The mechanisms behind this response are uncertain, but may involve activation of stretch-sensitive non-selective cation channels to depolarize the smooth muscle or epithelial cells. This response can account for the autoregulation of blood flow that occurs in some vascular beds. In portal veins, where there is only a small pressure drop along the length of the vessels, spontaneous oscillatory myogenic activity is seen, resulting in periodic contractions of the vessel that help blood flow (Fig. 8.15). Underlying these contractions are action potentials that occur in bursts, superimposed on a spontaneous slow depolarization of the cell membranes. Blood vessels may also alter their properties in response to denervation and develop more tone, but whether this is because they become more sensitive to local or circulating factors, or genuinely develop spontaneous tone, is not certain.

Locally produced vasoactive substances

These again may be of remarkable diversity, and induce different responses in different blood vessels. Vasoactive substances can be produced by metabolic processes in surrounding tissue (including lactic acid, CO_2, K^+ ions, adenosine diphosphate (ADP), adenosine monophosphate (AMP), inorganic phosphate, adenosine), and blood vessels can also respond to the subsequent changes in pH, local osmolarity and to hypoxia. The endothelium

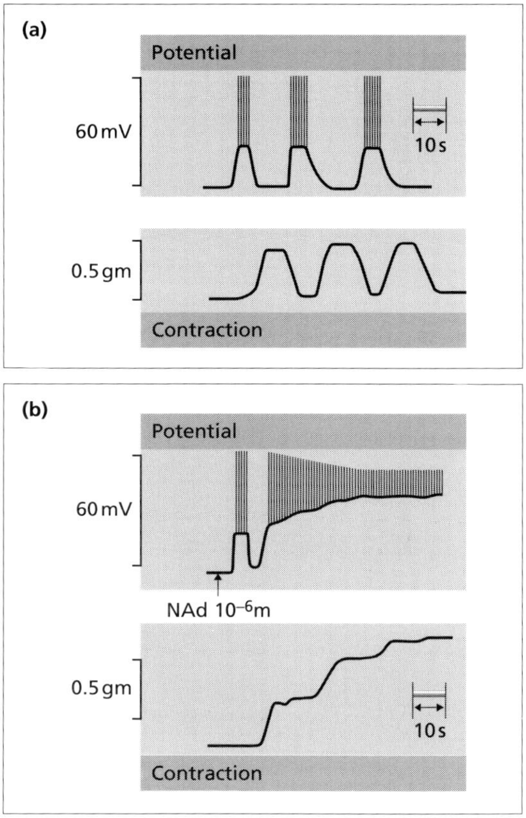

Fig. 8.15 Recordings of membrane potential (intracellular microelectrode) and contraction from strips of guinea-pig portal vein smooth muscle. This vein generates spontaneous rhythmic activity (a) consisting of rhythmic depolarizations with spike activity superimposed. The tissue also develops sustained depolarization with persistent spiking and tone in response to noradrenaline (b). Adapted from Golenhofen *et al.* (1973).

can produce endothelial-derived hyperpolarizing factor (EDHF), NO, (endothelium-derived relaxing factor (EDRF)), and endothelin (a peptide vasoconstrictor). Mast cells, white blood cells and local glands can produce many vasoactive substances (histamine, serotonin, kinins, leukotrienes, prostaglandins).

Circulating factors

These include adrenaline, vasopressin, angiotensin II and atrial natriuretic peptide (ANP). The response to adrenaline may be dilation or constriction, depending on whether β- or α-adrenoceptors predominate, vasopressin and angiotensin are powerful vasoconstrictors, and ANP mildly dilates resistance vessels. It should be pointed out that locally produced and circulating factors may not only have direct effects on the smooth muscle, but may also alter the activity of the endothelium and the nerves.

Innervation

Nearly all blood vessels are innervated by sympathetic adrenergic nerves

(Fig. 8.16), and the major reflexes use this system to control vascular smooth muscle tone. This ensures the maintenance of the blood pressure and enables the redistribution of blood flow necessary when other factors have caused alterations in flow to individual vascular beds. The nerves are tonically active at rest, and constriction can be induced through increased activity and dilation through reduced activity. This function is largely carried out

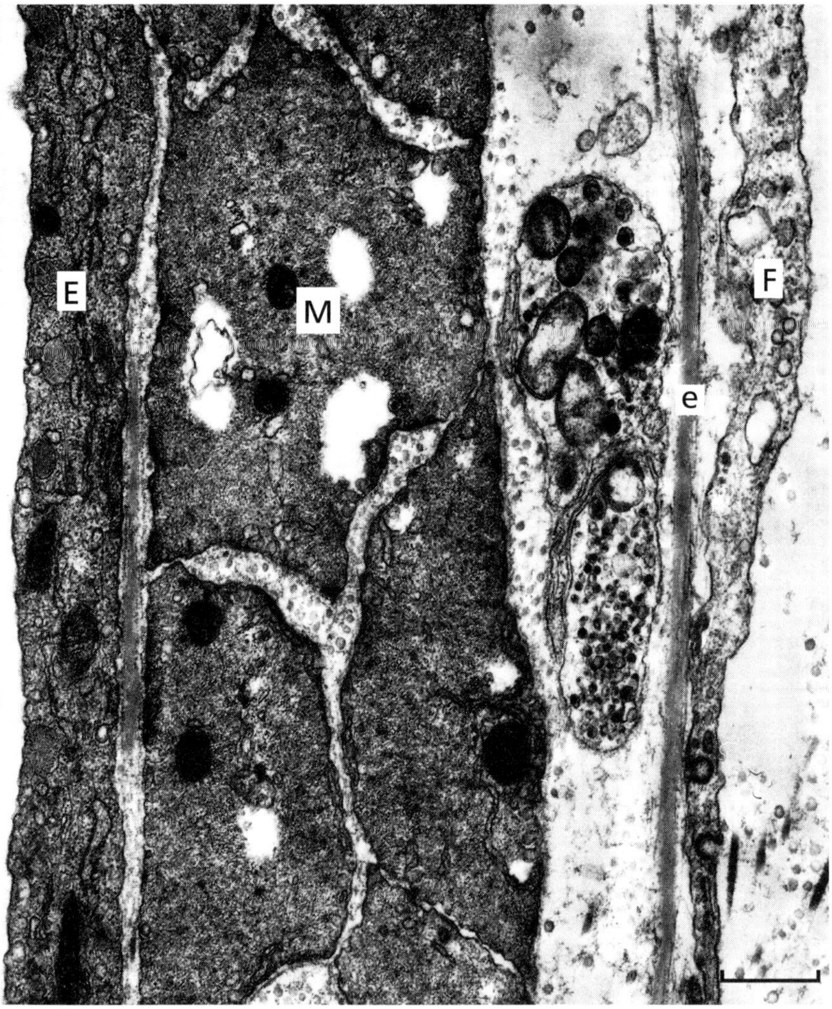

Fig. 8.16 Longitudinal section through an arteriole. The lumen is on the far left. This is lined by endothelium (E) which displays many organelles, and inside this are seen the larger smooth muscle cells of the tunica media (M). In the tunica adventitia to the right, there is a small nerve bundle with two axons, one packed with mitochondria and the other with small granular vesicles (an adrenergic nerve ending). To the right of the nerve bundle is an elastic fibril (e) and a fibroblast (F). The large clear areas in the muscle cells correspond to accumulations of glycogen which were dissolved during preparation. Scale bar: 1 μm. Micrograph kindly provided by G. Gabella.

at the level of the arterioles and veins; the former to regulate the peripheral resistance, and the latter to ensure the correct venous return, and thus cardiac output. As well as being involved in the overall reflex control of the circulation, the vascular beds can be individually controlled through the sympathetic adrenergic system, depending on the prevailing conditions.

The control of the individual vascular beds may, however, also involve inhibitory innervation. Inhibitory nerves may be sympathetic, parasympathetic or sensory, and unlike the excitatory nerves are not tonically active, but only activated when necessary. The inhibition is brought about not only through the action of transmitters on the vascular smooth muscle cells, but also by presynaptic inhibition of the excitatory sympathetic input to the vessels.

8.2.4 Excitatory innervation

Sympathetic adrenergic excitatory nerves

On stimulation, these may release not only noradrenaline, but also ATP, neuropeptide Y (NPY) and, under some circumstances, adrenaline. Although noradrenaline is the main transmitter in all cases, the amount of ATP and NPY released varies depending on the vessel innervated, the species of animal and the frequency of stimulation. In small mammals, ATP is an important co-transmitter with noradrenaline in many blood vessels, although it appears to be less important in humans. Where it is important, ATP is responsible for the fast excitatory junction potentials seen in resistance vessels, which can trigger spikes and a rapid constrictor response of the vessel. ATP activates P_{2x} purinoceptors, which are probably directly activated non-selective cation channels. Noradrenaline, on the other hand, has less effect on the membrane potential, although it can evoke slower membrane potential changes through activation of α-adrenoceptors (Fig. 8.17). The chief mechanism through which it contracts smooth muscle is through pharmacomechanical coupling involving second-messenger pathways and release of intracellular calcium. NPY on its own contracts vascular smooth muscle, but less potently than noradrenaline. It enhances the vasoconstrictor responses to noradrenaline and other excitatory agents, and has been shown to inhibit the opening of Ca^{2+}-activated K^+ channels in vascular smooth muscle cells. There is also evidence that the nerve terminals have autoreceptors for ATP or its metabolites and for catecholamines, which may be involved in feedback regulation of transmitter release. Presynaptic and postsynaptic receptors to the various transmitters may differ in their affinity for agonists and antagonists, and this can allow pharmacological manipulation of the release as well as the effect of the transmitters. For instance, α_1-adrenoceptors are predominantly postsynaptic and α_2-adrenoceptors presynaptic, although exceptions occur.

Sympathetic adrenergic nerves are also affected by changes in their local

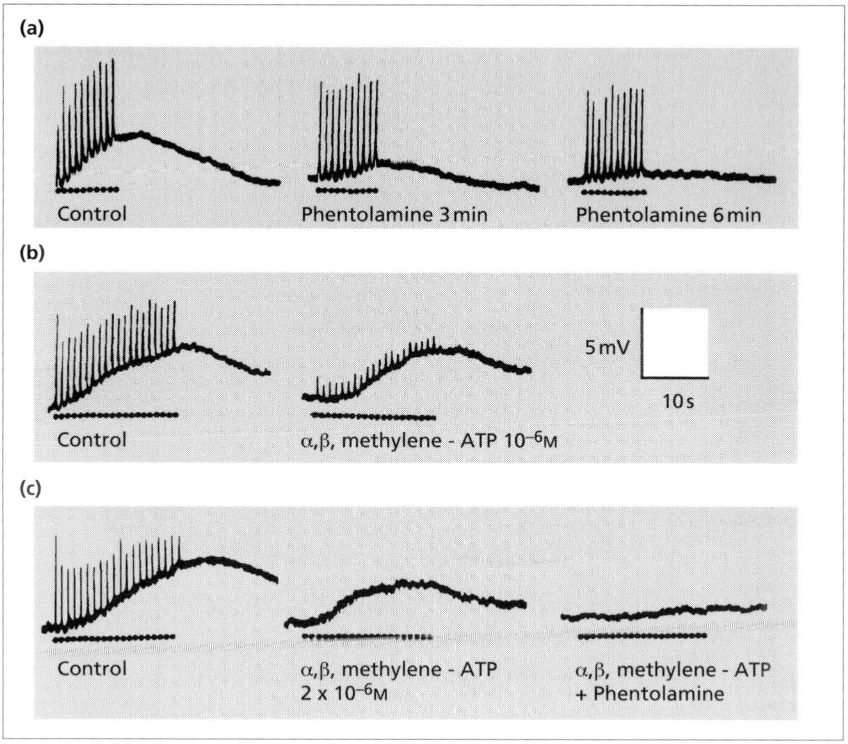

Fig. 8.17 Intracellular recordings of membrane potential of a rat tail artery smooth muscle cell, and its response to stimulation of its intrinsic nerves. Trains of pulses were delivered at 0.5 Hz, indicated by the dots. The control responses on the left show that stimulation induced a train of excitatory junction potentials (EJPs) superimposed on a slow depolarization. In (a), the tissue was then treated with the α-adrenoceptor blocker phentolamine (2×10^{-6} M), which eventually abolished the slow depolarization, leaving the EJPs unaffected. In (b), the tissue was exposed to α,β-methylene ATP which desensitizes the P_{2X} purinoceptors. This drug greatly reduced the EJP amplitude, without affecting the slow depolarization. In (c), application of both drugs abolished the response to nerve stimulation. This suggests that the EJPs are caused by release of ATP, and the slow depolarization by noradrenaline. Reproduced from Sneddon & Burnstock (1984).

environment, and release can be modulated by many substances (Fig. 8.18). Particularly important are the inhibitory effects of transmitters such as acetylcholine, released from inhibitory nerves. The nerve terminals also contain powerful uptake mechanisms for noradrenaline, which are important for limiting its postsynaptic action both in time and space. Pharmacological blockade of this mechanism can markedly enhance the effectiveness of the innervation. When the circulating levels of adrenaline are high, sympathetic nerves may take up and package adrenaline, which can then be subsequently released – presumably a mechanism that can prolong the 'flight or fight' response.

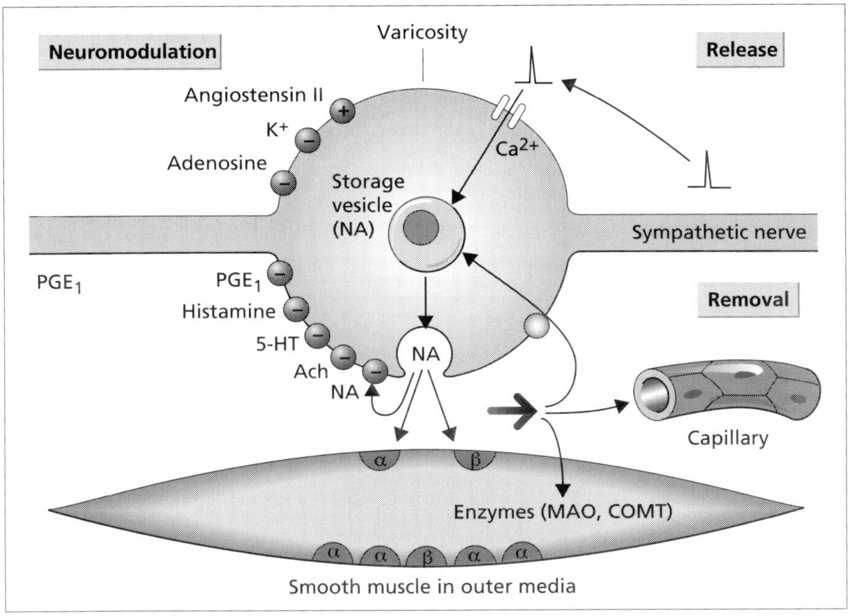

Fig. 8.18 Diagram of a varicosity in the sympathetic nervous system and the potential modulatory agents that can affect transmitter release. Noradrenaline itself has a feedback inhibitory action transmitter release.

8.2.5 Inhibitory innervation

Sympathetic cholinergic vasodilation

Sympathetic vasodilator nerves that release acetylcholine innervate the blood vessels of skeletal muscle in some animals, predominantly carnivores, and are also thought to occur in humans. The nerves are not tonically active, and are activated as part of the 'alerting response' to fear and danger. The response is short-lived, and probably causes the main increase in flow in shunt vessels that do not directly supply the skeletal muscle fibres. Its major role may be in allowing a rapid increase in cardiac output without a large increase in arterial pressure, to set the scene for later requirements in exercise. More prolonged skeletal muscle vasodilation occurs in response to local metabolites during exercise, and circulating adrenaline, which acts on β_2-adrenoceptors. The sympathetic cholinergic innervation to skeletal muscle has been implicated in psychogenic fainting in humans, and may play a role in the precipitous drop in blood pressure that can occur in syncope.

The response of blood vessels *in vitro* to applied acetylcholine is normally vasodilation, but this is largely mediated by release of NO from the endothelium (Fig. 8.19). Both the endothelium and the vascular smooth muscle

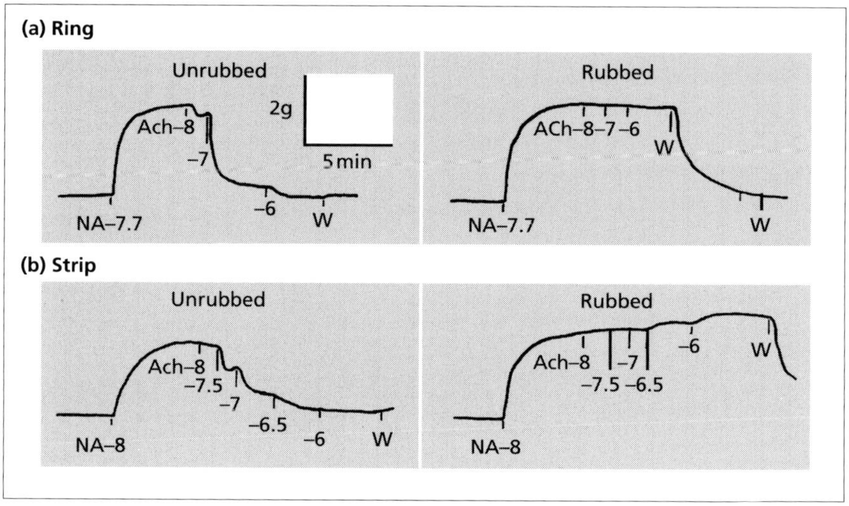

Fig. 8.19 The effect of the endothelium on the responses of rings (a) or strips (b) of rabbit aorta to acetylcholine (ACh). The endothelium has been removed from the preparations on the right by gentle rubbing. Both preparations contract in response to applied noradrenaline. Those with intact endothelium on the left, show a dose-dependent relaxation to ACh, those on the right without endothelium are insensitive to ACh. Later work has established that ACh releases endothelial-dependent relaxing factors such as NO. From Furchgott & Zawadzki (1980).

possess muscarinic receptors. If the endothelium is removed, the response to acetylcholine changes, and varies from vessel to vessel. In some blood vessels, the smooth muscle constricts in response to muscarinic receptor stimulation, in some there is little response, and in some the muscle relaxes. *In vivo*, there is no evidence that the cholinergic vasodilator innervation acts through the endothelium, and it is likely that the dilation is achieved by inhibition of the tonic excitatory sympathetic input, combined with a direct relaxing effect on the smooth muscle. It is of interest to speculate why the endothelium has muscarinic receptors, since acetylcholine is unlikely to reach them from nerves or through the main blood stream, since the plasma contains cholinesterase (although intravenous injection of acetylcholine will cause a transient drop in blood pressure through this mechanism). It has recently been shown that the endothelial cells themselves contain choline acetyltransferase, and may synthesise their own acetylcholine. Factors stimulating the endothelium may result in acetylcholine release that could act to produce dilation downstream of the stimulus.

Sympathetic cholinergic nerves also innervate sweat glands in humans, and their activation results not only in sweating, but also in the large increase in blood flow that accompanies it. Although some of this response is blocked by atropine, there is an atropine-resistant neurogenic vasodilation, which can be classified as non-adrenergic, non-cholinergic (NANC).

Many cholinergic vasodilator nerves contain vasoactive intestinal polypeptide (VIP), which will also cause relaxation of vascular smooth muscle. It is possible that this substance is the NANC transmitter.

Parasympathetic vasodilation

Some vascular beds are innervated by parasympathetic vasodilator nerves. Such nerves innervate blood vessels to many secretory tissues such as the salivary glands, the exocrine pancreas and the gastric and colonic mucosa. Parasympathetic vasodilator nerves also innervate some of the cerebral and coronary arteries, and the blood vessels supplying the erectile tissues of the external genitalia. Again, there is a significant NANC component of this innervation, and VIP has been implicated as a transmitter. In erectile tissue, the NANC relaxation of the trabecular smooth muscle that allows filling of the erectile tissue with blood uses nitric oxide as an inhibitory transmitter, although the parasympathetic relaxation of the arterial smooth muscle probably uses acetylcholine and VIP.

Sensory vasodilation

One class of sensory nerves, often called sensorimotor nerves, can also activate vasodilation. This was first demonstrated in the axon reflex vasodilation that can be initiated by antidromic stimulation of sensory nerves to the skin, and these nerves are responsible for Lewis's triple response of the skin to scratching with a blunt instrument. This class of sensory nerve has its cell body in the dorsal root ganglia, but *en route* from the periphery sends branches (axon collaterals) to innervate local blood vessels and mast cells, and probably also other smooth muscles and neurones on the way to the central nervous system (Fig. 8.20). These 'motor' terminals release substance P and calcitonin gene-related peptide (CGRP), both vasodilator peptides, but with excitatory activity on other tissues. Stimulation of mast cells results in release of other vasoactive and pain-sensitising agents, and also in an increase in vascular permeability, resulting in local oedema. The transmitters can be released locally by capsaicin, the ingredient in chillies that makes them 'hot'.

8.2.6 Types of blood vessel and properties of their smooth muscles

Arteries

These contain smooth muscle cells in their tunica media. Elastic arteries contain smooth muscle cells roughly circularly arranged, in layers interspersed with elastic fibres (Fig. 8.21a). These arteries are readily distensible, and can expand to receive the volume of blood delivered from the heart with each heartbeat. Their elastic recoil helps in maintaining the pressure

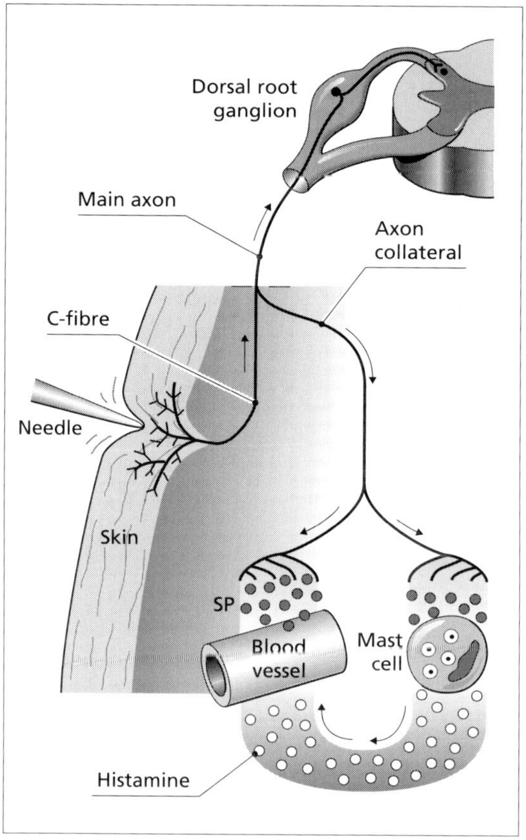

Fig. 8.20 Sensory vasodilation. A class of nociceptors in the skin sends axon collaterals back into the adjacent skin, and releases substance P and CGRP. These can act either directly on the local blood vessels, or by release of mediators from mast cells, resulting in vasodilation. This can also be induced by activation of the sensory nerve trunks through antidromic impulses.

gradient necessary for continuous blood supply to the tissues. Contraction of the smooth muscle will alter wall compliance more than narrowing of the lumen. In the smaller muscular arteries (Fig. 8.21b), the layers of smooth muscle cells are interspersed with less elastin and more collagen. The smooth muscle cells of most arteries are normally electrically inexcitable. Their cells are interconnected through low-resistance electrical pathways (gap junctions), and under normal conditions are developing tone, either spontaneously or in response to continuous activation of the sympathetic nerves innervating the vessels. Tone can be altered by changing the membrane potential (and thus altering the number of voltage-sensitive Ca^{2+}

Fig. 8.21 (*Opposite.*) Electron micrographs of longitudinal sections of the wall of small elastic (a) and muscular (b) arteries from the rat mesenteric bed. In both cases the smooth muscle cells (M) are arranged in layers, but in (a) these layers are interspersed with elastic laminae (E) and, in (b), with collagen (C). In both cases there is an elastic lamella under the endothelium (En) at the top of the section which is the lumen of the vessel (L). At the bottom of the muscular artery (b), at the intimal edge, are dense collagen fibrils and fibroblasts (F) Scale bars: 2 μm. Micrographs kindly provided by G. Gabella.

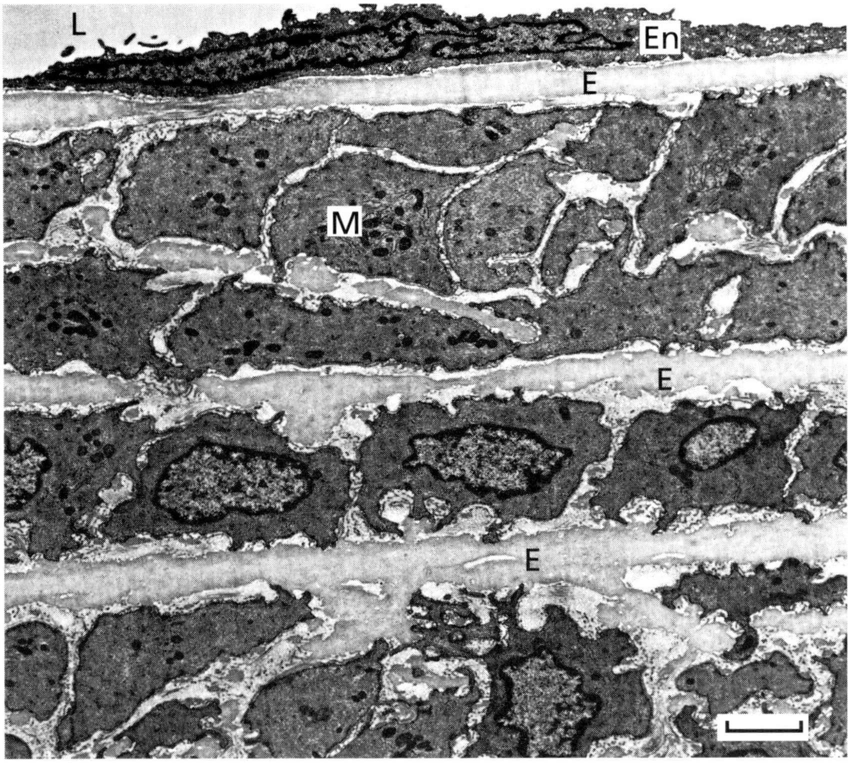

(a)

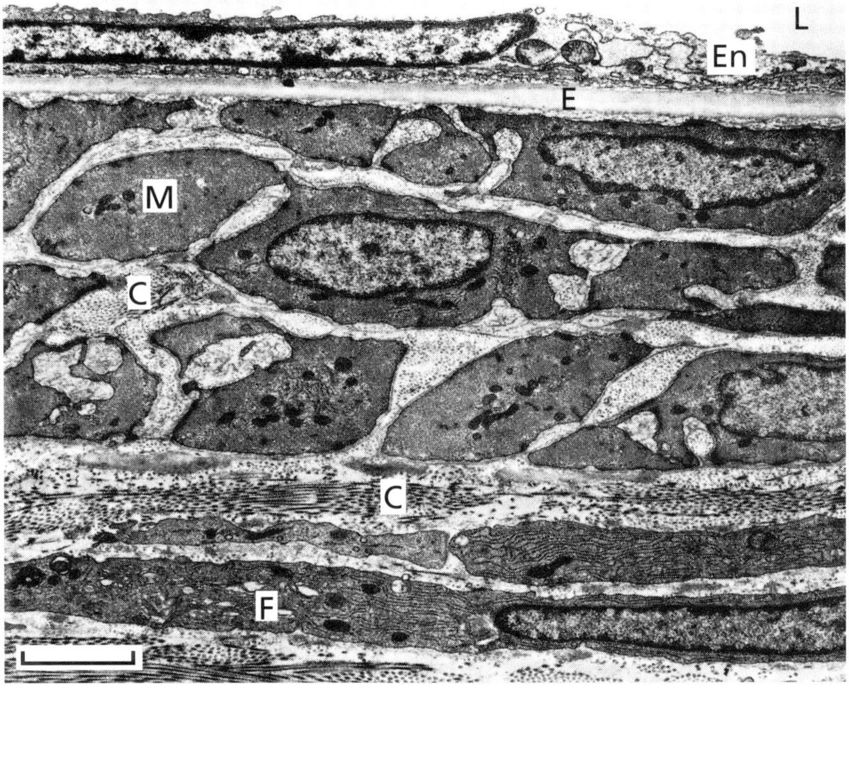

(b)

channels that are open, and Ca^{2+} entry into the cells), and also by receptor-mediated activation of second-messenger systems and release of Ca^{2+} from intracellular stores (pharmacomechanical coupling), which may be independent of potential changes. Sympathetic adrenergic nerves run in the adventitia, and varicose terminal branches penetrate the smooth muscle layers. Close connections can be made between varicosities where they lose their Schwann cell sheaths and individual smooth muscle cells. In the high-pressure arteries, the varicose terminal branches only penetrate a little way into the vessel wall, the majority of the innervation being on the outer layers of smooth muscle (Fig. 8.16). In response to damage and the local release of noradrenaline, the excitable properties of the membranes can change to allow regenerative spike-like activity to occur, which can produce sufficient synchronous contraction of the smooth muscle in the smaller muscular arteries to nearly occlude the lumen, and thus play a role in haemostasis. This type of activity is not often seen, the response to alterations in sympathetic nerve activity normally being a slow change in contraction that spreads passively from the outer towards the inner smooth muscle cells.

Arterioles

These contain a single layer of circularly arranged smooth muscle cells in their media (Fig. 8.22). In large arterioles, more than one smooth muscle cell may be needed to surround the arteriole, and in the small ones, a single smooth muscle cell may wrap completely around the vessel. In contrast to arteries, arteriolar smooth muscle is electrically excitable, and can fire action potentials in response to excitatory nerve input, although tone can also be developed through pharmacomechanical coupling. Again, the sympathetic innervation runs on the outside of the arterioles, and the terminal varicose branches innervate the outer surface of the smooth muscle cells. In the more proximal arterioles, the density of innervation is such that most smooth muscle cells will have a close varicosity, although the smaller, more distal arterioles may be less densely innervated, and more controlled by their local environment. Recent ultrastructural studies using serial electron microscopy have shown that each varicosity makes a very close connection to a smooth muscle cell (a gap of 35–75 nm with fused basal laminae). The diameter of the arterioles is finely controlled by the degree of sympathetic nerve activity; reduction of the activity leads to dilation of the arterioles, and increased activity to constriction. This is a major effector of the baroreceptor reflex control of the blood pressure.

Veins and venules

These have thinner walls with a wider diameter and contain less smooth muscle than their arterial counterparts. In venules, there are sparse smooth muscle cells interspersed with large amounts of collagen. As the diameter of

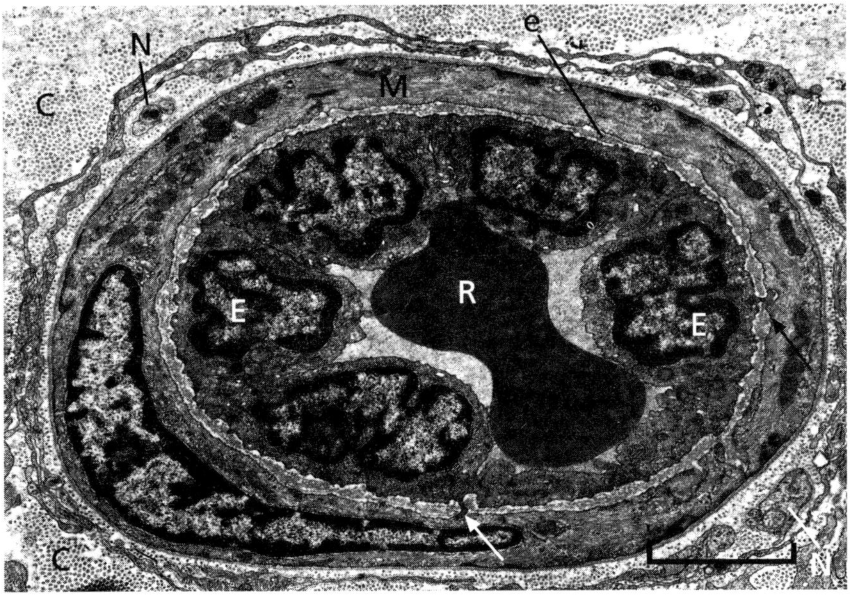

Fig. 8.22 In this electron micrograph an arteriole appears in transverse section. In the centre is a red blood cell (R) and some blood plasma, surrounded by a layer of endothelial cells (E), forming the innermost lining of the vessel (tunica intima). The endothelial cells, five of which display the nucleus, are firmly attached to each other by specialized junctions: over their abluminal surface is a continuous thin layer of elastic material (the inner elastic lamina) (e), less than 1 μm thick, and beyond it is a single muscle cell (M) which makes a full turn in the wall of the vessel. The muscle cell, clearly showing its nucleus, mitochondria and dense bands, forms the tunica media of the vessel, and at two sides (arrows) it is contacted by small finger-like processes arising from the endothelial cells, which may allow some communication between the two types of cell. Two small nerve bundles (N) run in the adjacent connective tissue; the latter is made of collagen fibrils, which are mainly in transverse section (C), and lamina processes of fibroblasts. Scale bar: 2 μm. Micrograph kindly provided by G. Gabella.

the vessels increases from the collecting to the muscular venules and small, medium and large veins, so the amount of smooth muscle also increases, although it may still be interspersed with collagen and elastic fibres. The smooth muscle progressively becomes arranged in more or less circular and longitudinal bundles (Fig. 8.23). The smooth muscle has less myogenic tone than is seen in the arteries, although portal veins have myogenic fluctuations in diameter. The smooth muscle of the muscular venules and veins is innervated by the sympathetic nerves, and again there is tonic activity of the innervation keeping a degree of tone in the vessel walls. Since about 60% of the blood volume is contained in the venules and veins, a decrease in their diameter can discharge large volumes of blood into the central veins, and play an important role in controlling venous return, stroke volume and cardiac output. The veins are the other important vascular effectors of the baroreceptor reflex, and are particularly important when postural changes

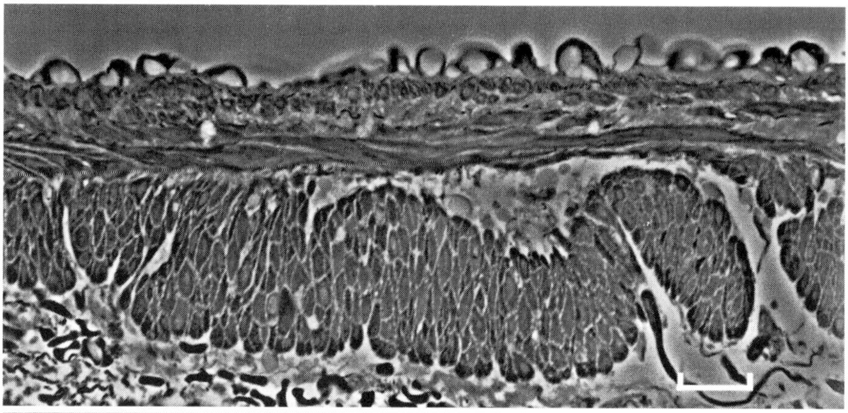

(a)

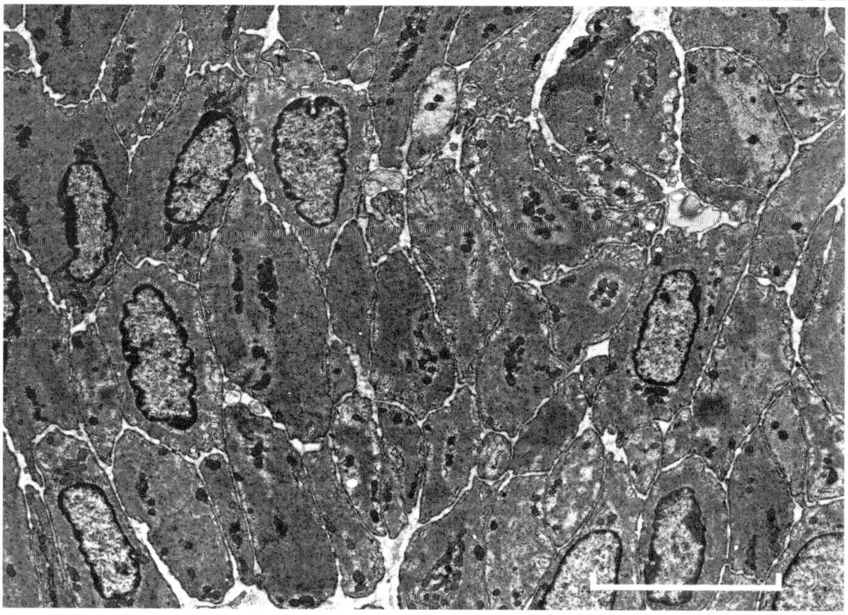

(b)

Fig. 8.23 Guinea-pig vein. (a) Light micrograph of a transverse section of the wall of a guinea-pig portal vein. The lumen is at the top and is lined with endothelium which has an irregular outline. The tunica media (muscle coat) is made of two distinct layers of musculature, a thinner internal one running circumferentially, and a thicker external one running longitudinally. At the bottom of the micrograph is the adventitia. Scale bar: 20 μm. (b) Electron micrograph of the longitudinal muscle layer. Note the similarity of this muscle layer to those of visceral muscles. Scale bar: 10 μm. Micrographs kindly supplied by G. Gabella.

alter the gravitational forces applying. Constriction of the veins prevents pooling of blood in the extremities, and ensures sufficient venous return. Veins running within striated muscle in the legs are less well innervated, and rely more on the 'muscle pump' action of the striated muscle, in combination with the valves in the veins, to ensure venous return (Fig. 8.24).

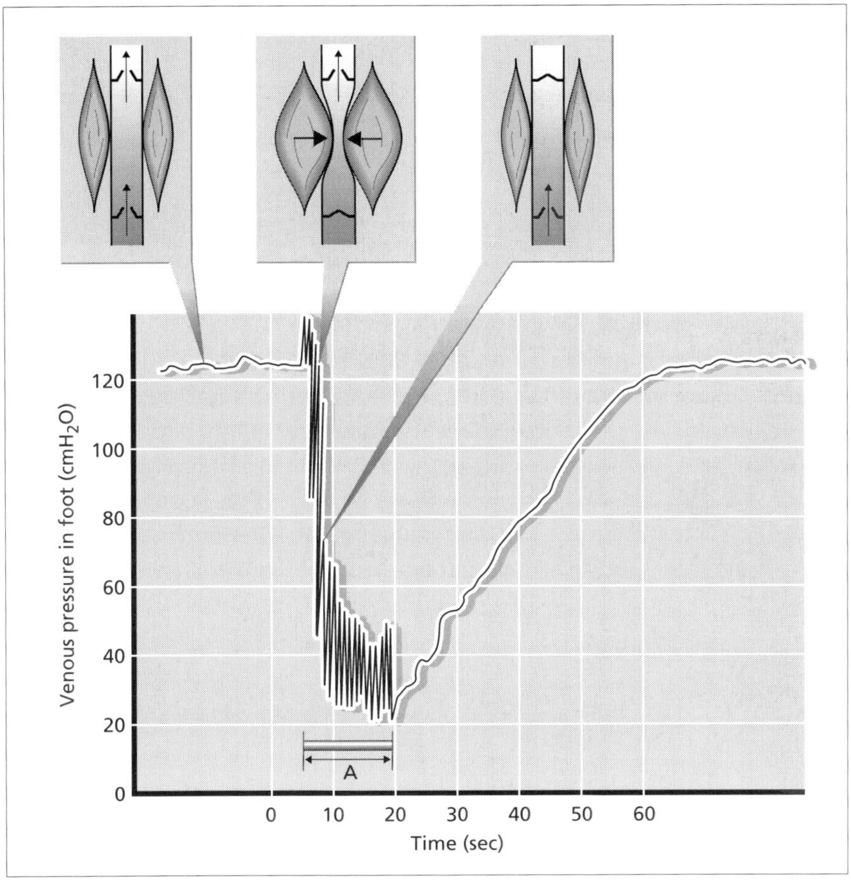

Fig. 8.24 A recording of the pressure in the dorsal vein of the human foot during quiet standing, interrupted by rhythmic contraction of the calf muscles (A). Inset above illustrates how the muscle pump operates. Activity of the calf muscle forces the blood towards the heart. Competent valves prevent backflow, resulting in a drop in the pressure recorded in the foot. Adapted from Levick (1991).

8.2.7 Reflex control of vasculature

The arteriolar and vein smooth muscles are the main targets of the baroreceptor reflex control of blood pressure, using the sympathetic nerves as the efferent arm of the reflex. Control of this reflex is discussed above (see Section 8.1.6). The overall neuronal control of the vascular system is determined in the hypothalamus, which receives and integrates input from relevant sense organs all over the body. Different classes of sympathetic neurones may be specifically activated to ensure that the overall response is appropriate, and to preserve blood supply to important organs. For instance, the reflex vascular constriction evoked in haemorrhage does not involve vasoconstriction of the mesenteric arterioles, since without medical intervention, the only way an animal has of replacing fluid volume lost in haemorrhage is through stimulation of drinking and uptake of fluids in the gut.

8.2.8 Relevant pharmacology

Drugs are commonly used to alter the tone of vascular smooth muscles and affect blood pressure or blood flow. The vast number of different classes of receptor that exist on vascular smooth muscles and the presynaptic nerve terminals and the variability of their distribution give considerable potential for pharmacological intervention and the development of selective drugs for treatment of different conditions. Substantial investments are currently being made by drug companies and medical charities in pursuing research in this area. Unfortunately, the degree of complexity is such that not many new clinically useful drugs have yet been produced. In this section, we will consider the main classes of drugs that are currently used clinically. Table 8.1 shows the main subtypes of adrenergic receptors, the agonists and antagonists acting on them and their medical uses.

Vasoconstrictor drugs

Local effects. The main clinical use for vasoconstrictors is for local

Table 8.1 Adrenoceptors in the cardiovascular system.

Receptor	Location	Effect	Agonists	Antagonists and their uses
α_1	Postjunctional—on vascular smooth muscle	Constricts	Noradrenaline Adrenaline Phenylephrine (S)	Phenoxybenzamine, phaeochromocytoma Phentolamine, Raynaud's vasospasm Ergotamine (PA), migraine Prazosin (S), hypertension
α_2	Prejunctional on adrenergic nerves Postjunctional on some vascular smooth muscles	Inhibits release of NAd (negative feedback) Constricts	Noradrenaline Adrenaline Clonidine (S)	Yohimbine (S), pharmacological tool
β_1	SA node Conducting tissue Myocardium	Increases heart rate Increases propagation rate Increases contractility	Noradrenaline Adrenaline Isoprenaline Dobutamine (S)	Propranolol, angina Atenalol (S), hypertension
β_2	Arterioles (specifically in skeletal muscle, heart and liver)	Vasodilation (bronchodilation)	Adrenaline Isoprenaline Salbutamol (S)	Butoxamine (S), pharmacological tool

S: Specific for receptor subtype; PA: partial agonist.

vasoconstriction – for example, as nasal decongestants or in combination with local anaesthetics to prolong the anaesthetic action by reducing the rate of removal from the injection site. An increase in local vascular tone can be achieved by use of drugs acting on α-adrenoceptors. Adrenaline, noradrenaline, phenylephrine and methoxamine will all achieve this, and are used as nasal decongestants. These drugs will have complex effects if given systemically, due to their ability to activate receptors throughout the circulatory system. This may cause changes in the systemic blood pressure and thus alter baroreceptor reflexes. Adrenaline should not be used with local anaesthetics when anaesthetising appendages such as fingers or toes, since the constriction of the arteries supplying them, combined with the increased metabolism that activation of adrenoceptors can cause, could lead to necrosis. Vasopressin is sometimes used as a vasoconstrictor with local anaesthetics. Indirectly acting sympathomimetic drugs (which cause release of noradrenaline from sympathetic nerve terminals), such as ephedrine, may also be used as nasal decongestants.

Systemic effects. Pure vasoconstrictors are not useful for increasing blood pressure. Under normal conditions, any increase in blood pressure achieved will trigger reflex responses, including bradycardia and a reduced activation of vasoconstrictor nerves, which will counteract the direct actions. When the blood pressure has dropped due to stimuli such as bacterial toxins, burns or haemorrhage, vasoconstriction will be triggered through the baroreceptor reflex, but this may lead to underperfusion of the tissues and local production of vasodilators, leading to a further drop in blood pressure and an increase in capillary permeability, resulting in the clinical condition of shock. The addition of vasoconstrictors can exacerbate this. In treating shock, the ideal approach is to balance vasoconstriction of vascular beds supplying non-essential organs with vasodilation of the supply to vital organs. This is not easy to achieve. Dobutamine, a β_1-adrenoceptor agonist, is sometimes used. This drug has positive inotropic effects on the heart, and enhances blood supply to the kidneys. It also has some α-adrenoceptor activity at higher concentrations, causing some systemic vasoconstriction. Currently, efforts are being made to evaluate the usefulness of a variety of antagonists to locally produced vasodilator substances in treating shock.

Vasodilator drugs

Vasodilator drugs have important therapeutic uses. In general, they will increase local tissue blood flow, reduce arterial pressure and reduce central venous pressure.

Cardiac effects. Vasodilators reduce the work-load of the heart. Reduced arterial pressure reduces the after-load on the heart (less intraventricular pressure development necessary for expulsion of the blood), and reduced central venous pressure reduces the pre-load (reduced filling, less stretch of the ventricles and, by Starling's law, less force development). Local vasodilation may also improve blood flow to the cardiac muscle. All three actions are valuable for the treatment of angina and heart failure. In angina, the intense pain from underperfusion of the heart can be relieved by vasodilators such as organic nitrates and calcium antagonists. Short-lasting organic nitrates, such as glyceryl trinitrate, are often taken as a tablet held under the tongue for sublingual absorption. This route can cause rapid relief, as it benefits from the fact that the blood leaving the buccal cavity does not enter the portal circulation, and the 'first pass' rapid destruction of the drug by the liver is avoided, allowing almost immediate access of the drug to the cardiac circulation. Longer-lasting isosorbide mono- or dinitrates are swallowed. These organic nitrates work by local production of NO and its activation of guanylyl cyclase (see Section 6.2.2) and subsequent smooth muscle relaxant effects. Calcium antagonists, particularly diltiazem and the dihydropyridines, cause both vasodilation and reduce the force of contraction of the cardiac muscle through the reduced Ca^{2+} entry into the muscles, and are thus effective in treating angina. In heart failure, vasodilators are used in combination with diuretics to further reduce the load on the heart, and cardiac glycosides are used to improve cardiac contractility.

Hypertension. Vasodilators are used in the treatment of hypertensive crises, and are frequently also used in the long-term management of systemic hypertension, although diuretics and β-blockers are also commonly used. Amongst the directly acting vasodilators are calcium antagonists and organic nitrates. K^+ channel-opening drugs are also potent vasodilators, and some, such as minoxidil and diazoxide – acting largely through this mechanism – are of use in hypertensive crises. Indirectly acting vasodilators include those drugs that somehow reduce the sympathetic drive on the vascular smooth muscles. Amongst these, α-adrenoceptor antagonists have some clinical use as antihypertensives, particularly in hypertensive crises, such as that caused by phaeochromocytoma (a catecholamine-producing tumour), but tend to cause postural hypotension. Another class of indirectly acting vasodilator drugs are the angiotensin-converting enzyme (ACE) inhibitors. Angiotensin I is formed from a plasma protein by the action of renin released from the juxtaglomerular apparatus of the kidney. This is converted to angiotensin II by the converting enzyme. Although in normal people the main function of angiotensin II is in the control of blood volume through its ability to release aldosterone from the adrenal cortex, it is also a powerful vasoconstrictor, and can be produced in blood vessel walls, which may contain the converting enzyme. In normal people, ACE inhibitors only cause a small fall in blood pressure, but in many hypertensive patients the ACE inhibitors are remarkably effective in lowering the blood pressure. They have little effect on the cardiac muscle.

8.3 The lymphatic system

8.3.1 Structure and function

The lymphatic system is a system of vessels that connects with the interstitial fluid, into which excess fluid and proteins leaving blood capillaries through Starling forces, reabsorbed fluid in the kidneys and fluid and chylomicrons absorbed across the gut wall all drain. The lymph is then returned to the venous blood through the thoracic and right lymphatic ducts, which enter the venous system between the internal jugular and subclavian veins on both sides of the body. The lymphatic system also picks up small particles, bacteria and viruses, and these are transported to the lymph nodes.

The vessels start as blind-ending lymphatic capillaries that arise near to the venous capillaries. These vessels have thin endothelial walls, similar to blood capillaries, but wider and with the junctions between the endothelial cells open, allowing easy passage of proteins and small particles into them (Fig. 8.25). The lymphatic capillaries coalesce to form progressively larger vessels. The medium-sized and larger vessels are divided into segments called lymphangions, separated by unidirectional valves and surrounded by a sleeve of smooth muscle (Fig. 8.26). Along the length of the larger vessels there are strings of lymph nodes. These have a fibrous capsule with

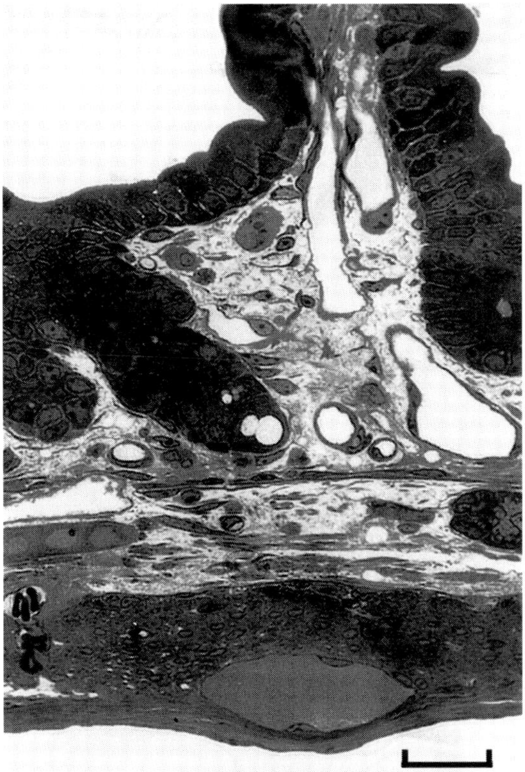

Fig. 8.25 Electron micrograph of a lymphatic vessel (lactea) in the guinea-pig ileum. Note the single endothelial layer with overlapping edges at the bottom, and a small nerve containing a dozen or so nerve fibres on the left. Collagen fibres are lying in the stroma on the right of the vessel. Micrograph kindly supplied by G. Gabella. Scale bar: 0.5 mm.

smooth muscle and underlying lymph sinuses surrounding a core composed of a fibrous stroma containing lymphoid tissue (reticulo-endothelial cells and lymphocytes) and blood vessels (Fig. 8.27). The entering lymphatic vessel divides up into a number of vessels that penetrate the capsule, delivering lymph to the sinuses. Lymph then passes through the lymphatic

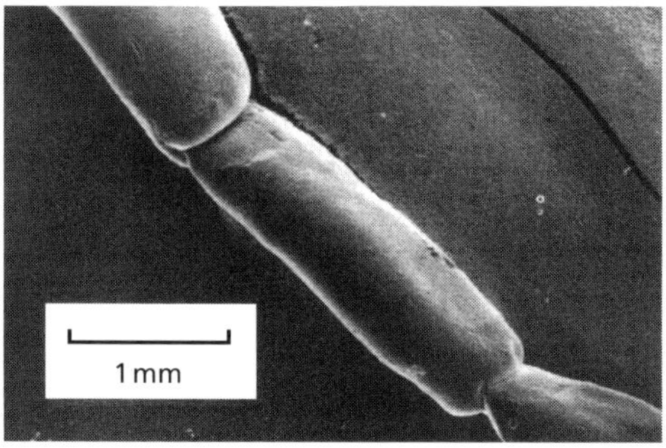

Fig. 8.26 Scanning electron micrograph of a cast of a segment of a lymphatic collecting vessel showing three lymphangions with their unidirectional valves. Kindly supplied by N. McHale.

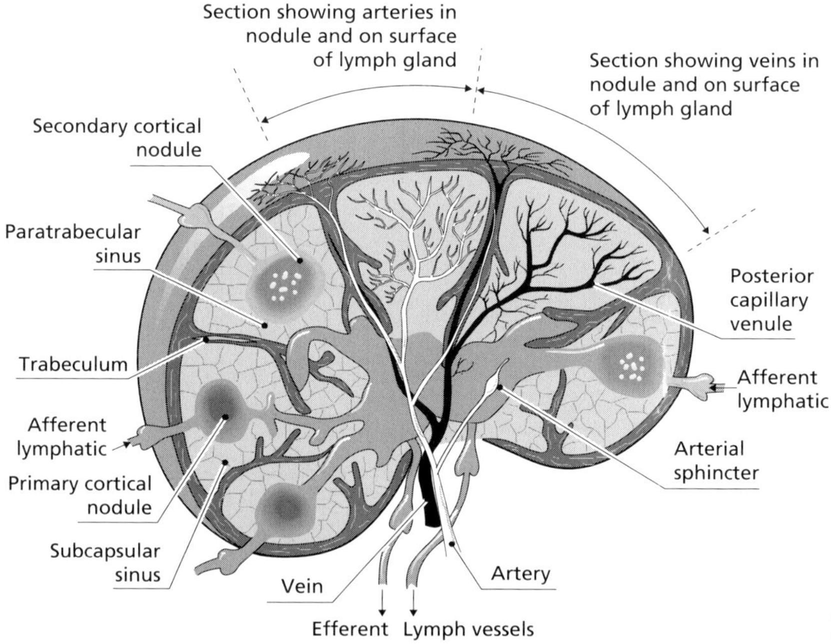

Fig. 8.27 Diagram of a typical lymph node. The lymph enters the node through many small vessels, each guarded by a valve. The lymph flows into the subcapsular lymph space that is lined with macrophages, and then diffuses through the cortex of the node which is densely packed with lymphocytes. These remove bacteria and foreign particles from the lymph. In the medulla, lymph is collected up into efferent lymph vessels which leave the node. Nodules of developing lymphocytes are present throughout the node. Adapted from Binns *et al.* (1970).

tissue and emerges in a single efferent lymphatic vessel. Within the nodes, bacteria and foreign particles are taken up by the reticulo-endothelial cells, and the immunological processes involved in antigen production and cell-mediated responses begin.

8.3.2 Regulation

The smooth muscle in the walls of the lymphatic vessels shows myogenic activity, each of the small lymphangions acting in isolation as a tiny pump, which because of the valves propels lymph along the vessels. There is a correlation between the lymph flow and the rate of contraction of the vessels. The smooth muscle cells within a lymphangion are well coupled electrically, although the coupling to neighbouring lymphangions is relatively poor. Action potentials underlie the contractile activity. The smooth muscle cells have slow pacemaker potentials leading to firing of an action potential complex, which in bovine lymphatics, at least, is composed of a series of spikes superimposed on a small plateau. This triggers a contractile response of the smooth muscle. This myogenic activity is abolished in Ca-free solution or by Ca antagonists. The frequency of the beat is determined by the fluid load delivered to the vessels. Increased distension increases the frequency and, up to a certain point, the force of contraction. The lymphatics and also the lymph glands are innervated by the sympathetic nervous system, and sympathetic stimulation in an intact animal increases the frequency of contractions and the lymph flow (Fig. 8.28).

The physiological role of the innervation is not entirely clear. Because of the autoregulation of the lymph vessels and the sympathetic innervation of the blood vessels, activation of sympathetic nerves could modify the functions of the lymphatic system not only by directly stimulating lymphatic pumping, but also by modifying the rate of lymph formation, or by changing the lymph composition in the lymph nodes. The most likely effect of sympathetic stimulation on the formation of lymph would be a reduction, due to a fall in capillary pressure subsequent to constriction of the arteriolar

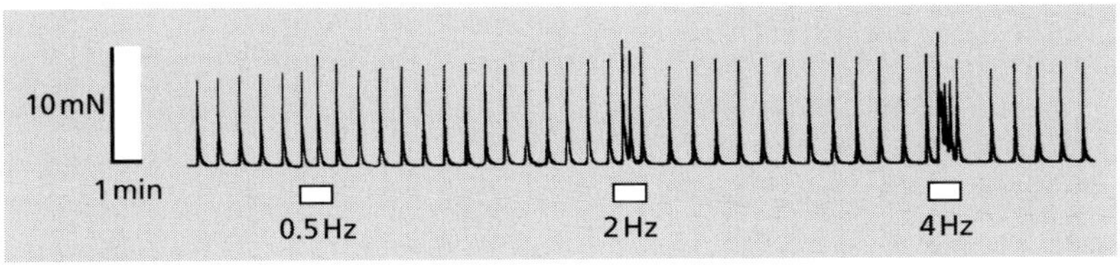

Fig. 8.28 Spontaneous pulsatile activity in a bovine lymph vessel, and the effect of stimulating the intrinsic sympathetic nerve endings at different frequencies. Note that sympathetic stimulation increases the frequency of the pulsatile activity. Adapted from McHale *et al.* (1980).

smooth muscle. This combined enhanced lymphatic pumping and reduced lymph production would tend to reduce interstitial fluid, and increase circulating fluid volume in the blood stream. The effects of sympathetic stimulation on the lymph nodes are contraction of the capsule and increased lymphocyte output. These effects can be mimicked by application of noradrenaline, and are mediated by α-adrenoceptor activation, at least in bovine lymphatics. The lymphatic activity can also be suppressed by β-adrenoceptor activation.

8.4 The lungs

The lungs have an extensive sensory innervation, and activation of sensory receptors of various types is involved in regulating the rate and depth of breathing, and in activating autonomic reflexes. The autonomic motor innervation of the lungs plays an important role not only in determining the calibre of the airways through effects on the airway smooth muscle, but also in the secretion of the various cells of their mucosal lining.

The airways receive both parasympathetic and sympathetic innervation. The parasympathetic system provides the most important innervation of the airway smooth muscle. The sympathetic system plays a role in controlling secretions, and can modulate the parasympathetic system. There are also non-adrenergic, non-cholinergic nerves running in the vagus and present in the airways.

8.4.1 Neuroanatomy

Parasympathetic

The preganglionic parasympathetic nerves have their cell bodies in the dorsal motor nucleus of the vagus. On each side, the axons run in the vagus to the ganglion cells, situated both in the walls of the airways and in the pulmonary plexus around the hilum of the lungs, the trachea and bronchi. The ganglion cells in this plexus process signals directed at airway smooth muscle, secretory cells, vascular smooth muscle and epithelium. There is an extensive cholinergic innervation of the airways, with the nerves running primarily between the smooth muscle bundles, with little penetration within them. The density is fairly uniform in the trachea, but decreases distally in the bronchial tree, so that there are relatively few cholinergic nerves in the terminal bronchioles, and none in the alveolar sphincters. The cholinergic innervation is excitatory on the smooth muscle cells, reducing the diameter of the airways.

Sympathetic

The sympathetic innervation arises from the thoracic outflow, and the preganglionic fibres probably synapse with ganglia in the paravertebral chains, and enter the lungs along with the blood vessels, as well as through the pulmonary plexus. Postganglionic adrenergic neurones are much sparser in the airways than cholinergic neurones, and evidence suggests that, in humans, there is little or no adrenergic innervation of the airway smooth muscle. Sympathetic innervation of the epithelium and the blood vessels is more important. Although they may have little direct effect on airway smooth muscle, it is probable that sympathetic nerves can modulate the parasympathetic innervation, since there is evidence of postganglionic sympathetic fibres innervating the parasympathetic ganglion cells. Adrenergic and cholinergic nerve fibres are also seen running together between the smooth muscle bundles, opening the possibility of presynaptic interactions between them.

NANC innervation

Apart from the classical sympathetic adrenergic and parasympathetic cholinergic innervation of the lungs, there is much evidence to suggest that there is a considerable amount of non-adrenergic, non-cholinergic (NANC) innervation. Functional studies show responses of airway smooth muscle to stimulation of intrinsic nerves that are resistant to muscarinic and adrenergic blockade. Both bronchodilator and bronchoconstrictor responses are seen, and it is likely that there is also NANC innervation of the epithelium. Possible transmitters are peptides such as VIP (which causes inhibition of airway tone) and tachykinins (peptides such as substance P and its relatives), which are excitatory. These peptides may be present in a population of nerve fibres that have sensorimotor function. Many of the peptides have been identified in the autonomic nerves in the lungs, and in some cases they have been shown to co-exist in the same neurone as one of the classical transmitters.

8.4.2 The effector systems and their innervation

The nerves innervate the epithelium and the smooth muscle. The arrangement of these is shown in Fig. 8.29, which shows a cross-section of the trachea from a guinea-pig.

Epithelium

The epithelium of the airways is shown in more detail in Fig. 8.30. It is a ciliated epithelium and contains glands. The submucosal glands contain serous cells and goblet cells. The serous cells are the primary defensive cells of the mucosa, and secrete bactericidal compounds which make up about 60% of the volume of the secretion. Goblet cells secrete mucus. Fluid is secreted by the epithelial cells themselves, and this is important in mucocil-

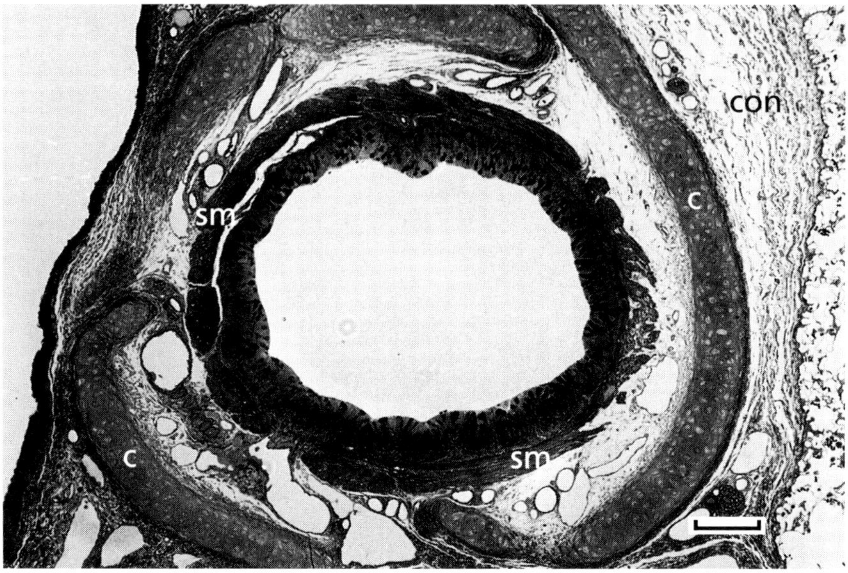

Fig. 8.29 Cross-section of the dorsal wall of the guinea-pig trachea. The ring had been relaxed in calcium-free solution before fixation. The smooth muscle (sm) forms a narrow band which, in this specie, inserts onto the inner surfaces of the C-shaped cartilage (c). The trachea is lined with epithelium, and between it and the smooth muscle is the tunica propria which is rich in elastic fibres. Collagen fibres run in the connective tissue (con) dorsal to the smooth muscle, and ganglion cells are embedded in the connective tissue. Scale bar: 1 mm. From Amiri & Gabella (1988), with permission from the publisher, Springer-Verlag.

iary clearance. The function of the submucosal glands and the epithelial cells is influenced by autonomic agonists, both with direct effects and through changes in the blood flow. The predominant innervation is adrenergic. Catecholamines lead to increased fluid secretion. They cause opening of apical Cl^- channels and basolateral K^+ channels, and lead to secretion of Cl^-. Na^+ diffuses by the paracellular route, resulting in an isotonic NaCl secretion. The beat rate of the cilia is also increased by activation of β-adrenoceptors.

Smooth muscle

Airway smooth muscle is unusual in many respects. It is electrically inexcitable, due to the strongly rectifying properties of the cell membranes. In some species, it can maintain a small degree of spontaneous myogenic tone, which may be associated with slow wave activity in the cell membranes (Fig. 8.31). The cells are well connected electrically, and have a long length constant. Gap junctions can be seen in electron micrographs. Mechanical activity is regulated by changes in membrane potential, and depolarizations of only a few millivolts can trigger contraction.

In spite of the network of cholinergic nerve fibres running in the intra-

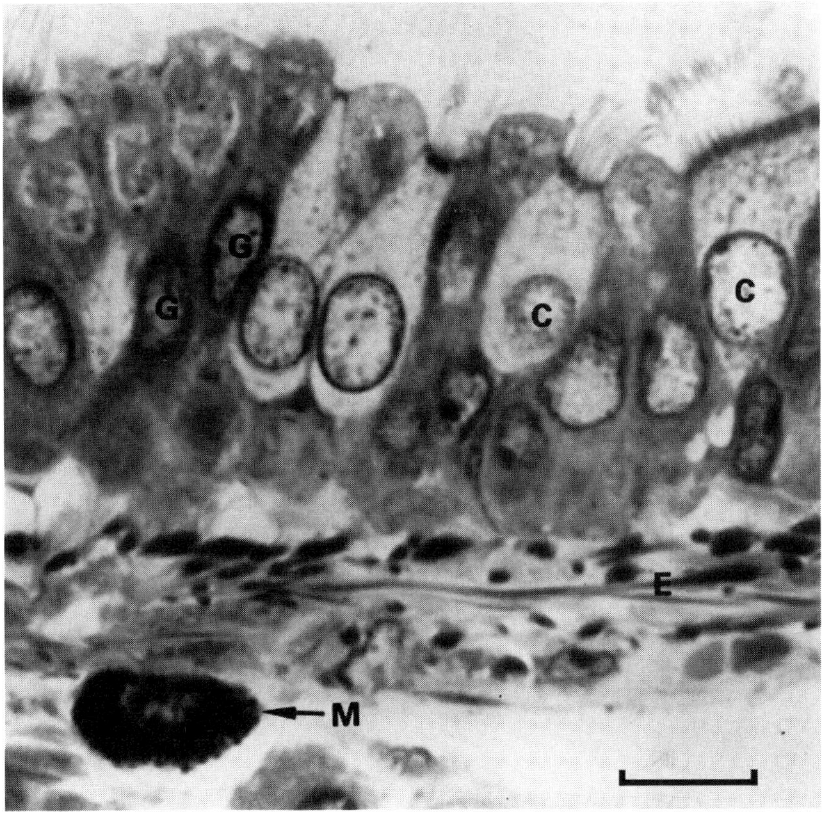

Fig. 8.30 Light micrograph of a thin section of the bronchial epithelium from a rat. The epithelium is pseudostratified – that is the bases of all the cells extend down to the basement membrane, but not all the cells reach the luminal surface. The epithelium contains goblet cells (G), which contain mucous and stain darkly, and ciliated cells (C) with large nuclei. The underlying lamina propria contains elastin and mast cells (M). Scale bar: 20 μm. From Burkett (1993), with permission from the publisher, Churchill Livingstone.

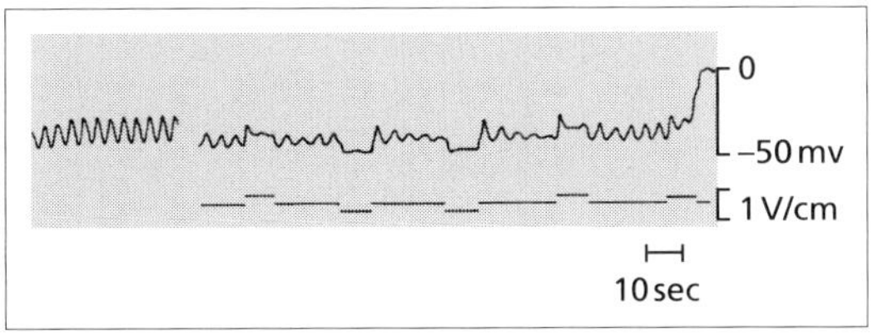

Fig. 8.31 Microelectrode recording of spontaneous electrical activity in bovine tracheal smooth muscle, and the effects of conditioning hyperpolarization and depolarization. These slow waves are sensitive to the membrane potential. Hyperpolarization reduces the amplitude, and depolarization triggers a slow wave. Adapted from Kirkpatrick (1981).

muscular septa, the penetration of varicose nerve endings into the smooth muscle bundles is sparse. In humans, there is less than one axon per 100 muscle cell profiles in electron-microscopic sections in the trachea, and only 18 in the more densely innervated bronchi. The majority of the axon profiles seen are some distance (100 nm–1 μm) from the smooth muscle, although examination of serial sections would be necessary to exclude some close junctions. Since the activity of the nerves seems to be the most important regulator of smooth muscle tone, it is perhaps a little surprising that the innervation is so sparse in comparison with other smooth muscles; but the good electrical connectivity between the cells, and their sensitivity to depolarization, may make the neural control more efficient than it would appear.

Stimulation of the intrinsic nerves in bovine tracheal smooth muscle causes muscarinic excitatory junction potentials, each of which is associated with a slow, phasic contraction (Fig. 8.32). Application of excitatory agonists is also always associated with depolarization, where it has been studied. In humans, there is a small excitatory response to stimulation of α-adrenoceptors in the trachea, which can be revealed after blockade of the β-adrenoceptors, but the predominant response of the smooth muscle to catecholamines is a β-adrenoceptor-mediated relaxation, accompanied by hyperpolarization of the membrane. This is effective at reducing the con-

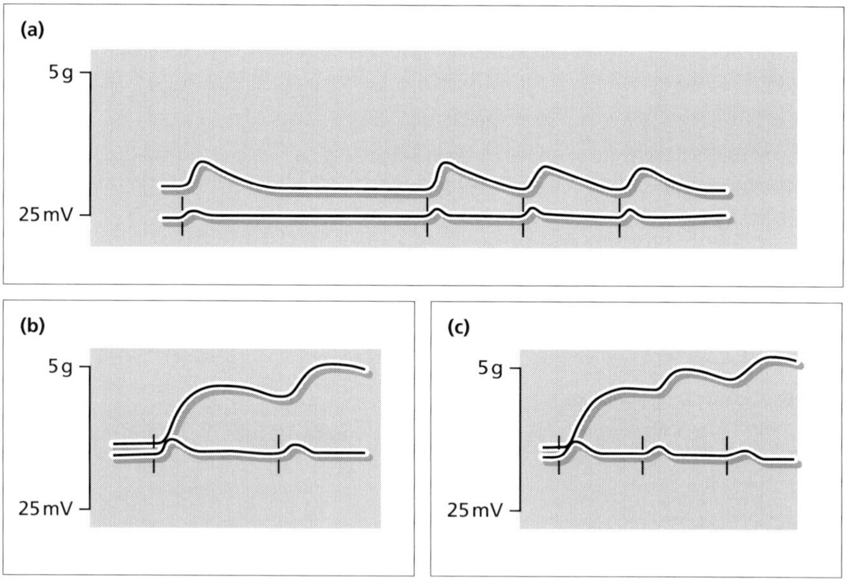

Fig. 8.32 Effect of stimulation of intrinsic parasympathetic nerves on the membrane potential (lower traces) and contractile activity (upper traces) of bovine tracheal smooth muscle. (a) Single shocks are associated with discrete excitatory junction potentials (EJPs) and phasic contractions, (b) and (c). At higher frequencies of stimulation the EJPs remain separate, but the contractions fuse. Note that no action potentials are evoked. Both types of activity are abolished by muscarinic receptor blockade with atropine. Adapted from Kirkpatrick (1981).

tractile response to activation of the cholinergic nerves. As there is no evidence of inhibitory sympathetic innervation of the smooth muscle, these receptors are presumably normally activated by circulating catecholamines.

8.4.3 Functions of smooth muscle innervation

The diameter of the airways has important implications for the functioning of the lungs. Constriction of the upper airways reduces the airway conductance, whilst constriction of the terminal airways and alveolar sphincters reduces the lung compliance by closing off groups of alveoli.

The overall level of contraction will determine the dead space of the lungs, and this is known to be regulated as the tidal volume changes to give maximum efficiency – thus, in the resting state, where the tidal volume is low, efficiency is increased with a reduction in the dead space, since at constant tidal volume, the smaller the dead space, the greater the alveolar ventilation. With small tidal volumes, and thus relatively low flow rates, there can be significant decreases in airway diameter without too much of an increase in frictional resistance. In exercise, on the other hand, where the necessity for a large alveolar ventilation means that there is a high air flow through the tubes, greater efficiency is achieved with a wider diameter, even at the expense of a larger dead space. Thus, there is decreased vagal activity during exercise, and increased activity during quiet breathing. There are also breath-by-breath changes in vagal activity in quiet breathing, with a rhythmic cycle of reflex dilation and constriction during inspiration and expiration.

Protective reflexes involving secretion and smooth muscle activity can be triggered by irritation of the mucosa, and in many disease states, such as asthma, anaphylaxis and bronchitis, sensitisation of afferent nerve endings and enhanced reflex activation of the smooth muscle, leading to bronchoconstriction, have been shown to occur.

8.4.4 Relevant pharmacology

Pharmacological intervention is frequently appropriate in various diseases of the respiratory system. The various systems targeted are as follows.

Airway smooth muscle

Relaxation is produced by administration of β_2-specific adrenoceptor agonists, in particular salbutamol (marketed as Ventolin). This can be given either orally or by inhalation. The drugs may act indirectly by reducing the effectiveness of vagal activity, or directly on the smooth muscles to elevate cellular cAMP, resulting in activation of various A kinases. The smooth muscle relaxing effects of these kinases include the enhanced Ca extrusion from the cell, and the reduction of the affinity of myosin light chain kinase for Ca. Cardiovascular side effects are a problem, and for patients who cannot tolerate these, another smooth muscle relaxant, theophylline – a methylxanthine – is often used. This is usually administered chelated with ethylenediamine (forming aminophylline), which increases its solubility. The precise mechanism of action is uncertain. The methylxanthines are known to inhibit phosphodiesterase in smooth muscle cells, and elevate the levels of cAMP, thus mimicking the actions of the β-adrenoceptor agonists, but they also have other actions – for instance, they can block some purinoceptors. Unlike the β-adrenoceptor agonists, the methylxanthines cross the blood–brain barrier, and may have useful effects at the level of the brainstem, where they tend to enhance autonomic output (both sympathetic and parasympathetic). It is noticeable that many people who find salbutamol intolerable can tolerate aminophylline.

Mucosa

Inflammation can be reduced by inhalation of steroids. This will be effective not only through reduction of oedema and excess secretory activity, but also by reducing the sensitivity of the nerve endings and reducing reflex activation of the vagus. Codeine can be used to reduce the central cough-generating effects of stimulation of the irritant nerves. Expectorants and mucolytics are used to promote the removal of secretions, and antibiotics to control infections. Prophylactic protection against anaphylactic reactions to antigens (for instance in asthma) can be achieved by inhalation of disodium cromoglycate (Intal), although its mechanism of action is unclear.

Further reading

Di Francesco, D. (1993) Pacemaker mechanisms in cardiac tissue. *Ann. Rev. Physiol.* **55**, 455–72.

Hutter, O.F. (1961) *Nervous Inhibition*. Pergamon Press, Oxford.

Janig, W. & McLachlan, E.M. (1992) Characteristics of function-specific pathways in the sympathetic nervous system. *Trends in Neuroscience* **15** (12), 475–81.

Kirkpatrick, C.T. (1981) Tracheobronchial smooth muscle. In: *Smooth Muscle: An Assessment of Current Knowledge* (eds E. Bülbring, A.F. Brading, A.W. Jones & T. Tomita). Edward Arnold , London.

Levick, J.R. (1991) *An Introduction to Cardiovascular Physiology*. Butterworths, London.

Luff, S.E. (1996) Ultrastructure of sympathetic axons and their structural relationship with vascular smooth muscle. *Anat. Embryol. Berl.* **193**, 515–31.

McHale, N.G. (1993) Nervous control of the lymphatic system. *Vascular Medicine Review* **4**, 307–19.

Rang, H.P., Dale, M.M. and Ritter, J.M. (1995) *Pharmacology*, 3rd edn, Churchill Livingstone, Edinburgh.

Vizi, E.S. (1984) *Nonsynaptic Interaction Between Neurones*. J. H. Wiley, Chichester.

References

Amiri, M.H. & Gabella, G. (1988) Structure of the guinea-pig trachea at rest and in contraction. *Anat. Embryol.* **178**, 389–97.

Binns, R.M., Gillman, T. & Ruskin, J. (1970) Aspects of the microanatomy of the structures and microcirculation in the calf's lymph nodes. *J. Physiol.* **210**, 117–18.

Bramich, N.J., Brock, J.A., Edwards, F.R. & Hirst, G.D. Iontophoretically applied acetylcholine and vagal stimulation in the arrested sinus venosus of the toad, *Bufo marinus*. *J. Physiol.* **478** (2), 289–300.

Burkett, H.G., Young, B., Heath, J.W., Wheater, P.R. & Deakin, P.J. (1993) *Wheater's Functional Histology*. Churchill Livingstone, Edinburgh.

DiFrancesco, D. & Mangoni, M. (1994) Modulation of single hyperpolarization-activated channels (If) by cAMP in the rabbit sino-atrial node. *J. Physiol.* **474**, 473–82.

Furchgott, R.F. & Zawadzki, J.V. (1980) The obligatory role of endothelial cells in the relaxation of arterial smooth muscle by acetylcholine. *Nature* **288**, 373–6.

Furness, J.B. & Marshall, J.M. (1974) Correlation of the directly observed responses of mesenteric vessels of the rat to nerve stimulation and noradrenaline with the distribution of adrenergic nerves. *J. Physiol.* **239**, 75–88.

Giles, W. & Noble, S.J. (1976) Changes in membrane currents in bullfrog atrium produced by acetylcholine. *J. Physiol.* **261**, 103–23.

Gillman, T., Binns, R.M. & Ruskin, J.J. (1970) Aspects of the micro-anatomy of the structures and microcirculation of the calf's lymph nodes. *J. Physiol.* **210**, 117.

Golenhofen, K., Hermstein, N. & Lammel, E. (1973) Membrane potential and contraction of vascular smooth muscle (portal vein) during application of noradrenaline and high potassium and selective inhibitory effects of iproveratril (verapamil). *Microvascular Research*, **5**, 73–80.

Hutter, O.F. & Trautwein, W. (1956) Vagal and sympathetic effects on the pacemaker fibers in the sinus venosus of the heart. *J. Gen. Physiol.* **39**, 715.

Jalife, J. & Moe, G.K. (1979) Phasic effects of vagal stimulation on pacemaker activity of the isolated sinus node of the young cat. *Arc Res.* **45**, 595–608.

Johnson, P.C. & Intaglietta, M. (1976) Contributions of pressure and flow sensitivity to autoregulation in mesenteric arterioles. *Am. J. Physiol.* **231**, 1686–98.

McHale, N.G., Roddie, I.C. & Thornbury, K.D. (1980) Nervous modulation of spontaneous contractions in bovine mesenteric lymphatics. *J. Physiol.* **309**, 461–72.

Sarnoff, S.J., & Mitchell, J.H. (1962) *Handbook of Physiology, Cardiovascular System,* Vol. 1, *Circulation*. American Physiological Society, Baltimore.

Sneddon, P. & Burnstock, G. (1984) ATP as a co-transmitter in rat tail artery. *European J. Pharmacol.* **106**, 149–52.

9 : Gastrointestinal Systems

9.1 Introduction

The autonomic innervation of the gut is extremely complicated. The intrinsic neurones of the enteric nervous system (the nerve plexuses in the gut wall) are as numerous as the neurones in the cerebellum, and of sufficient complexity to ensure that the gut can perform the vast majority of its functions in a co-ordinated manner totally independent of the central nervous system. The central nervous system can, however, influence the enteric nervous system, and it does this through the other divisions of the autonomic nervous system, the parasympathetic and sympathetic systems, which supply what could be called the 'extrinsic' as opposed to the 'intrinsic' innervation of the gut (see Figs 2.15–2.18, pp. 35–7). The extrinsic control of the gut is concerned with such things as the preparation of the gut for the receipt of food, the evacuation of the faeces at a convenient time and place, and the shutting down of the activity of the gut when the body has more important demands on its energy resources.

We will deal first here with the general properties of the enteric nervous system and the extrinsic control of the gut by the sympathetic and parasympathetic systems. We will then examine in more detail the role of the autonomic nervous system in the motility and secretory/absorptive activity of the individual regions of the gut.

9.2 The intrinsic innervation of the gut

The enteric nervous system controls motility of the gut and the transport of water and electrolytes across the gut wall. It also modulates blood flow to the gut, and plays a role in the secretion of some gastrointestinal hormones, gastric acid secretion and mucous production.

Most of the intrinsic innervation is found in two networks of interconnected ganglia, the myenteric plexus (Auerbach's plexus) and the submucous plexus (Meissner's plexus), the details of which are given in Chapter 2. The neurones in these plexuses make up complex reflex pathways containing sensory neurones, interneurones and motor neurones within the gut. Figures 9.1–9.3 show some details of the structure. The axons of some neurones run between the two plexuses, interconnecting them, and axons of the motor neurones extensively innervate the smooth muscle layers and the mucosa, often forming separate but non-ganglionated plexuses. The sensory neurones may also project out of the gut and interconnect with the prevertebral ganglia as part of entero-enteric reflex pathways that can influence more distal and proximal parts of the gut, and yet bypass the central nervous system (Fig. 9.4).

The myenteric plexus is found between the longitudinal and circular muscle layers throughout the gut, from the oesophagus to the anal canal. It is a continuous network surrounding the gut circumferentially (Fig. 2.17, p. 37). The submucous plexus is only fully developed in the small and large intestines. Scattered ganglia may occur near the mucosa of other organs.

9.2.1 Identification of neuronal types

Recent histological techniques have enabled the layout of the various plexuses to be seen in whole-mount preparations (Fig. 2.18, p. 37), and in any one species the networks have characteristic patterns in each segment of the gut (Fig. 9.5).

The anatomical details of the innervation of the small intestine of the guinea-pig are being studied in exquisite detail in Australia by J.B. Furness,

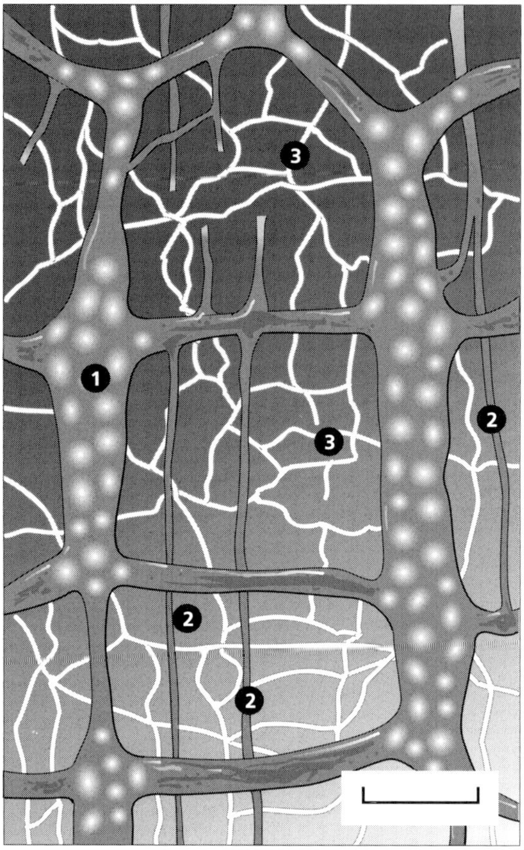

Fig. 9.1 This figure shows the three components of the myenteric plexus in the guinea-pig small intestine. The primary plexus (1) consists of the ganglia and the internodal strands. The secondary component (2) consists of nerve bundles that arise from the primary plexus and run parallel to the circular smooth muscle, between it and the internodal strands. These nerve fibres supply the circular smooth muscle. The third component (3) is a network of small nerve fibres running between the primary meshes at the interface between longitudinal and circular smooth muscle. Adapted from Furness & Costa (1987). Scale bar: 100 μm.

M. Costa and their co-workers. It turns out that populations of neurones with similar structures, anatomical positions and functions usually contain antigenic proteins in combinations that are unique to each type. The antigens provide precise markers for populations of neurones, and their visualisation can be achieved using specific antibodies coupled to various labels. These immunohistochemical techniques are thus a powerful tool for identifying classes of neurones, and have enabled many interesting experiments to be designed that have thrown light on the physiological properties and functions of each class.

Initially, the antibodies used were raised against enzymes known to participate in either the synthesis or breakdown of established classical neurotransmitters, such as choline acetyltransferase (the enzyme synthesising acetylcholine) or tyrosine hydroxylase (involved in the synthesis of catecholamines). Later, antibodies raised against a host of biologically active peptides have been utilised. Multiple staining of the same cells with several antibodies linked to different fluorescent labels has shown that many neuronal classes can be uniquely identified by the expression of a group of antigens, many of which are located on neuropeptides that have been shown to have either a neurotransmitter or neuromodulator function. For example, in

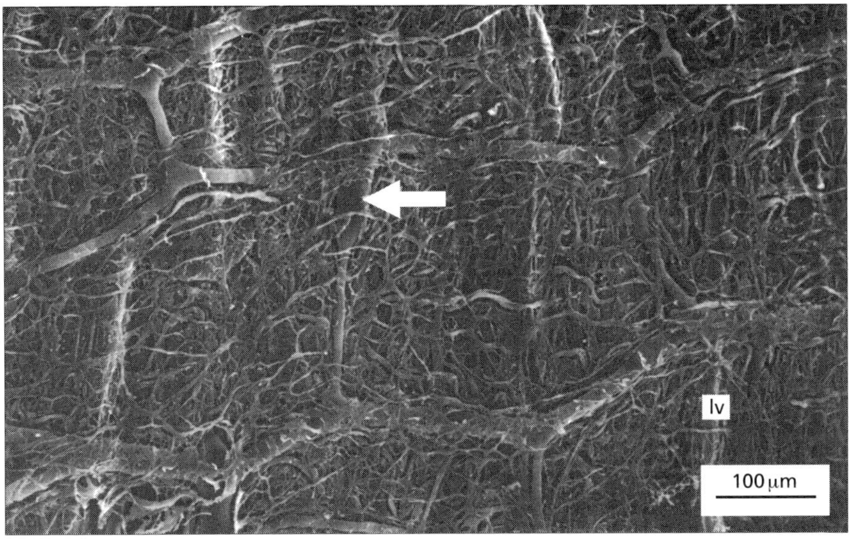

Fig. 9.2 Enzymatic digestion followed by fixation and scanning electron microscopy reveals details of the intermuscular layer between the longitudinal and circular smooth muscles of the guinea-pig small intestine. The meshes of the myenteric plexus are seen covered with a dense network of connective tissue cells. The ganglia are exposed at intervals, for instance at the arrow. This layer also contains blood vessels and lymphatic vessels (one of which (lv) runs across the figure from top to bottom on the right). Bar: 100 μm. From Baluka & Gabella (1987).

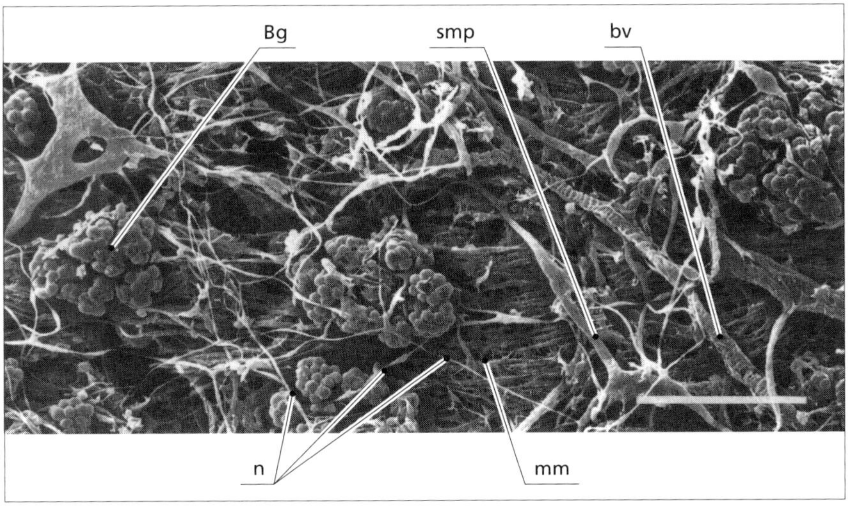

Fig. 9.3 Scanning electron micrograph of the submucosa of the guinea-pig duodenum. Elements visible are the ganglia and connecting strands of the submucous plexus (smp), the grape-like clusters of Brunner's glands (Bg), blood vessels (bv), smooth muscle cells of the muscularis mucosa (mm) and fine nerve fibres (n) innervating the latter three. Scale bar: 100 μm. From Baluka & Gabella (1987).

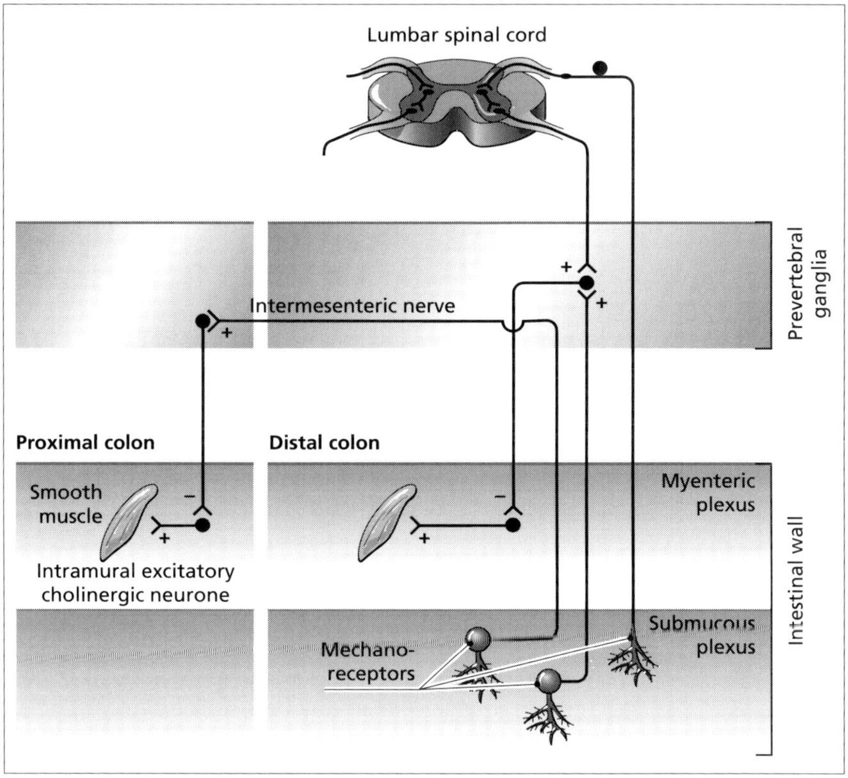

Fig. 9.4 Diagram of sensory pathways. Sensory neurones in the submucous plexus leave the gut and synapse with neurones in the prevertebral ganglia, setting up local reflexes that do not involve the CNS. Other sensory neurones have their cell bodies in the dorsal root ganglia, and their axons enter the spinal cord, taking information to the CNS.

the submucous ganglia in the guinea-pig small intestine, 54% of neurones are putative cholinergic neurones, judged from the fact that they contain choline acetyltransferase (ChAT). However, these can be divided into three groups: some 29% also contain cholecystokinin (CCK), calcitonin gene-related peptide (CGRP), neuropeptide Y (NPY) and somatostatin (SOM); some 11% also contain substance P (SP); and the rest contain ChAT alone of these substances.

With reference to the neurochemistry of the enteric neurones, the fact that the cell bodies contain neuropeptides does not, of course, mean that they necessarily release them at their nerve terminals – it is equally possible that the cell bodies may take up neuropeptides released by axons innervating them. Nevertheless, pharmacological studies of the response of neurones and smooth muscle cells to the stimulation of intrinsic nerves and application of putative neurotransmitters and neuromodulators have identified more than 20 substances that could be potential neurotransmitters. A list of the more important of these is given in Table 9.1. It is clear that there is a very considerable degree of complexity of this system, reminiscent of the

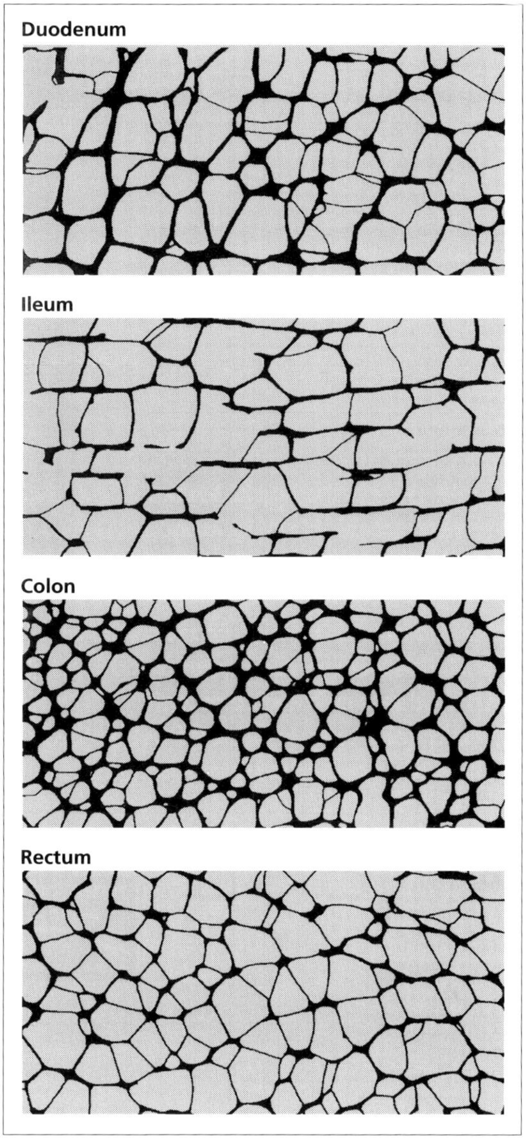

Fig. 9.5 Patterns of the myenteric plexus from various parts of the guinea-pig intestine. Kindly supplied by G. Gabella.

situation in the central nervous system. In fact, the enteric nervous system is often used for experiments that can shed important light on the functions of the central nervous system, and a large number of the important central transmitters have first been discovered in the enteric nervous system.

9.2.2 Functional classes of enteric neurones

Motor neurones

Excitatory muscle motor neurones. These innervate the longitudinal and

Table 9.1 Potential transmitters and neuromodulators in the enteric nervous system.

Excitatory motor neurones	Inhibitory motor neurones	Secretomotor neurones	Interneurones
Acetylcholine*	Nitric oxide*	Acetylcholine*	Acetylcholine*
Substance P*	Vasoactive intestinal polypeptide*	Vasoactive intestinal polypeptide*	Serotonin*
Neurokinin A	ATP	Dynorphin	Substance P*
Neuropeptide γ	Dynorphin	Galinin	At least 15 peptides
Neuropeptide κ	Galinin	Neuromedin U	
Dynorphin	Neuropeptide Y	Cholecystokinin	
Enkephalin	Gastrin-releasing peptide	Calcitonin gene-related peptide	
		Somatostatin	
		Neuropeptide Y	
		Gastrin-releasing peptide	

There are several subclasses of neurones in each group, each of which contains a primary transmitter and a subset of peptides.
* There is evidence that these substances are primary transmitters.

circular muscles, and the muscularis mucosa (the muscle layer under the mucosa). The principal transmitter is acetylcholine, acting through muscarinic receptors. Several peptides are also released from these neurones, and may have longer term actions than acetylcholine. These are principally the tachykinins (substance P and neurokinin A).

Inhibitory muscle motor neurones. These innervate circular and longitudinal smooth muscles. The neurotransmitters vary between regions and species, but it is becoming clear that an important inhibitory transmitter is nitric oxide (NO). Vasoactive intestinal polypeptide (VIP) is also released from several inhibitory neurones, and it is possible that adenosine triphosphate (ATP) may be involved in inhibitory transmission, but this is not well established.

Secretomotor neurones. These enhance the secretion of salts and water across the gut wall into the lumen. There are two classes: cholinergic neurones, which act through muscarinic receptors, and non-adrenergic, non-cholinergic (NANC) neurones, which probably act by releasing VIP, with a similar effect. Another class of cholinergic neurones act on the parietal cells of the gastric mucosa and play a role in gastric acid secretion.

Vasodilator neurones. These act as inhibitory motor neurones on vascular smooth muscle, and probably release VIP.

Interneurones

These act in reflex pathways, and may be ascending or descending. They may be excitatory or inhibitory. Some are cholinergic, some non-cholinergic. Some may use 5-hydroxytryptamine (5-HT) as a transmitter.

Sensory neurones

These may have their cell bodies in the submucosa or in the myenteric plexus. They may be cholinergic or NANC (the transmitters are unknown, but substance P and CGRP are probably important).

9.3 The extrinsic innervation of the gut

9.3.1 The sympathetic system

Structure

The extrinsic sympathetic nerves enter the gut mostly from the prevertebral ganglia and plexuses. The postganglionic axons usually run into the gut wall along with the blood vessels. These fibres form varicose nerve endings, which innervate several different elements in the gut wall.

1 The myenteric plexus contains large numbers of sympathetic axons, with nerve terminals forming synapses on intrinsic neurones. Some cholinergic neurones in particular receive a dense sympathetic input (Fig. 9.6).

2 The submucosal plexus also has a moderately dense sympathetic input, with synaptic connections to some specific neurones.

3 The mucosa receives sympathetic input, with synaptic connections to the mucosal glands.

4 There is a dense sympathetic innervation surrounding the intramural arteries.

There is little, if any, direct sympathetic innervation of the longitudinal smooth muscle cells in most areas of the gut wall, although there may be a sparse sympathetic input to the taeniae and the rectum. There is also only a sparse sympathetic innervation to the majority of circular smooth muscles, and to the smooth muscle in the stomach. Sympathetic relaxation is mediated by inhibition of the cholinergic motor neurones. The only gut smooth muscles that receive a dense sympathetic innervation are the sphincters, where the innervation is excitatory. These include the lower oesophageal sphincter, the pylorus of the stomach, the sphincter of Oddi, the ileocolic sphincter and the internal anal sphincter.

Functions

The main role of the extrinsic sympathetic nerves is inhibition of the activity of the gut. Motility is inhibited by constriction of the sphincters and relaxation of the longitudinal elements of the gut, and secretion is inhibited (with

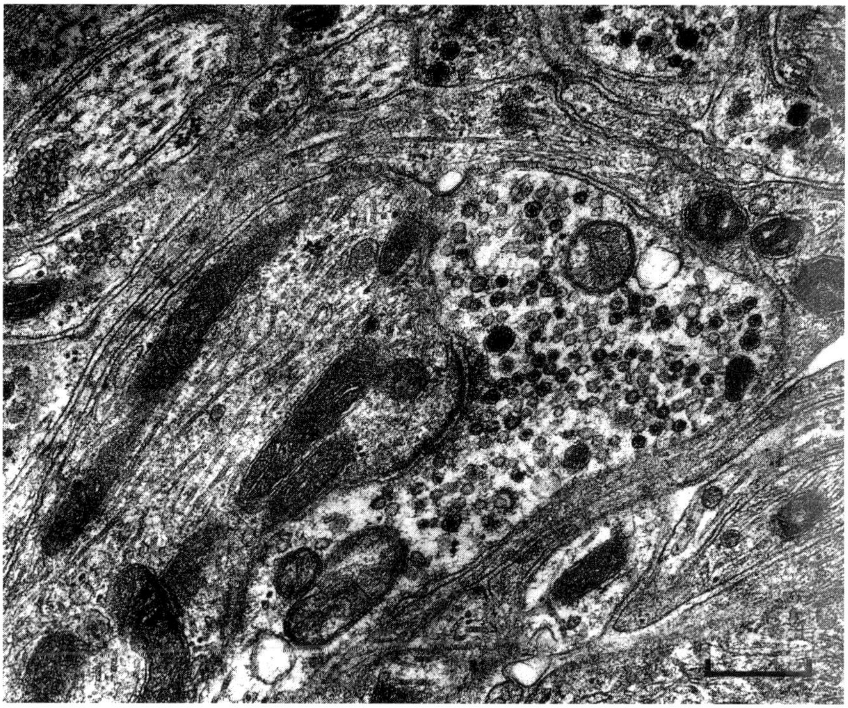

Fig. 9.6 Electron micrograph of an axo-dendritic synapse in a myenteric ganglion in the guinea-pig. The nerve terminal contains small dense-cored vesicles characteristic of postganglionic sympathetic nerves, and is synapsing onto a dendrite of a myenteric neurone containing mitochondria and microtubules. Scale bar: 0.5 μm. Kindly supplied by G. Gabella.

enhanced reabsorption of fluids and electrolytes). Blood flow is reduced and blood is expelled from the splanchnic circulation.

Postganglionic adrenergic fibres inhibit cholinergic motor neurones in the myenteric plexus, reducing ongoing excitation of the smooth muscle. Inhibition may also occur through direct activation of α-adrenoceptors on the longitudinal smooth muscle cells, which hyperpolarise and inhibit these smooth muscles. Circulating adrenaline will activate α- and β-adrenoceptors, both of which are inhibitory, and will also activate presynaptic receptors on cholinergic motor neurones, leading to a reduction in acetylcholine release. In the sphincters, tonic contraction is evoked through activation of excitatory α-adrenoceptors, preventing movement of the gut contents from one part to another.

Activating sympathetic nerves to the gut has profound effects on the blood vessels, due to their dense innervation. Arteries are constricted, increasing the resistance to flow, and veins are also constricted, reducing the volume of blood in the splanchnic vasculature. Since about 20% of the total blood volume of the body may be in the splanchnic circulation, and about 40% of this can be expelled by moderate sympathetic activity, this mechanism can be of considerable use in enhancing blood flow to more important areas of the body in an emergency. Circulating adrenaline has a similar effect, suggesting that α-adrenoceptors mediating the contractile response are more important in this part of the circulation than β-adrenoceptors.

Sympathetic nerves inhibit the secretion of water and electrolytes from the mucosa of the small intestine and probably also the large intestine, and also enhance reabsorption. They exert tonic activity on the secretory mechanisms, so that sympathetic blockade results in a net secretory response of the gut. The sympathetic nerves have their effects mainly on the secretomotor neurones in the submucosal plexus, which they inhibit through activation of α-adrenoceptors. The epithelial mucosal cells are also directly inhibited by noradrenaline, again mainly through α-adrenoceptors. Reduced secretion and enhanced absorption in response to sympathetic activity and circulating catecholamines are clearly appropriate in many emergency situations, such as haemorrhage, or in heavy exercise, when replacement of body fluids and electrolytes is essential. It is interesting that blood vessels supplying the mucosa and secretory and absorptive cells may be dilated through neural and hormonal pathways independent of the catecholamine system, which is presumably necessary to ensure adequate perfusion for fluid absorption in spite of sympathetic vasoconstriction.

9.3.2 The parasympathetic system

Structure

Extrinsic parasympathetic input to the gut comes through the facial and glossopharyngeal nerves (which supply salivary glands opening into the buccal cavity), the vagus, which supplies the upper part of the gut, and the sacral outflow, which controls the distal part of the gut. The vagal fibres enter the gut wall in the region of the stomach as preganglionic neurones. Some of these neurones run down into the small intestine in the myenteric plexus, but the vagal influence falls off with distance down the length of the gut. The sacral input runs through the pelvic plexus. It is not yet known whether the nerves entering the lower gut are preganglionic or postganglionic.

Functions

Vagal input causes receptive relaxation of the stomach, promotion of acid secretion, promotion of gastrin secretion, and enhanced peristalsis in the stomach and possibly also the proximal small bowel. It also enhances secretion in the small intestine. Input from the pelvic nerves enhances motility, secretion and blood flow in the distal colon and rectum. It is involved in the initiation of defecation, particularly causing the peristaltic contractions that evacuate the lower bowel. Preganglionic cholinergic fibres synapse on many of the motor neurones in the intrinsic nerve plexuses, and have excitatory effects, mainly through nicotinic receptors. There is evidence that some of the preganglionic neurones in the vagus may be non-cholinergic.

9.4 Myogenic activity of the smooth muscles

Although the enteric nervous system is essential for the generation of the complex motility patterns in the gut, the majority of the smooth muscles have an underlying myogenic activity, i.e. they possess mechanisms for the generation of rhythmic contractions. In most gut muscles, these are best studied with electrical recordings of the membrane potential, which undergoes regular depolarisations called slow waves (Fig. 9.7). If these are large enough, they can initiate contractions, either by themselves reaching a voltage at which net Ca^{2+} entry occurs, or by triggering action potentials that may both involve Ca^{2+} entry and cause Ca^{2+} release from internal stores (Fig. 9.8). In many parts of the gut, the slow waves may initially be produced by specialised pacemaker cells, the interstitial cells of Cajal, which lie just outside some of the muscle layers, and interconnect both with enteric nerves and with smooth muscle cells. These cells generate large slow waves by unknown mechanisms. They last between two and five seconds, and vary in frequency from three to 30 per minute, depending on the part of the gut and the species studied. Currents associated with the slow waves then spread through gap junctions into the adjacent smooth muscle layers, and activate voltage-sensitive ion channels, resulting in slow waves in the muscle cells with a configuration characteristic of the part of the gut they are recorded from. In Fig. 9.9 examples of electrical activity recorded from the interstitial cells are shown and from the adjacent smooth muscle cells when

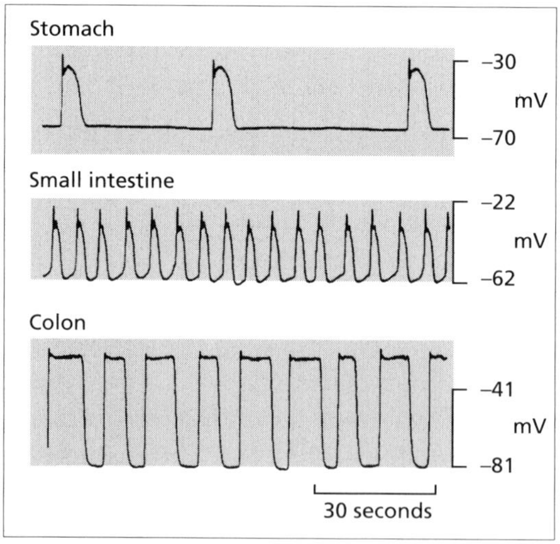

Fig. 9.7 Slow wave activity recorded with intracellular electrodes from the stomach, small intestine and colon of the dog. Although the resting potentials, frequencies and amplitudes of the slow waves differ, each consists of a rapid upstroke with a spike-like top, repolarizing to a plateau depolarization followed by rapid repolarization to the baseline. Adapted from Sanders (1992).

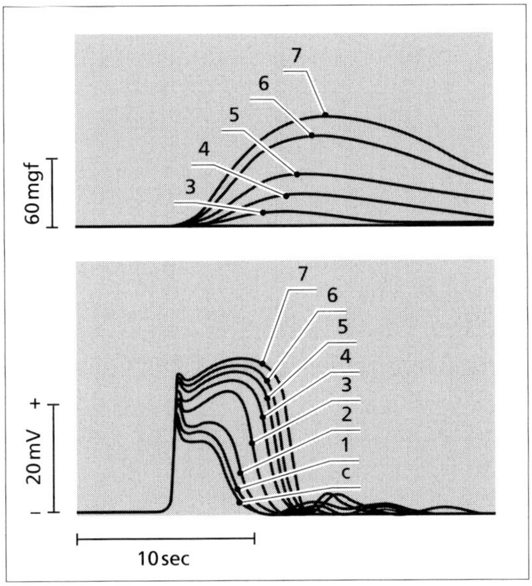

Fig. 9.8 The effects of acetylcholine on the slow waves (lower traces) and their evoked contractions (upper traces) recorded from the antrum of the dog stomach. In the lower trace, c labels the control slow wave, which did not evoke a mechanical response. Increasing concentrations of acetylcholine (traces 1–7) increased the amplitude and duration of the electrical slow waves, and from traces 3 onwards, a contractile response was evoked, which also increased with increasing acetylcholine concentration. Adapted from Szurszewski, (1975).

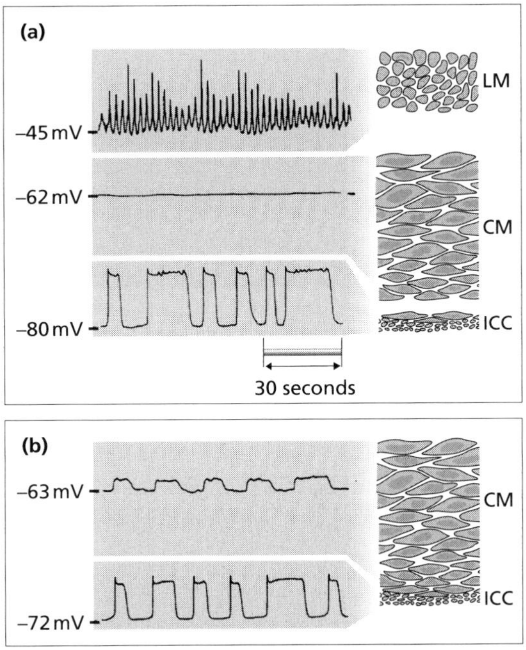

Fig. 9.9 Electrical activity recorded from isolated segments of the dog colon. On the right the cells are shown. (a) The muscle layers have been experimentally isolated from each other. Under these conditions the longitudinal smooth muscle (LM) shows spike-like activity, the circular smooth muscle (CM) is silent, and the interstitial cells of Cajal (ICC) produce large slow waves. (b) The CM layer remains attached to the ICC. Under these conditions the superficial cells of the CM show regular slow waves of the same rhythm as the ICC. Cells nearer to the ICC will show larger slow waves. Adapted from Liu & Huizinga (1993).

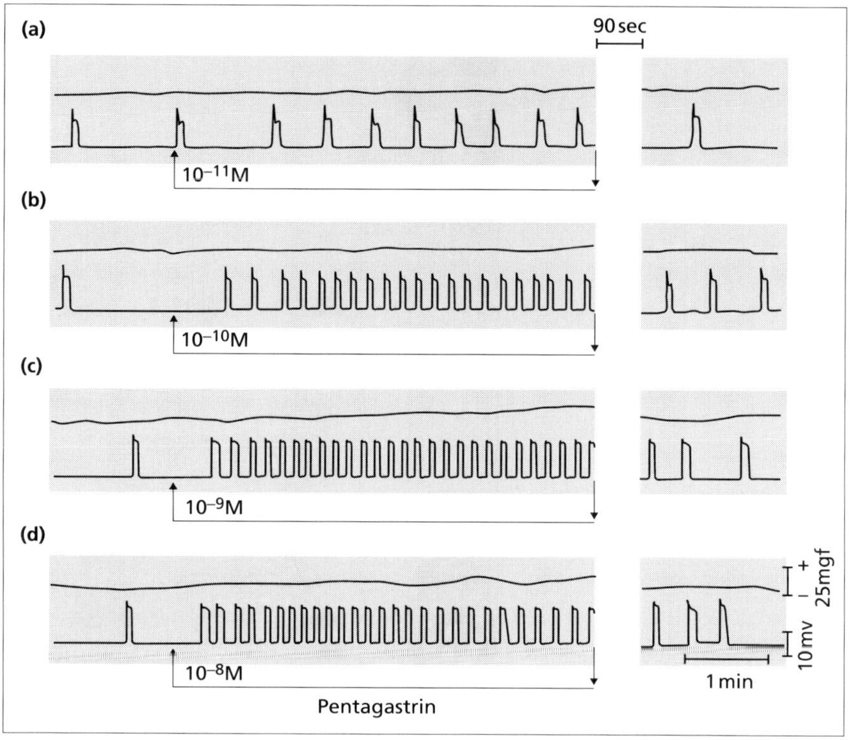

Fig. 9.10 The effects of increasing concentrations of the peptide pentagastrin on the slow wave frequency in the dog stomach. Note that, regardless of their frequency, the slow waves are not initiating contractions. Adapted from Szurszewski (1975).

they are either experimentally isolated from the interstitial cells or with their normal contact. Each area of gut also tends to have slow waves of a characteristic frequency. In the small intestine, the intrinsic frequency decreases from the duodenum to the terminal ileum, and because the cells are electrically coupled, their interactions result in propagation of activity in the oral-to-anal direction. The effects of the enteric nervous system on motility operate on these basic mechanisms. The underlying frequency of the slow waves is very insensitive to changes in the membrane potential of the smooth muscle cells (see Fig. 7.13), and thus classical autonomic transmitters that cause alterations of the membrane potential of the smooth muscles have little effect on the frequency of the slow waves. Such transmitters can, however, easily alter the magnitude of the slow waves, and determine whether or not they initiate action potentials, so altering the size of the contraction triggered. The activity of neuropeptides and hormones may, on the other hand, alter the frequency of the slow waves, presumably acting at the level of the cells of Cajal (Fig. 9.10).

9.5 The role of the autonomic nervous system in gut motility

9.5.1 Oesophagus

The oesophagus is a particularly interesting organ, as it is controlled voluntarily both by striated muscle in the striated region and also by smooth muscle. Particularly interesting is the fact that peristaltic waves in the smooth muscle are activated in response to the voluntary initiation of swallowing, which triggers the primary peristaltic response. The striated muscle of the oesophagus is controlled by somatic motor neurones, which run from the brainstem to the oesophagus with the vagus. Swallowing, triggered by activation of sensory fibres in the oropharynx, begins a sequence in which the tonic activity of the upper striated sphincter is inhibited, and the oesophageal body is sequentially activated, producing a contractile wave, which then passes into the smooth part of the oesophagus, initiating a true peristaltic wave involving the circular and longitudinal elements of the smooth muscle, as described below for the small intestine (Fig. 9.11). Distension of the upper oesophagus by a food bolus triggers secondary peristalsis via sensory pathways passing to the brainstem, and vagal efferents, which co-ordinate with the primary wave to ensure the smooth passage of the bolus towards the stomach.

The isolated smooth section of the oesophagus can produce a peristaltic reflex in response to distension without involvement of the extrinsic innervation. Since there are no submucous ganglia, the cell bodies involved in the reflex must all lie in the myenteric plexus.

The lower oesophageal sphincter is a circular smooth muscle sphincter, which is normally tonically contracted through myogenic mechanisms. It is densely innervated by excitatory and inhibitory neurones, and will contract further in response to increases in gastric pressure through a vagovagal reflex to prevent reflux. Passage of food into the stomach is by relaxation of the sphincter, mediated through inhibitory nerves that are predominantly nitrergic (using NO as a transmitter).

9.5.2 Stomach

The stomach can be divided into different parts, the smooth muscles and innervation of which have different properties. The divisions of the stomach are shown in Fig. 9.12. The proximal parts of the stomach, the fundus and corpus, show less slow wave activity than the distal part, the antrum and pylorus. The proximal parts of the stomach are involved in reception and storage of the food, and are characterised by receptive relaxation to a bolus of food entering the stomach from the oesophagus, and further relaxation to increasing volumes of food. During digestion in the

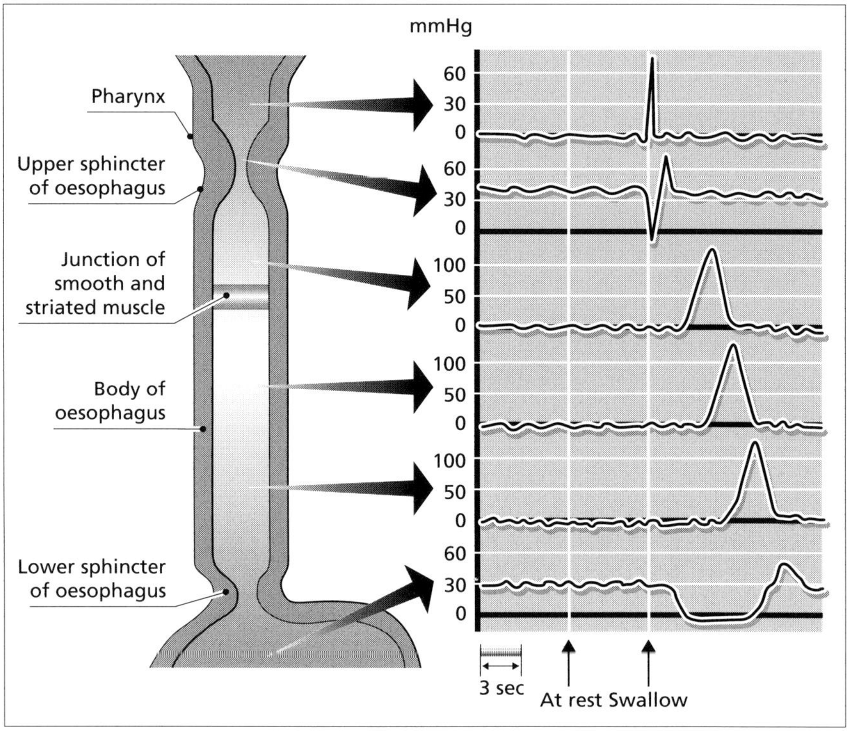

Fig. 9.11 Diagram of the pharynx, oesophagus and oesophageal sphincters and the changes in pressure recorded during a swallow. Note the reflex reduction in pressure (relaxation) of the sphincters initiated by swallowing, the rapid activation of the striated muscle and the peristaltic wave progressing along the smooth muscle segment of the oesophagus. Adapted from Berne and Levy.

stomach, the proximal smooth muscle can produce sustained tone. This tonic activity and the receptive relaxation involve activation of extrinsic nerves (in isolated preparations, activation of the vagus initiates contraction through cholinergic mechanisms and NANC relaxation, which can be demonstrated after blocking the cholinergic excitation with atropine), but the input is relayed through the intrinsic ganglia. The more distal stomach can use the myogenic slow waves to initiate peristaltic waves that run over the pyloric end of the stomach, and which produce mixing and break-up of the food contents, and finally, in combination with relaxation of the pyloric sphincter, expulsion of the liquid chyme into the duodenum (Fig. 9.13). This peristaltic activity can be sustained entirely through the intrinsic innervation of the stomach. The activity is also controlled by production of local hormones – gastrin markedly enhances the frequency of the slow wave production (Fig. 9.10) – and intrinsic reflex nerve pathways between the duodenum and stomach. Extrinsic input can, however, modulate this activity.

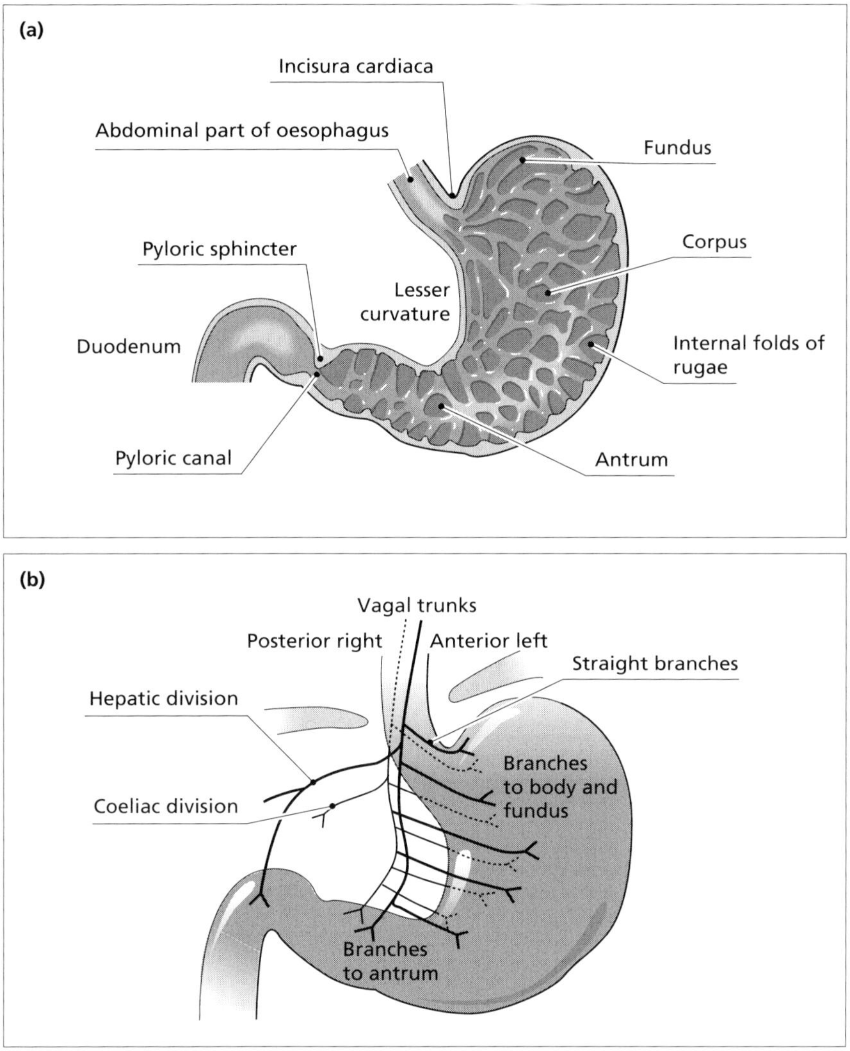

Fig. 9.12 Diagrams of the stomach. (a) Shows the different regions (fundus, corpus, antrum and pylorus) in a bisected stomach, and the foldings of the epithelium (rugae). (b) The vagal innervation of the stomach.

9.5.3 Small intestine

Motility in the small intestine is designed to allow mixing of the semiliquid chyme with digestive enzymes, its exposure to the absorptive surfaces of the small intestine and its net aboral movement.

Segmentation and pendular activity

After feeding, the main type of activity seen in the small intestine is segmentation. This is alternate contraction and relaxation of short segments (bands)

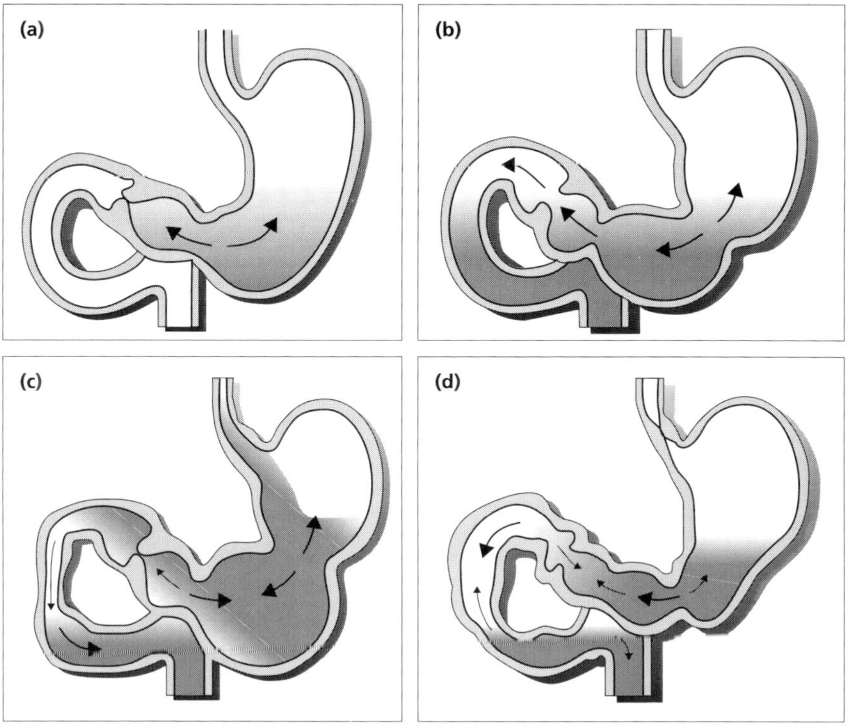

Fig. 9.13 Diagrams showing the activity in the stomach during filling and emptying. (a) Peristaltic waves mix the contents. (b) Transient relaxation and opening of the pyloric sphincter allows emptying of some of the contents. (c) Closure of pyloric sphincter and more vigorous peristalsis in the antrum and pylorus. (d) Late emptying with relaxed pyloric sphincter and strong peristaltic contractions in the antrum.

of circular muscle. Adjacent segments are coupled, so that when one segment contracts, the adjacent segments relax (Fig. 9.14). This activity divides and mixes the contents of the intestine. The frequency of the contractions and relaxations is determined by the underlying slow wave activity, but it is reflex activity in the intrinsic nervous system that results in the waxing and waning of the effectiveness of the slow waves in triggering mechanical activity. Presumably, some form of reciprocal innervation of adjacent parts of the gut is involved. This type of activity is also responsible for the slow propulsion of the gut contents along the intestine, since each part has its own inherent rhythmicity, the slow wave frequencies being higher orally and progressively declining in the aboral direction. Models show that the coupling of out-of-phase oscillatory circuits can result in a progressive movement of activity. Coupling in the gut is thought to occur through the gap junctions between the smooth muscle cells, and results in the slow aboral movement of the food contents (0.5–2 cm/min) without peristaltic activity. Rhythmic activity in the longitudinal muscle is also seen,

Motility pattern	Site	Function
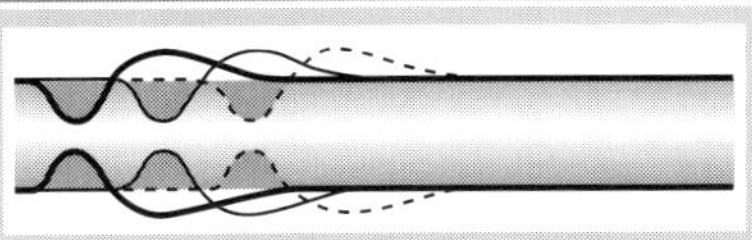 Peristalsis	Oesophagus Stomach Small intestine	Propulsive, causes transport, non-propulsive causes mixing
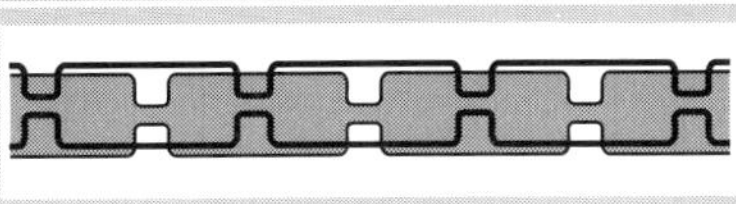 Rhythmic segmentation	Small and large intestines	Mixing and slow propulsion
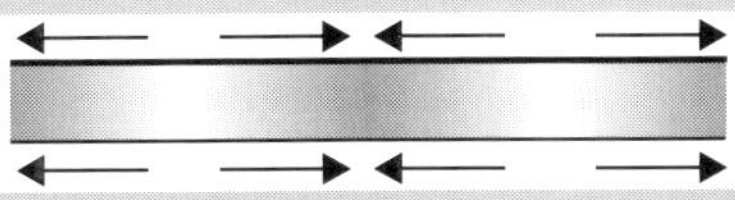 Pendular activity	Small and large intestines	Longitudinal movement of bowel wall over column of chyme
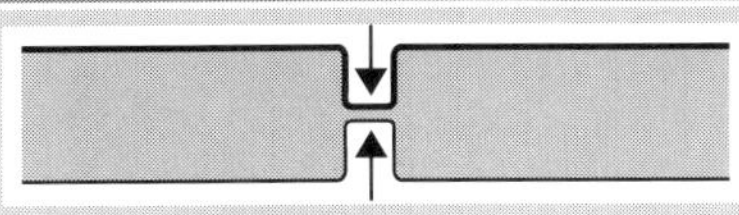 Tonic contraction	Gastrointestinal sphincters	Blocking passage Separation

Fig. 9.14 Different types of mechanical activity in the gastrointestinal tract. Peristalsis is triggered by reflex activity in the enteric plexuses. Segmentation and pendular activity are triggered myogenically through the electrical slow waves. Sphincters have myogenic tone, which may be re-enforced by excitatory nerve activity from the enteric nervous system, and relaxed by inhibitory nerves.

usually called pendular activity, and, again, slow waves in the smooth muscle membranes underlie the activity (Fig. 9.14).

Peristalsis

Fast propulsive movements caused through the peristaltic reflex are seen less often than segmentation and pendular activity in the normal small intestine, but may occasionally occur over restricted lengths of the intestine. Peristalsis can move the food contents at the rate of 3–4 cm/s. It is a complex reflex involving the intrinsic nervous system, and can be triggered by local stretching of the small intestine. The threshold of the sensory nerves initiating the peristaltic reflex is subject to modulation by locally produced inflammatory agents and bacterial toxins, and in some types of food poisoning the whole of the small intestine can become activated by peristaltic rushes, which result in the emptying of the small intestine, and which progress through the large intestine, resulting in diarrhoea.

The sequence of muscular events in the peristaltic reflex predominantly concerns the circular muscle, although there is evidence in guinea-pig intestine for synchronous but opposite response of the longitudinal muscle. Ahead of the point of stimulus (anally), relaxation of the circular muscle is triggered and activation of the longitudinal muscle, resulting in a drop in pressure of the gut contents. Behind the stimulus (orally), contraction of the circular muscle occurs, with a reduction in longitudinal muscle tone and an increase in pressure resulting in the anal propulsion of the chyme.

The circuitry underlying the peristaltic reflex has been studied intensively for many years, and is still not yet entirely resolved. In the small intestine there may be built-in circuits of reciprocal excitatory and inhibitory innervation of the longitudinal and circular smooth muscles at the same location, since there is evidence that they are never normally activated together, and also there may be a similar reciprocal innervation to adjacent parts of the ileum, since in segmentation, as well as peristalsis, adjacent areas constrict or dilate. Excitation of both longitudinal and circular smooth muscles is largely through cholinergic motor neurones and muscarinic acetylcholine receptors, although other excitatory transmitters may be involved. Direct inhibition of the smooth muscle cells is seen more often in circular smooth muscle than longitudinal smooth muscle, and is NANC. Candidates for the transmitter are NO, ATP and VIP. Inhibition may also be through reduction of tonic excitatory input. The cell bodies of the sensory neurones lie in the myenteric plexus; some have their sensory nerve terminals in the mucosa, and some in the muscle layers. The sensory neurones project both orally (ascending projection) and anally (descending projection). The descending inhibitory pathway to the circular smooth muscle is polysynaptic, with excitatory cholinergic (nicotinic) synapses on the interneurones. The descending excitation of the longitudinal smooth muscle is probably activated by the same sensory neurones, and also involves a polysynaptic pathway, possibly with 5-HT as an excitatory synaptic transmitter onto the motor neurone exciting the longitudinal smooth muscle. The ascending pathway also involves polysynaptic excitation of cholinergic motor neurones to the circular smooth muscle and inhibition of the longitudinal smooth muscle – the latter predominantly through reduction in the cholinergic input to the muscle.

In the colon, however, during peristalsis the longitudinal and circular smooth muscles are activated or inhibited together, stretch at a point initiating co-ordinated excitation of both layers of muscle oral to the stimulus, and relaxation of both layers in the aboral direction. A tentative circuit is shown in Fig. 9.15. This pattern may be useful for the propulsion of faecal pellets.

9.5.4 Gall-bladder and sphincter of Oddi

The gall-bladder wall is composed of smooth muscle with an endothelial lining (see Fig. 9.16). The sphincter of Oddi, which controls the release of bile into the duodenum, is also composed of smooth muscle. Although hormones play a major role in the expulsion of bile, the gall-bladder and the

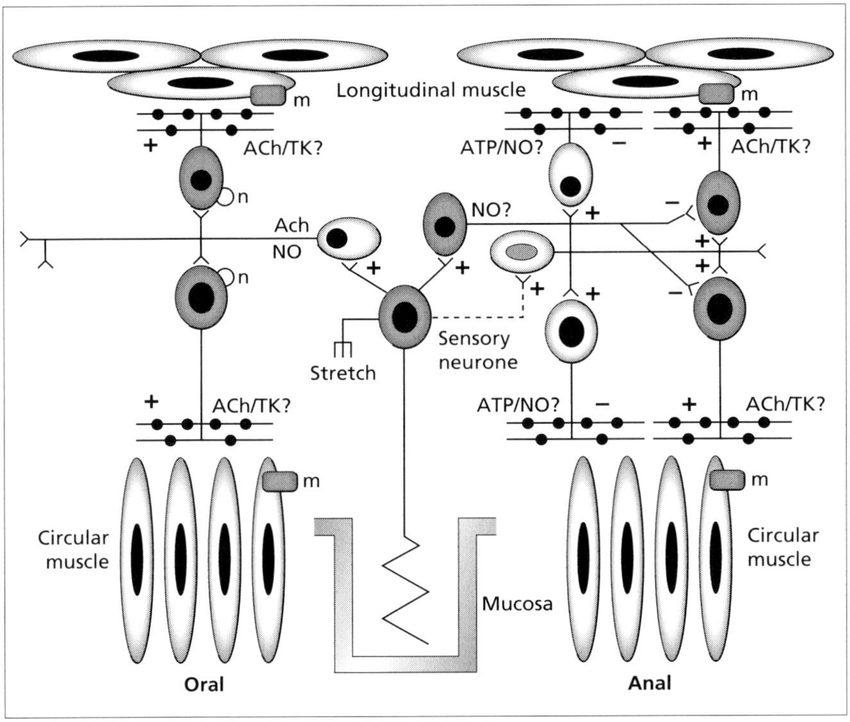

Fig. 9.15 A tentative circuit for the peristaltic reflex in the guinea-pig colon. Sensory neurones in the myenteric plexus have their sensory terminals in the mucosa and/or the smooth muscle layer, and are responsive to stretch and chemical stimuli. These activate both ascending and descending pathways. The ascending pathways activate motor neurones to both circular and longitudinal smooth muscles. The descending pathways excite inhibitory interneurones to the circular and longitudinal smooth muscles, and inhibit excitatory interneurones. The more powerful contractions of the circular smooth muscle orally combined with the relaxation anally will tend to propel the faecal pellet towards the anus. The simultaneous contraction of the longitudinal muscle orally will pull the intestine over the rear of the pellet. From Smith & Robertson (1998). n, nicotinic receptor; m, muscarinic receptor; TK, tachykinin; ACh; acetylcholine; NO, nitric oxide; ATP, adenosine triphosphate.

sphincter of Oddi are densely innervated by autonomic nerves (see Fig. 9.17), with intramural ganglia present. These neurones can be classified as part of the enteric nervous system, and are involved in the co-ordination of the secretory and motor activity of the gut, including the migrating motor complex. Immunocytochemistry demonstrates the presence of many peptidergic neurones which may be involved in modulating both contractile activity and the reabsorptive and secretory activity of the gall-bladder (see Section 9.6.7). The gall-bladder is innervated by the vagus which activates the smooth muscle through muscarinic receptor stimulation and helps in expulsion of the bile, and also by the sympathetic nerves which appear to act on the vagal terminals to inhibit acetylcholine release by activation of presynaptic α_2-adrenoceptors. There are also non-adrenergic, non-cholinergic inhibitory nerves present. The sphincter of Oddi has sponta-

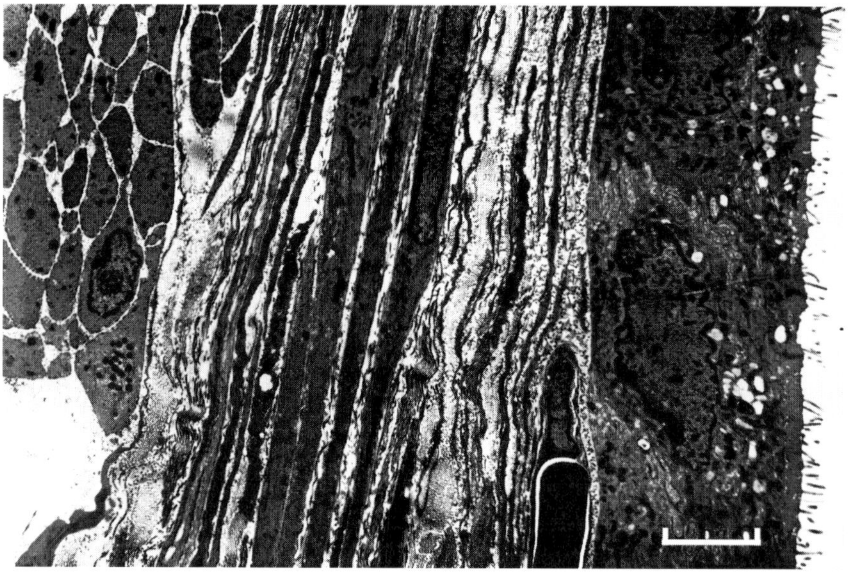

Fig. 9.16 Full thickness section of the gall-bladder from a guinea-pig. Note from the right the epithelium with a capillary in the stroma under it containing a red blood cell. Then two layers of smooth muscle cells in different orientations separated by connective tissue containing collagen. Scale bar: 5 μm. Micrograph kindly provided by Giorgio Gabella.

neous myogenic tone, which can be increased or decreased by activity of intramural neurones. The vagus acting through muscarinic receptors can increase the contractile activity of the sphincter, as can activation of opiate receptors. Neurones containing enkephalin-like immunoreactivity are present. Relaxation of the sphincter of Oddi appears to be due mainly to release of NO from inhibitory nerves, but sympathetic innervation may also play a role in generating relaxation of the sphincter.

9.5.5 Large intestine

Activity in the large intestine is designed to allow the absorption of water and electrolytes from the chyme to form the solid faeces, to allow the development and maintenance of the micro-organisms that are involved in the breakdown of food, and to allow the evacuation of the faeces in the process of defecation.

Ileocaecal junction

The small and large intestines are linked through the ileocaecal junction – this is a 4-cm long segment that acts as a sphincter, with the circular muscle in a state of tonic contraction. Dilation of the terminal ileum results in reflex relaxation of the sphincter, whereas a rise in pressure in the colon causes a

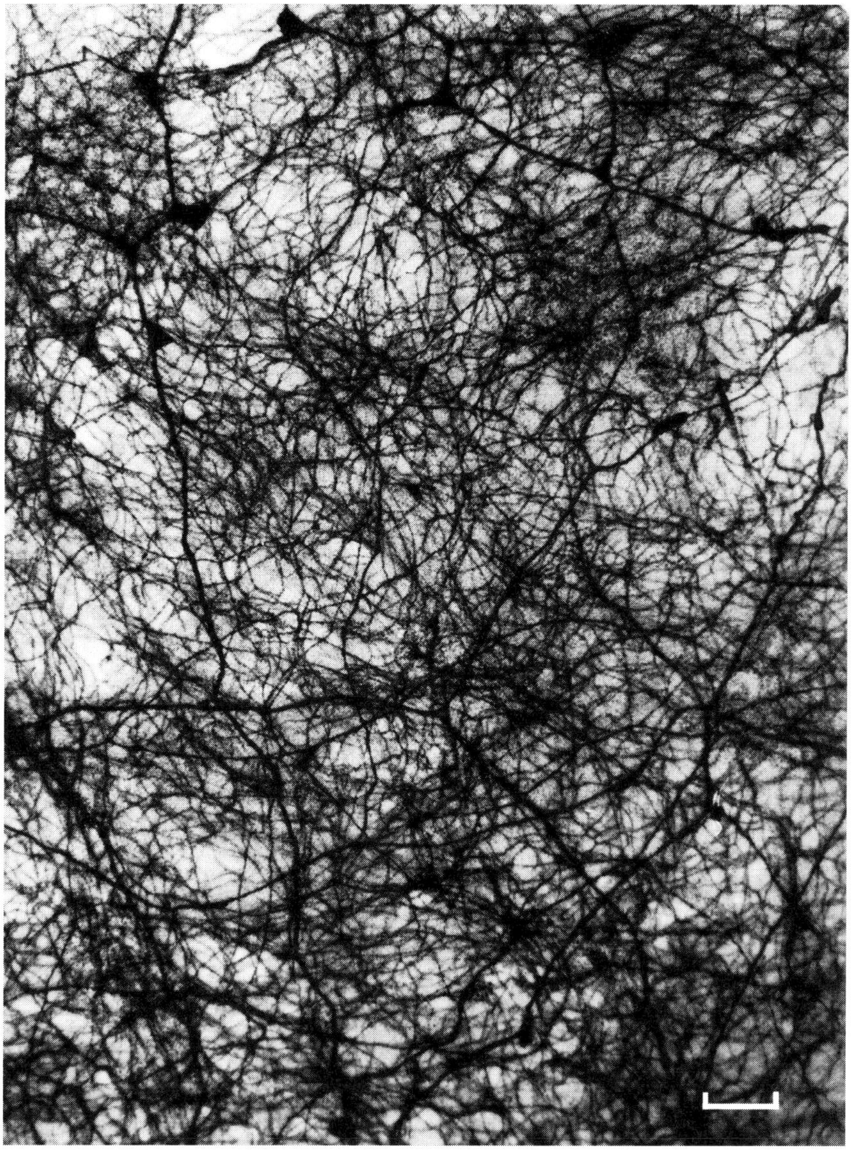

Fig. 9.17 Whole-mount stretch preparation of the gall-bladder stained to demonstrate the cholinergic innervation. There is a ganglionated plexus on the outer (serosal) surface of the smooth muscle with numerous small ganglia and interconnecting nerves. There is also a mucosal nerve plexus under the epithelium, containing cholinergic, adrenergic and peptidergic nerve fibres. Scale bar: 200 μm. From Cai & Gabella (1983).

reflex increase in tone (see Fig. 9.18). The circular smooth muscle has myogenic tone, which can be maintained in the absence of any nervous input, but the reflex decrease in tone is neurogenic and mediated by NANC innervation, probably using NO as a transmitter. The reflex increase in tone may be mediated through adrenergic nerves. These reflexes involve the intrinsic

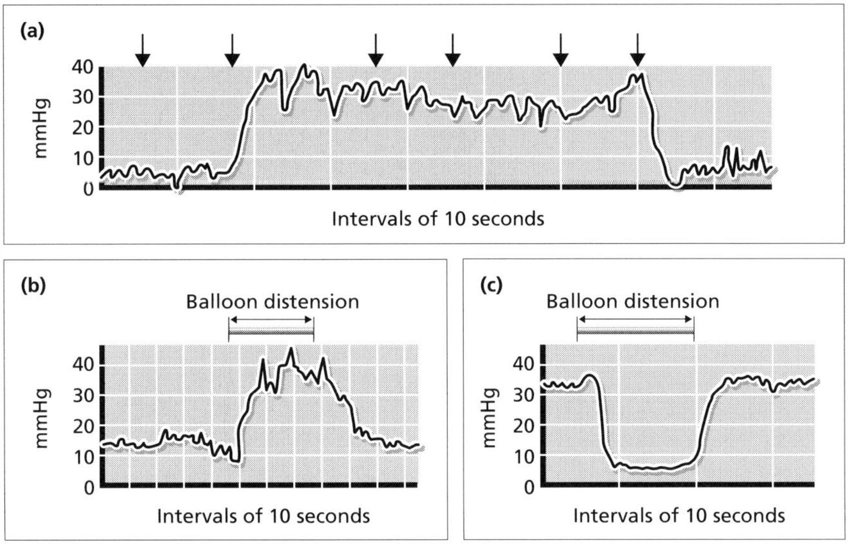

Fig. 9.18 Pressure recordings from the ileocaecal region in humans. (a) The recording device was moved from the colon into the ileum. The arrows represent 1 cm movements of the device. Note low pressure in the colon and ileum, and high pressure between. (b) The effect on the pressure in the ileocaecal junction of distending a balloon in the colon. There is a prompt increase in pressure. (c) The effect on the pressure in the ileocaecal junction of distending a balloon in the ileum. The pressure falls rapidly. Adapted from Cohen *et al*. (1968).

nervous system. The sphincter also receives extrinsic innervation, and an increase in tone can be induced by stimulation of the sympathetic input to this region – it is mediated through α-adrenoceptors.

Proximal large bowel

The caecum and the ascending colon undergo peristaltic activity, which is oriented towards the caecum and can therefore be considered as anti-peristalsis. These progressing waves of circular muscle constriction occur relatively slowly, and function to mix the gut contents and keep them in the proximal colon for long periods – as much as several days – to allow fluid absorption and provide time for micro-organisms to work.

Transverse and descending colon

In this middle part of the large bowel, rings of tonic contraction of the circular muscle appear, which divide the gut contents into a series of masses (Fig. 9.19). The constrictions seem to be similar to the segmental contractions in the ileum, and can move the faecal masses for short distances in either direction, but with an overall slow movement in the direction of the rectum. Occasionally, mass movements occur in which there is a sudden shift of the

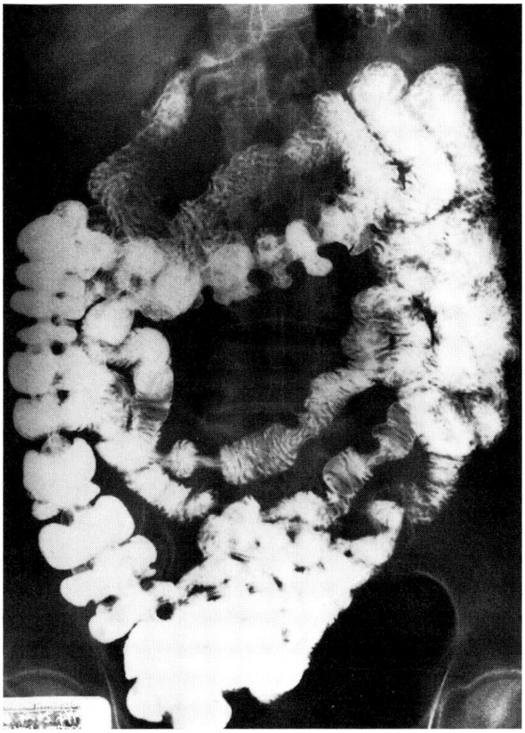

Fig. 9.19 X-ray of a human normal bowel after a barium meal. The small intestine (on the right) and the ascending and transverse colon are filled with barium. This shows the indentations or 'haustrations' in the column of barium caused by the tonic contractions of the circular smooth muscle. These vary in number and position from time to time.

faecal masses over about one-third of the length of the colon. In the sigmoid colon, peristaltic activity moves the contents of the colon into the rectum preceding defecation. These patterns of motility are again built on the spontaneous slow waves of the smooth muscle cells, with intrinsic nerves determining the degree of activation triggered by each slow wave, and on the peristaltic reflex, again relying on intrinsic innervation. There is good evidence that reflex activity can occur between different segments of the gut, in which the sensory nerve axons leave the gut and activate neurones in the paravertebral ganglia that return to a different part of the gut, thus allowing co-ordination of activity.

9.5.6 Defecation

Normally, the faeces are kept in the large intestine by high pressure in the anal canal. This is the result of striated muscle activity in the external anal sphincter and the pelvic floor, controlled by constant activity in somatic motor nerves, and tone also in the circular smooth muscle of the internal anal sphincter (Fig. 9.20). Rectal distension may trigger defecation, which involves relaxation of the anal sphincters and initiation of peristalsis in the colon and rectum. Relaxation of the striated muscles involves reflex pathways running to the central nervous system, as does the increased peri-

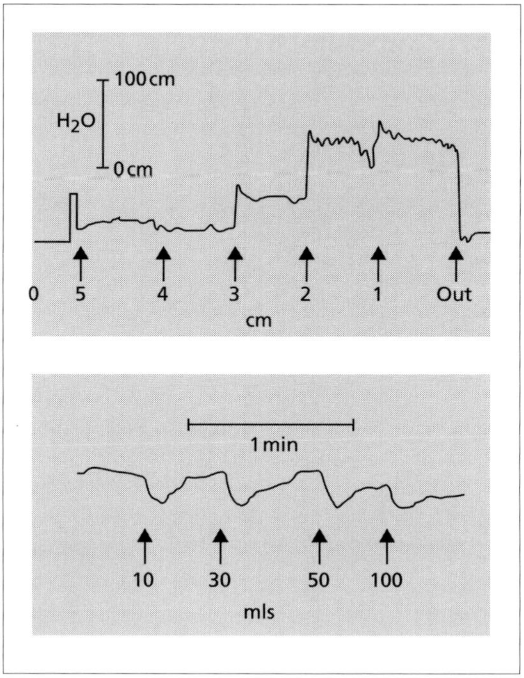

Fig. 9.20 Pressure recordings from the ano-rectum. In the upper panel, the pressure profile along the anal canal is demonstrated by withdrawing a balloon tipped catheter from the rectum a centimetre at a time and recording the resting pressure. In the lower panel, the responses of the internal anal sphincter to progressive distension of an air-filled balloon in the rectum are recorded. The internal anal sphincter relaxes transiently at each inflation, and the overall tone is progressively lowered. The transient relaxations are evidence of the recto-sphincteric reflex.

staltic activity of the lower bowel. The intrinsic innervation co-ordinates the peristaltic contractions responsible for evacuation of the rectum and often part of the descending colon, but initiation of the activity is through reflex parasympathetic input to the intrinsic nervous system. Relaxation of the internal anal sphincter is, however, brought about by reflexes that are entirely within the intrinsic nervous system. When defecation is triggered, a descending inhibitory reflex from the rectum relaxes the circular muscle of the internal anal sphincter. This muscle normally generates myogenic tone, but receives a dense inhibitory innervation, a substantial amount of which uses NO as the inhibitory transmitter (Fig. 9.21). The internal anal sphincter is also innervated by adrenergic neurones, and activation of sympathetic nerves increases the tone. Parasympathetic input to the muscle is weak, and activation of muscarinic cholinergic receptors may lead to relaxation of the sphincter (Fig. 9.22). The anal canal has an outer longitudinal layer of smooth muscle, which is also probably involved in defecation. This develops little myogenic tone, but it receives both excitatory cholinergic and adrenergic input. It relaxes on activation of β-adrenoceptors.

Personal experience will rapidly reveal that defecation is a sophisticated and complex process. Defecation can normally be inhibited or initiated at will, and it is possible for the sensory receptors in the anal canal to distinguish whether distension is caused by solid faeces or gas, since it is rare for the passing of gas (flatus) to cause any evacuation of faeces as well. The frequency of defecation varies greatly between individuals. Those that have

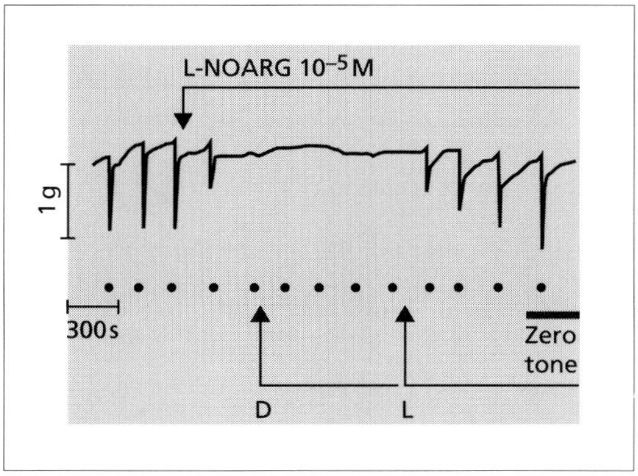

Fig. 9.21 Relaxant responses of the internal anal sphincter to intrinsic nerve stimulation. Relaxant responses are abolished by *N*-nitro-L-arginine (L-NOARG) which competes with the normal substrate (L-arginine) for the nitric oxide synthase enzyme preventing synthesis of NO. The inhibition can be reversed by increasing the concentration of L-arginine (L), but not D-arginine (D). Adapted from O'Kelly *et al.* (1993a).

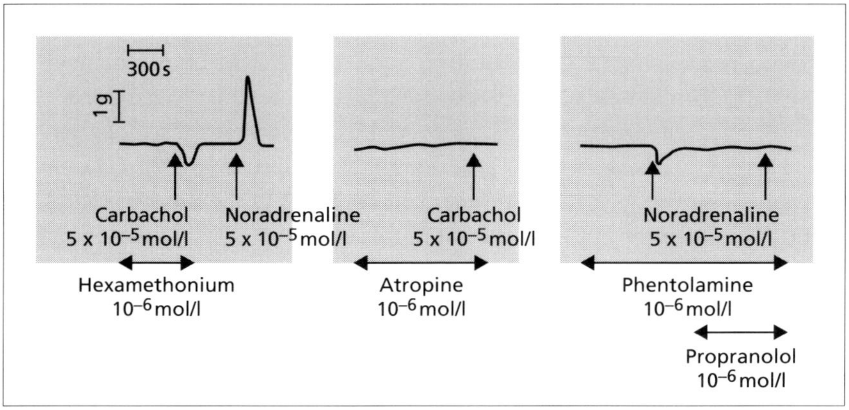

Fig. 9.22 Effects of carbachol and noradrenaline on the contractile activity of a strip of human internal anal sphincter. The muscle generates spontaneous tone which is relaxed by activation of muscarinic receptors (response blocked by atropine) and contracted by noradrenaline. Blockade of α-adrenoceptors with phentolamine abolishes the contractile response and reveals an underlying relaxation that is mediated by β-adrenoceptors (blocked by propranolol). Adapted from O'Kelly *et al.* (1993b).

been brought up to defecate daily are uncomfortable and often consider themselves constipated if a daily bowel movement is not achieved. Others may only defecate once or twice a week, with no discomfort or adverse consequences.

9.5.7 Vomiting

Vomiting is a complex reflex action, requiring control of both smooth and striated muscles, and integration with respiration. This control is achieved through a centre in the medulla oblongata of the brain that can be triggered through neuronal signals coming from the gastrointestinal tract, the visual and labyrinthine pathways and higher centres, or through blood-borne chemicals. The output of the vomiting centre triggers reverse peristalsis in the upper part of the small intestine, returning its contents to the stomach, and also relaxation of the stomach wall, oesophageal sphincter and oesophagus. Expulsion of the stomach contents is achieved through contraction of the abdominal striated muscles, working in conjunction with fixation of the chest wall through cessation of breathing in mid-inspiration. Under these circumstances, contraction of the abdominal muscles rapidly increases intra-abdominal pressure, which is transmitted to the stomach, compressing it. The respiratory tract is protected from vomitus by closure of the glottis, and the soft palate rises to prevent vomitus entering the nose. The reflex also results in copious secretion of the salivary and lachrymal glands and activation of other autonomic pathways, producing pallor, slowing of the heart rate and sweating.

Vomiting functions to protect the body from ingesting harmful substances, and this function can be triggered by stimulation of the mucosa by chemical or mechanical stimuli and by abnormal distension of the gastrointestinal tract or gall-bladder. It can also be triggered by circulating substances, which interact with neurones in the chemoreceptor trigger zone of the medulla. This is in the area postrema of the medulla, which lies close to the fourth ventricle, and is characterised by being functionally outside the blood–brain barrier, the structure of its circulation allowing more intimate contact between blood-borne substances and the neurones than is normally possible. Nausea and vomiting are also triggered by other sensory stimuli, such as pain, abnormal motion, smell and emotionally charged visual inputs.

9.5.8 Migrating motor complex

In the fasting animal, or between periods of feeding, another type of activity is seen, both in the stomach and the rest of the gut – the migrating motor complex (MMC). This is seen as a periodic appearance of increased electrical activity in the smooth muscle, which occurs every few minutes if recording at one site. Recording from several sites demonstrates that the activity actually propagates from one end of the gut to the other at a rate of a few centimetres per minute (Fig. 9.23). It is often said to have a 'housekeeping' role, being able to remove the undigested solids from the stomach and sweep them down the gut. It is also thought to play a role in preventing the build-up of bacteria in the fasting gut.

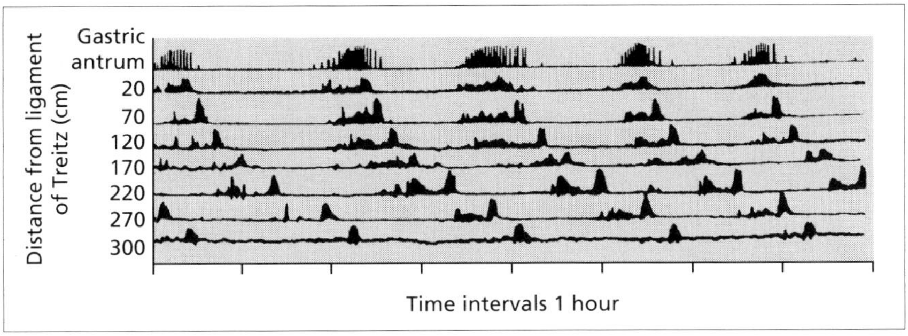

Fig. 9.23 Recordings of contractile activity in the stomach and small intestine of a fasting dog, showing the migrating myoelectric complex. The contractions consist of several phases, the first phase being quiescent, the next characterised by irregular contractions that build up into a more intense phase, and then fade away. The early contractile phase resembles that in the digesting state and would therefore mix the gut contents; the more intense contractions squeeze and expel the contents in a caudal direction. Adapted from Itoh & Sekiguchi (1983).

9.6 The role of the autonomic nervous system in glandular and epithelial secretion and absorption

9.6.1 Mechanisms

The mechanisms for the secretion and absorption of fluids by epithelia and glands, and the ways in which these can be regulated through activation of receptors, are described in Section 7.3.2. Briefly, secretion is caused by Cl^- entering the epithelial cells through the basolateral membranes via electrically neutral co-transport or counter-transport processes, and leaving through luminal Cl^- channels, thus achieving net electrogenic secretion of Cl^-. This generates a luminally directed transepithelial electrochemical gradient for Na^+, which normally flows via the paracellular route, water following passively down the osmotic gradient generated (Fig. 9.24). Absorption results from entry of Na into the cells through the apical membrane, and its active extrusion through the basolateral membrane using the electrogenic Na^+,K^+-ATPase. This Na^+ absorption will generate a net serosally directed current, allowing Cl^- to follow down its transepithelial electrochemical gradient, either through the cellular or paracellular pathway. Water will again follow (Fig. 9.24). Neuronal or hormonal activation of secretion or absorption depends on switching the ionic mechanisms involved on or off. This may involve several different intracellular systems. Some bacterial toxins can cause massive secretion by activating second-messenger pathways, which result in switching on luminal Cl^- channels. They may act at the level of the epithelial cells, or by activation of sensory nerve terminals and reflex pathways. Cholera toxin, for example, permanently activates G_s, the G protein responsible for stimulating adenylyl

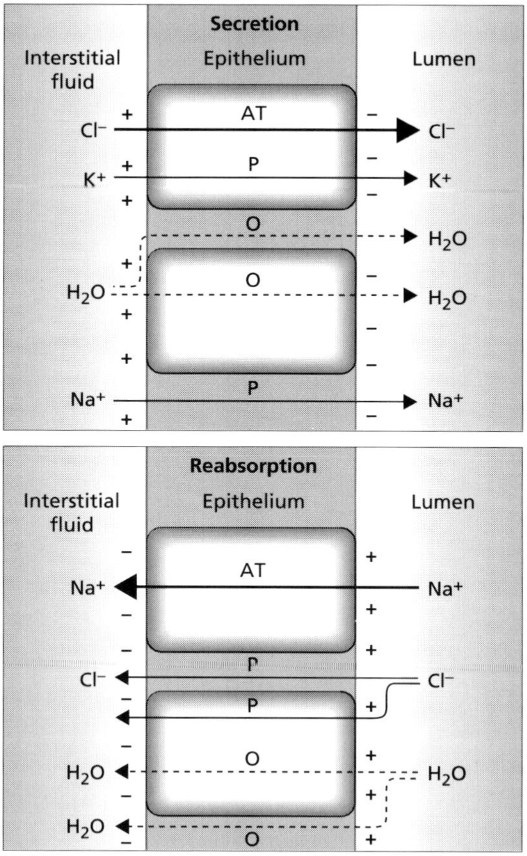

Fig. 9.24 Main mechanisms for secretion and reabsorption of fluid and electrolytes. In secretion the active mechanism (AT) is an electrogenic secretion of Cl^-. This is achieved by Cl^- entry into the cells through a variety of co- or counter-transport mechanisms (fuelled ultimately by the Na^+ gradient) and Cl^- exit to the lumen through Cl^- channels that can be regulated by a variety of mechanisms. When the Cl^- channels are open, a net Cl^- current flows, generating a transepithelial potential. Na^+ ions flow down this electrical gradient passively (P) largely through the paracellular route, and water follows using the osmotic gradient (O) generated by the ions. In reabsorption, the active process is Na^+ reabsorption. This is achieved by Na^+ entering the luminal border through a variety of co- and counter-transport processes down its electrochemical gradient, and being expelled to the interstitial fluid by the Na pump. This generates a current and a lumen-positive transepithelial gradient. Cl^- and water follow passively down the electrical and osmotic gradients.

cyclase, and activates Cl^- channels through a cAMP-dependent protein kinase (Fig. 9.25).

9.6.2 Mucous secretion

This occurs throughout the length of the gut, mucus being secreted from a variety of different cells and glands. Most show histological evidence of

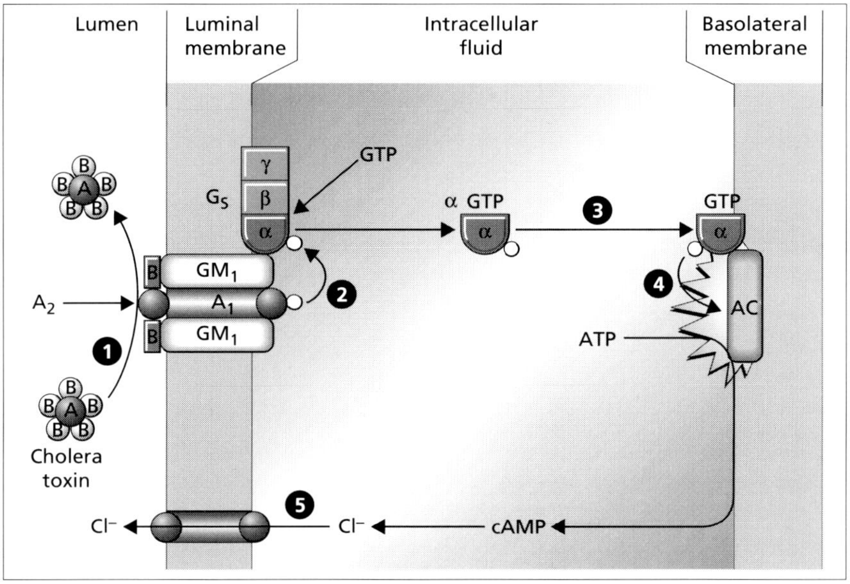

Fig. 9.25 Mechanism of action of cholera toxin. (1) The toxin binds to a monoganglioside in the cell membrane (GM_1) through the B subunits. (2) This results in a conformational change and triggers release of the α-subunit of the G protein G_s, and its ADP-ribosylation which permanently activates this subunit. (3) The activated subunit interacts with adenylate cyclase (AC), activating it (4), resulting in the continuous production of cAMP from ATP. cAMP then triggers the opening of Cl^- channels in the luminal membrane and thus switches on secretion.

innervation. There is evidence in different species for both cholinergic and non-cholinergic innervation leading to mucous secretion, and for activation both through local reflexes and through parasympathetic stimulation, although there are differences between areas of the gut and between species.

9.6.3 Mucosal endocrine secretion

At least 15 types of mucosal endocrine cells have been identified histologically in the walls of the gut. The cells contain a range of substances (including 5-HT, gastrin, cholecystokinin, secretin, somatostatin, gastric inhibitory polypeptide, motilin, neurotensin and glucagon) which have local paracrine or true endocrine function. In many instances, it can be shown histologically that nerve fibres come into close contact with such cells, and it is probable that they play a role in endocrine secretion. Certainly, in the case of the enterochromaffin cells, which contain 5-HT, stimulation of adrenergic fibres can cause degranulation of the cells. One of the peptides, motilin, is secreted during the migrating motor complex described in Section 9.5.8, and this secretion is blocked by atropine.

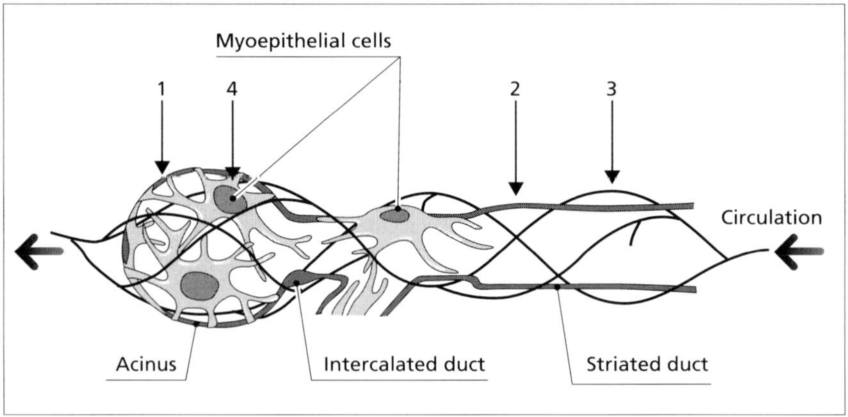

Fig. 9.26 A salivary acinus showing the possible sites of action of the autonomic nerves. (1) The primary endothelial secretory cells, (2) the tubular cells that can modify the primary secretion, (3) the capillaries supplying the acinus, (4) the myoepithelial cells.

9.6.4 Salivary glands

Salivary glands produce about 1 l of saliva over 24 h. The glands consist of acini (groups of secretory acinar cells surrounding a central cavity), which are drained by a complex of ducts. These ducts are surrounded by myoepithelial cells. The acini produce the primary secretion, which can be modified by the cells in the ducts, and the myoepithelial cells can contract, probably to support the delicate ducts during secretion (Fig. 9.26). The glands are innervated both by the parasympathetic and sympathetic nervous systems (Fig. 9.27). Parasympathetic stimulation causes secretion of copious amounts of a low-protein watery secretion; it also enhances blood flow to the glands, possibly by release of VIP, and constricts the myoepithelial cells, whereas activation of the sympathetic nervous system causes production of smaller volumes of more viscous saliva. Activation of α-adrenoceptors and muscarinic receptors causes secretion of fluid through a mechanism involving an increase in cytosolic calcium, whereas β-adrenoceptor activation stimulates enzyme secretion via elevation of intracellular cAMP. Sympathetic stimulation will also cause vasoconstriction through α-adrenoceptor activation, which may account for the smaller volume of fluid secreted in response to sympathetic stimulation.

9.6.5 Gastric secretions

The stomach secretes 2–3 l per day of gastric juice. This is neutral or alkaline during fasting, when only a small amount is secreted, but strongly acidic (pH 0.8–1.5) after eating, when it is nearly isotonic with plasma, and it contains proteolytic enzymes, mucus and intrinsic factor, as well as HCl. Stimulation of the vagus nerve increases secretion of acid and enzymes. Acid and

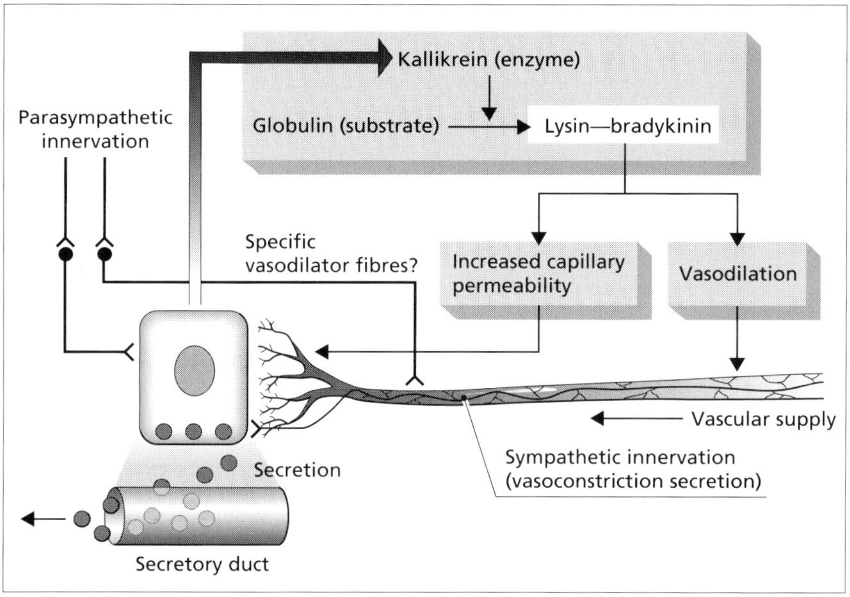

Fig. 9.27 Innervation of the salivary glands. Activation of the sympathetic nerves causes secretion of a low volume viscous saliva. The sympathetic innervation enters the gland along the blood vessels. It can cause vasoconstriction, thus reducing the volume of saliva produced, and acting on the secretory cells it can stimulate secretion of enzymes. The parasympathetic innervation stimulates copious secretion of a watery saliva. The nerves directly activate the secretory cells, and trigger the secretion, and also the release of the enzyme kallikrein, which cleaves lysin–bradykinin from its globular protein substrate. Bradykinin increases capillary permeability, and causes vasodilation. The parasympathetic system also probably directly innervates the blood vessels with vasodilator nerves.

intrinsic factor are secreted from the parietal cells, and the inactive pepsinogen precursors of the proteolytic enzymes are secreted from the chief cells. Three agonists are involved at the level of the acid-secreting parietal cells: acetylcholine, acting through M_1 muscarinic receptors and released from the parasympathetic nerve endings; histamine, acting through H_2 receptors and probably released from mast cells; and gastrin, released by a non-cholinergic agonist (probably gastrin-releasing peptide) acting on gastrin cells. Factors affecting blood flow may also be involved. The mechanisms controlling acid secretion at the level of the parietal cell are complex, and are shown in more detail in Box 9.1.

Vagal stimulation probably acts by direct activation of muscarinic receptors on the parietal cells as well as through stimulation of gastrin release from the gastrin cells and histamine release from the enterochromaffin cells. The effects of vagal stimulation are blocked by hexamethonium, the ganglion-blocking drug, suggesting that nicotinic synapses occur in both the vagal pathways. Gastrin also stimulates release of histamine from the ente-

Box 9.1 Mechanisms and control of gastric acid secretion

The parietal cells of the gastric glands are responsible for the production of gastric acid. Secretory canaliculi within the cells communicate with the lumen of the gland. H^+ and HCO_3^- ions are made in the cell from water and CO_2 using the enzyme carbonic anhydrase. H^+ is secreted into the canaliculi using the H^+,K^+-ATPase, and HCO_3^- is exchanged for Cl^- across the basolateral membranes on the antiporter. Cl^- is secreted to accompany H^+ into the lumen through Cl^- channels (Fig. B9.1.1).

Regulation of acid secretion can occur through insertion of proton pumps into the apical membrane. The pumps are present within the cell in the form of intracellular vesicles, and on activation of the cells, the vesicles are incorporated. The precise mechanisms involved are unclear, but activation of M_1 muscarinic receptors and gastrin receptors increases intracellular Ca^{2+}, and activation of H_2 histamine receptors increases cAMP formation. The intracellular messengers probably activate kinases that are involved in insertion of the pumps, and may also indirectly control pump activity through regulation of the secretion of Cl^- or fluids by opening appropriate ion channels. The agonists interact such that one agonist may potentiate the activity of another. Acetylcholine and gastrin also act on mast cells to trigger release of histamine (Fig. 9.28).

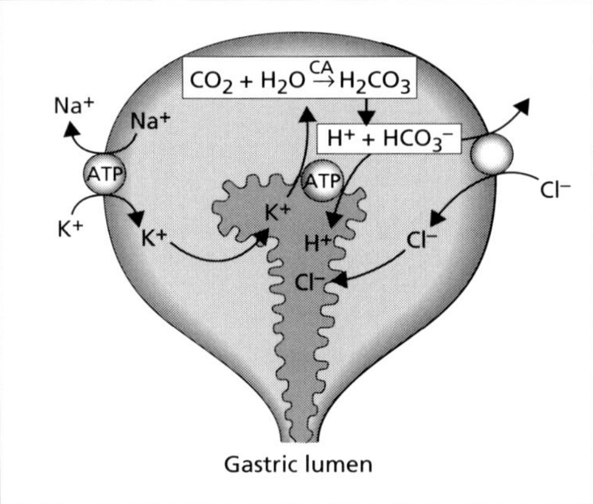

Fig. B9.1.1 Gastric acid secretion by a parietal cell.

rochromaffin cells, and somatostatin, secreted from endocrine cells in the fundus and antrum, switches off histamine release.

The vagus is important in the cephalic phase of secretion, in which secretion is stimulated by the taste and smell of food and conditioned reflexes, but there is also evidence that the intrinsic nervous system of the gut may play a role in controlling secretion. During the gastric phase, local reflex stimulation of gastric juice is initiated by stretching of the stomach wall,

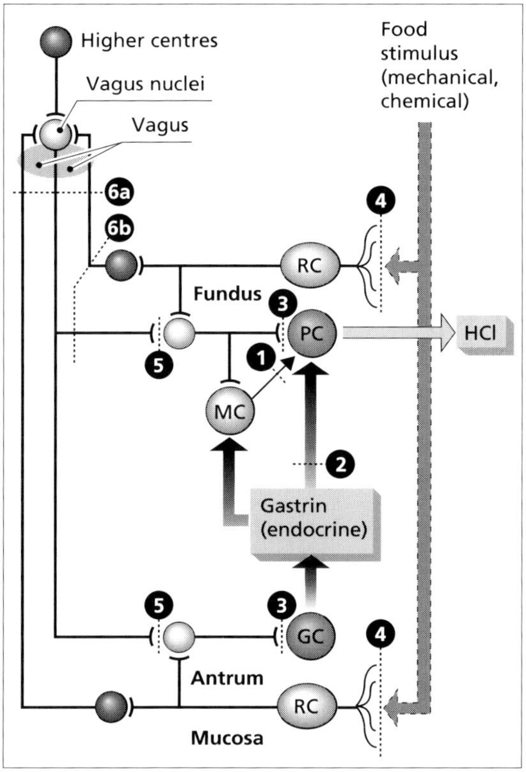

Fig. 9.28 Control of gastric acid secretion, and methods of inhibiting secretion. The postganglionic vagal fibres innervate the parietal cells (PC), mast cell-like histamine-secreting cells (MC) and the gastrin-secreting cells (GC) of the stomach wall. Receptors in the gut wall (RC) activate reflex pathways which can directly or indirectly trigger vagal activity. Acetylcholine acting through muscarinic receptors, histamine acting through H_2 receptors and gastrin act synergistically to trigger HCl secretion. Gastrin also triggers histamine release from MCs. Possible mechanisms to suppress secretion are: (1) H_2-receptor antagonists, (2) gastrin antagonists, (3) muscarinic blockers, (4) sensory receptor blockade, (5) ganglion-blocking drugs, (6) transection of vagal pathways.

both involving the intrinsic nervous system and also vagovagal reflexes (Fig. 9.28). In the intestinal phase of gastric secretion, various stimuli in the duodenum can modulate the secretion of gastric juice. It is certain that this involves gastrointestinal hormones, but it is difficult experimentally to eliminate the possibility that there is also involvement of neuronal reflexes. Stimulation of the splanchnic sympathetic input to the stomach reduces acid secretion and mucosal blood flow, but has no effect on enzyme secretion.

9.6.6 Pancreatic secretion

Pancreatic juice consists of isotonic fluid, which varies in its bicarbonate or Cl content depending on the flow rate. During peak secretion, the bicarbonate concentration can reach 130–140 mmol/l, whereas with low flows, the major anion is Cl. Pancreatic juice contains many digestive enzymes (peptidases, phospholipase, lipases, amylase, ribonuclease). Secretion of pancreatic juice is controlled largely by the hormones secretin and cholecystokinin, but the exocrine pancreas is innervated by the vagus, and activation leads to an enzyme-rich secretion. This is probably mediated by co-release of acetylcholine and VIP, since these agents have additive effects on pancreatic secretions and blood flow in the gland.

9.6.7 Gall-bladder

Bile (containing water and electrolytes, mucus, cholesterol, lecithin, bile acids and bilirubin) is secreted by the liver, and stored in the gall-bladder. The mucosa can reabsorb water to concentrate the bile, secrete water to dilute it and also acidify it by secretion of hydrogen ions. The dilution of the bile occurs during periods of bile expulsion when there is activity of the smooth muscle. This activity can be initiated by hormones such as CCK and enhanced by vagal activity. Concentration of bile by reabsorption of water seems to occur during periods of low contractile activity. Hydrogen ion secretion can be enhanced by activity in the sympathetic nerves. Release of bile into the duodenum is governed by a complex set of controls involving the secretion of bile by the liver, the activity of the smooth muscle in the gall-bladder and the contractions and relaxations of the sphincter of Oddi. Hormones and neuronal pathways are involved (see Fig. 9.29).

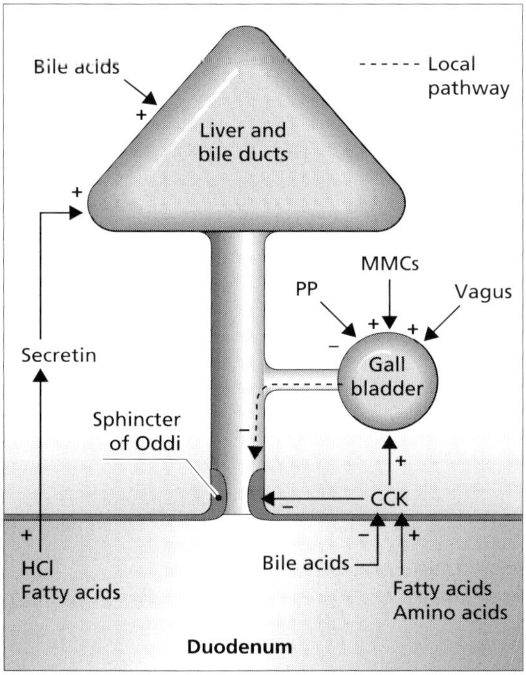

Fig. 9.29 Control of the bile flow into the duodenum. The secretion of bile from the liver is dependent on the extraction of bile from the blood and *de novo* synthesis from cholesterol by the hepatocytes, and also the secretion of electrolytes and water triggered by secretin (released into the blood in response to acids in the duodenum). The gall-bladder contracts in response to vagal stimulation, and to the neuronal pathways involved in the migrating motor complex (MMC). It can also be inhibited, for instance via a pancreatic polypeptide (PP). CCK secreted from the upper small intestine in response to bile acids and products of digestion also constricts the gall-bladder and dilates the sphincter of Oddi. There is evidence for a local reflex from the gall-bladder that is involved with sphincter relaxation.

9.6.8 Intestinal secretion and absorption

The intestine receives about 5 l of chyme from the stomach, receives a further 1.4 l of pancreatic secretion and bile, and secretes about 2.6 l of fluid, but also absorbs virtually all of this 9 l, in 24 h – only about 100 ml of fluid being lost in the faeces (Fig. 9.30). Both secretion and absorption can be modulated by the autonomic nervous system. Figure 9.30 gives an overview of the fluid balance in the gastrointestinal tract.

There are several classes of secretomotor neurones that apparently innervate the mucosa. In the guinea-pig, there are cholinergic and non-cholinergic neurones in the submucous plexus innervating the mucosa, and there are some cholinergic neurones in the myenteric plexus that also project there. Substance P-containing nerve terminals (presumably sensori-motor) are found in the mucosa, with their cell bodies in the myenteric

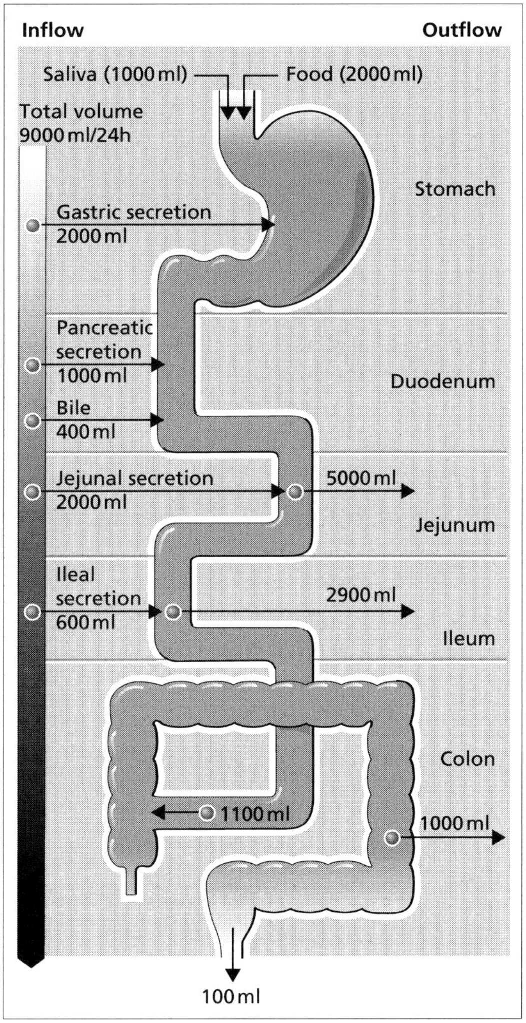

Fig. 9.30 Gastrointestinal fluid balance. Under normal conditions saliva and gastrointestinal secretions add some 7 l of fluid to the gut, in addition to a liquid intake of 2 l. The vast majority of this is reabsorbed by the gut, with only 100 ml leaving in the faeces.

plexus. Postsynaptic neurones of the sympathetic pathway, with their cell bodies in the prevertebral ganglia, also project directly to the mucosa and to the intrinsic neurones in the submucous plexus. At present, evidence suggests that the intrinsic neurones can all enhance secretory activity in various ways, there being no evidence for neurones that inhibit secretion. The excitation is predominantly cholinergic (hence the reduction of secretion produced by muscarinic blockade), but there is also a non-cholinergic excitatory transmitter, which is probably VIP. Presumably, the mechanisms in the epithelial cells, when not activated by the intrinsic neurones, are set to produce net absorption of fluids. The intrinsic neurones receive much input from interneurones in the enteric nervous system, giving them a tonic excitatory tone that would promote secretion. This is normally balanced by continuous activity in the extrinsic input from postganglionic sympathetic neurones. Increased sympathetic input promotes absorption; this can be seen, for instance, in the reflex response to a drop in body fluid volume (Fig. 9.31). When the sympathetic input to the gut is removed, enhanced secretion is seen which is abolished by atropine, supporting the above scenario. Vagotomy does not affect these responses, although activation of the vagus can cause enhanced secretion. There is thus wide scope for reflex control of secretion and absorption. It is known, for instance, that the presence of glucose in the intestine can trigger a specific reflex secretion of water and electrolytes via non-cholinergic neurones. The sensory nerve terminals involved may also be activated by bacterial toxins. The secretion induced by cholera toxin, for instance, although atropine-insensitive, is partially

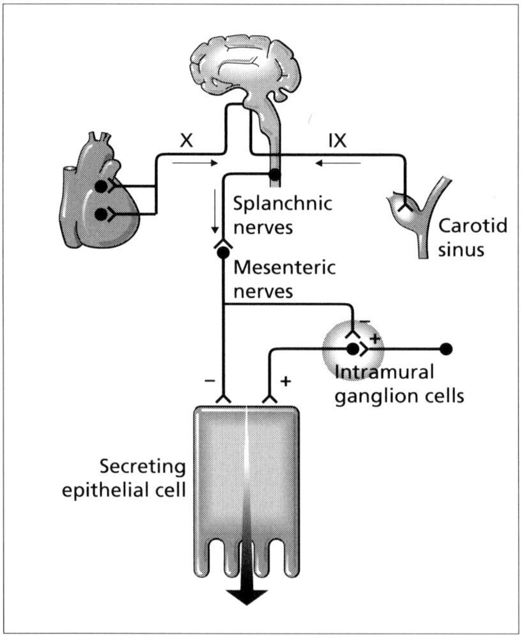

Fig. 9.31 Cardiovascular reflex control of jejunal fluid secretion. A drop in body fluid and blood volume will lower diastolic blood pressure and reduce discharge of the pressure receptors in the carotid sinus and cardiopulmonary baroreceptors (travelling to the brainstem in the IXth and Xth cranial nerves). This will cause a reflex activation of the sympathetic outflow to the intestine which will directly (acting on the epithelial cells) or indirectly (through inhibition of the secretomotor cells in the myenteric plexus) reduce secretion, and promote reabsorption of fluid.

blocked by hexamethonium, suggesting that it activates the same reflex pathway as glucose.

9.7 Relevant pharmacology

Gastrointestinal tract disorders are common, and many drugs are targeted at the autonomic nervous system and its effectors to control over-activity or under-activity in the smooth muscles and glands. Perhaps the most important are those controlling gastric acid secretion, those inhibiting or inducing vomiting, and those affecting intestinal motility (i.e. drugs used for the treatment of constipation and diarrhoea).

9.7.1 Drugs reducing gastric acid secretion

The main pathways for pharmacological control of gastric acid secretion are shown in Fig. 9.32. The synthesis of antagonists to the H_2 histamine receptors provided the first revolution in the treatment of gastric ulcers (the second revolution being the discovery that eradication of *Helicobacter pylori* infection results in long-term ulcer remission). H_2 antagonists such as cimetidine and ranitidine can antagonise acid secretion initiated not only by histamine, but also by gastrin and acetylcholine, and thus decrease both basal secretion of HCl and secretion stimulated by food intake. They promote healing of duodenal ulcers, and are also useful in the treatment of heartburn

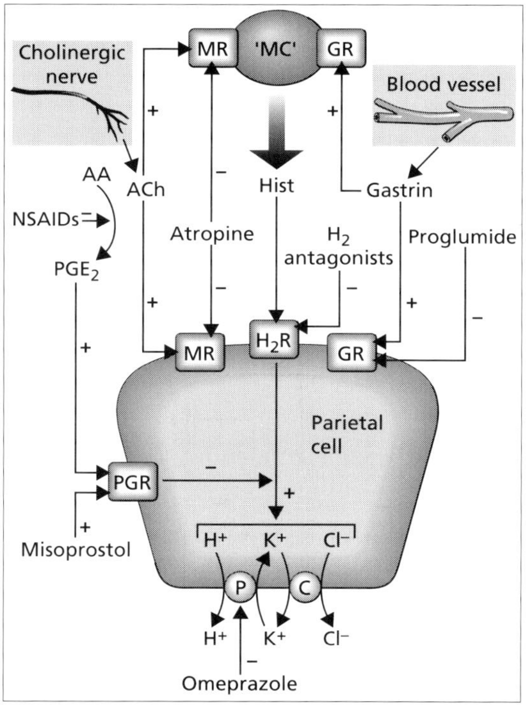

Fig. 9.32 Diagram of possible mechanisms of action of secretagogues and drugs on acid secretion from the parietal cells of the stomach. Acetylcholine released from the vagus and gastrin carried in the blood may act directly on their receptors (MR-muscarinic receptor; H_2R-histamine H_2 receptor, GR-gastrin receptor) on the parietal cells or indirectly through the mast-cell-like histamine secreting cells ('MC'). PGE_2 synthesised from arachidonic acid (AA), acting through prostaglandin receptors (PGR), inhibits acid secretion. Drugs acting at the various sites as indicated. NSAIDs, non-steroidal anti-inflammatory drugs. Adapted from Rang *et al.* (1995).

and dyspepsia due to excess acid secretion. The main advantage of the H_2 antagonists is their comparative lack of side-effects, to such an extent that they are now available to the public in packs of a limited number of tablets without prescription. Muscarinic receptor antagonists are equally effective in reducing acid secretion and promoting ulcer healing, but have many side-effects. The M_1-specific antagonist pirenzepine is more specific in its actions, and can be useful.

Proton-pump inhibitors provide a more direct method of reducing acid secretion. These block the H^+,K^+-ATPase involved in proton secretion across the parietal cells of the stomach. Omeprazole is the main drug of this type, and it has the advantage of being inactive at neutral pH, although it is accumulated in an acid environment and activated at a pH of less than 3, so that it has relatively specific effects on gastric acid secretion in the body – although a wide range of side-effects is occasionally seen.

Prostaglandins E and I have been shown to inhibit gastric acid secretion, and to be produced normally in the stomach. Stable prostaglandin analogues, such as misoprostol, can be used clinically, especially for people receiving non-steroidal anti-inflammatory drugs, which block the normal synthesis of prostaglandins.

9.7.2 Emetics and anti-emetic drugs

Vomiting can be stimulated, and is sometimes useful to rid the stomach of recently ingested poisons. Ipecacuanha is normally used, causing irritation of the stomach mucosa and triggering the vomiting reflex. Drugs that can trigger nausea as a side-effect often work by activating the chemoreceptor trigger zone (see Section 9.5.7 above).

There are several classes of anti-emetic drugs, only some of which are effective against nausea triggered through activation of the chemoreceptor trigger zone. The most common clinical uses are in the treatment of motion sickness, vestibular disorders (e.g. Ménière's disease), chemotherapy and radiation therapy, and drug-induced nausea. H_1-receptor antagonists and muscarinic receptor antagonists are effective against motion sickness, sickness caused by stimulation of the gastric mucosa and often vestibular disorders, although they cannot prevent sickness from stimulation of the trigger zone. Commonly used are the H_1-receptor antagonists cyclizine and cinnarizine and the muscarinic antagonist hyoscine. For the treatment of sickness caused by agents stimulating the trigger zone, the neuroleptic phenothiazines are effective, probably through their D_2-receptor antagonism. These include chlorpromazine, prochlorperazine and trifluoperazine. The drugs are useful in drug-induced emesis, diffuse neoplastic disease and radiation sickness. They are ineffective against emetic stimuli in the gut. In addition, metoclopramide can be effective against gastrointestinal sickness and is effective in high doses against sickness caused by cytotoxic drug therapy, as is domperidone. 5-HT_3 receptor antagonists such as ondansetron are useful in the treatment of severely emetic cytotoxic drugs.

9.7.3 Drugs affecting intestinal motility

Although acute diarrhoea is best treated by maintaining fluid and electrolyte balance using oral rehydration fluids, drugs reducing gastrointestinal motility can be useful in adults. The main agents used are the opiates (in particular codeine, a morphine congener, and diphenoxylate and loperamide, synthetic pethidine-like drugs), and muscarinic receptor antagonists. The opiates act on neurones in the enteric plexuses and directly on smooth muscle to increase the tone, but decrease the propulsive activity of the gut. Low doses can be useful, but they can cause nausea, vomiting and abdominal cramps, as well as drowsiness.

Antimuscarinic drugs can suppress activity in the gut wall through their blocking effects on the excitatory muscarinic receptors of the smooth muscles. However, they will also reduce secretion by blocking the tonic stimulatory effects of the vagus on secretory activity, and they are not often used to block motility. Low concentrations are sometimes included in antidiarrhoeal products containing diphenoxylate. They are also occasionally used for their antispasmodic activity in the treatment of inflammatory bowel syndrome and diverticular disease.

Drugs increasing motility of the stomach are used in the treatment of gastric reflux and disorders of gastric emptying, and drugs increasing intestinal motility are used as laxatives to cure constipation. Domperidone is used to increase gastric motility. It is thought to do this by blocking the effects of the tonic inhibitory activity of the sympathetic nerves. Although the drug is a dopamine receptor antagonist, it also blocks the α_1-adrenoceptors that mediate inhibition at the level of the ganglia and nonsphincteric smooth muscle. Another drug increasing gastric motility is metoclopramide; this may also be a dopamine antagonist, although its precise mechanism of action is unclear. It causes marked acceleration of gastric emptying without increasing acid secretion. Both of these drugs are also powerful anti-emetics.

Purgative laxatives increase intestinal motility by their stimulatory effects on the mucosa of the colon and rectum. This triggers local peristaltic reflexes and can stimulate defecation. The most commonly used drugs are bisacodyl, sodium picosulphate and preparations of senna and other products containing anthracene derivatives. In senna, these substances are combined with sugars, and have no effect until bacterial actions in the colon hydrolyse the glycoside bond and release the free anthracene derivative.

Further reading

Davison, J.S. (1989) *Gastrointestinal Secretion.* Wright, London.

Furness, J.B. & Costa, M. (1987) *The Enteric Nervous System*. Churchill Livingstone, Edinburgh.
Gabella, G. (1976) *Structure of the Autonomic Nervous System*. Chapman & Hall, London.
Hersey, S.J. & Sachs, G. (1995) Gastric acid secretion. *Physiol Rev* **75**, 155–89.
Holman, M.E. (1981) The intrinsic innervation and peristaltic reflex of the small intestine. In: *Smooth Muscle: An Assessment of Current Knowledge* (eds E. Bülbring, A.F. Brading, A.W. Jones & T. Tomita), pp. 311–38. Edward Arnold, London.
Miolan, J.P. & Niel, J.P. (1996) The mammalian sympathetic prevertebral ganglia: integrative properties and role in the nervous control of digestive tract motility. *J Auton Nerv Syst* **58**, 125–38.
Sanders, K.M. (1992) Ionic mechanisms of electrical rhythmicity in gastrointestinal smooth muscles. *Ann Rev Physiol* **54**, 439–53.
Suprenant, A. (1994) Control of the gastrointestinal tract by enteric neurons. *Ann Rev Physiol* **56**, 117–40.

References

Baluka, P. & Gabella, G. (1987) Scanning electron microscopy of the muscle coat of the guinea-pig small intestine. *Cell Tissue Res* **250**, 551–61.
Berne, R.M. & Levy, M.N. (1990) *Principles of Physiology*. Wolfe, London.
Cai, W.-Q. & Gabella, G. (1983) Innervation of the gall-bladder and biliary pathways in the guinea-pig. *J Anat* **136**, 97–109.
Cohen, S., Harris, L.D. & Levitan, R. (1968) Manometric characteristics of the human ileocecal junctional zone. *Gastroenterology* **54**, 72–5.
Itoh, Z. & Sekiguchi, T. (1983) Interdigestive motor activity in health and disease. *Scand J Gastroenterol* (Suppl.) **82**, 121–34.
Liu, L.W. and Huizinga, J.D. (1993) Electrical coupling of circular muscle to longitudinal muscle and interstitial cells of Cajal in canine colon. *J Physiol* **470**, 445–61.
O'Kelly, T., Brading, A.F. & Mortensen, N. (1993a) Nerve mediated relaxation of the human internal anal sphincter: the role of nitric oxide. *Gut* **34**, 689–93.
O'Kelly, T.J., Brading, A. & Mortensen, N.J.M. (1993b) *In vitro* response of the human anal canal longitudinal muscle layer to cholinergic and adrenergic stimulation: evidence of sphincter specialization. *Br J Surg* **80**, 1337–41.
Rang, H.P., Dale, M.M. & Ritter, J.M. (1995) *Pharmacology*. Churchill Livingstone, Edinburgh.
Sanders, K.M. (1992) Ionic mechanisms of electrical rhythmicity in gastrointestinal smooth muscles. *Ann Rev Physiol* **54**, 439–53.
Smith, T.K. & Robertson, W.J. (1998) Synchronous movements of the longitudinal and circular muscle during peristalsis in the isolated guinea-pig distal colon. *J Physiol* **506**, 563–77.
Szurszewski, J.H. (1975) Mechanisms of action of pentagastrin and acetylcholine on the longitudinal muscle of the canine antrum. *J Physiol* **252**, 335–61.

10 : Renal, Urinary and Reproductive Tract Systems

10.1 Kidney

Neuroanatomy

In relation to its size, the kidney receives a richer innervation than almost any other organ. It is thought that the innervation is exclusively sympathetic, and the presynaptic fibres leave the spinal cord from roots T5 to L3. The innervation takes many different routes to the kidney, and there is an extensive renal plexus in association with the aorticorenal ganglion at the junction of the renal artery and the aorta. Fibres enter the kidney along the renal artery and vein at the hilum.

Sympathetic nerves supply the blood vessels in the kidney, in particular the afferent and efferent arterioles, and intrarenal arteries. In the afferent arterioles, nerves supply both smooth muscle and the granular cells of the juxtaglomerular apparatus (Fig. 10.1). In addition, sympathetic nerve endings are found in the proximity of tubular cells along most of the nephron segments: the proximal and distal tubules, the thick ascending

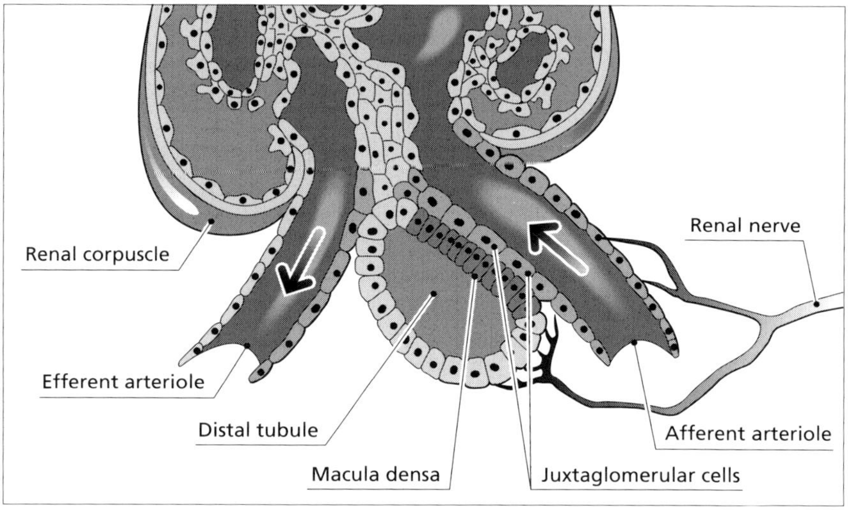

Fig. 10.1 Diagram of the arrangement of the juxtaglomerular apparatus, and its innervation. The juxtaglomerular apparatus consists of granule containing cells in the wall of the afferent arteriole, and specialized cells in the adjacent wall of the distal tubule belonging to that nephron. Renal nerves (sympathetic) supply the afferent arteriole and the cells of the juxtaglomerular apparatus. Stimulation can evoke release of renin from the juxtaglomerular cells directly or indirectly through alterations in the afferent arteriolar pressure or the composition of the tubular fluid.

limb of the loop of Henle, the macula densa and the collecting duct. Although intact innervation is not necessary for normal kidney function – a fact that is fortunate for kidney transplant patients – there is mounting evidence that the innervation plays an important role in the modulation of urine production and in salt and water homeostasis.

Functions of innervation

Sympathetic stimulation has several possible functions.

1 Through its constrictor effects on the vasculature, it can regulate the glomerular filtration rate and determine the relative blood flow through the salt-losing cortical nephrons and the salt-retaining juxtamedullary nephrons.

2 It can control secretion of renin from the juxtaglomerular cells of the afferent arteriole through several mechanisms: firstly, through its haemodynamic effects using the renal vascular baroreceptor mechanism (changes in pressure in the afferent arteriole, brought about by varying the afferent and efferent arteriolar tone, alter renin release); secondly, indirectly through the macula densa mechanism (alterations in the glomerular filtration rate result in alterations in the distal tubular content, which can affect renin release through the macula densa connecting the distal tubule with the granular cells of the juxtaglomerular apparatus in the afferent arterioles); and thirdly, through direct innervation of the granular cells.

3 It can have direct effects on tubular reabsorptive mechanisms.

Under normal conditions, there is tonic activity in the sympathetic nerves innervating the kidney. Denervation of the kidney leads to an increased urine flow, and stimulation of the sympathetic input causes an increased reabsorption of salt and water. The activity in the renal nerves is tonically inhibited by activity in the stretch receptors of the heart and lungs, and the carotid sinus and aortic arch. Increase in activity of these receptors, which reflects an increase in blood volume or pressure, thus reduces activity in the renal sympathetic nerves, and results in an increased urine production, whereas decreased activity in these peripheral systems results in increased activity and an enhanced salt and water reabsorption.

Effectors

Little is known about which of the various effector systems of the sympathetic nerves in the kidney is activated by which normal stimuli. Careful experimentation has, however, led to the conclusion that increased salt and water reabsorption in the proximal tubule can occur through a direct tubular mechanism, independent of any changes in the blood flow or glomerular filtration. There is normally a tonic sympathetic input to the tubules, which enhances salt and water reabsorption. This seems to be mediated by activation of α-adrenoceptors, as it is blocked by α-adrenoceptor-blocking drugs, and mimicked by application of noradrenaline.

In contrast, noradrenaline triggers release of renin from the granular cells of the juxtaglomerular apparatus through activation of β_1-adrenoceptors. α-Adrenoceptors, which are also present, are not essential for renin release, but may play a modulatory role in the release process. The mechanism of renin release is interesting, since it is associated with a reduction in free intracellular calcium.

Sensory innervation

The kidney also possesses afferent nerves. Intrarenal small myelinated A fibres are seen with endings near vascular or pelvic structures in the kidney. There are also nerve fibres present in the kidney which show immunoreactivity for substance P and calcitonin gene-related peptide (CGRP), peptides characteristically found in nociceptive neurones in the periphery, as would be expected from the severe pain that can be experienced on damage to the kidneys. Renal sensory neurones have been identified in the lower and upper thoracic dorsal root ganglia by anterograde transport (in which marker substances are injected into the kidney and taken up and transported by the sensory fibres to the cell bodies, where they can be visualised by histochemical techniques). Small and medium-sized neurones are seen, connecting respectively to C fibres or thin myelinated A fibres. Evidence suggests that the kidney possesses mechanoreceptors and chemoreceptors. The mechanoreceptors respond to increases in arterial and venous pressures, as well as ureteropelvic pressures. Chemoreceptors appear to be of at least two types – some are normally silent and only respond to complete renal ischaemia, others can be activated by back flow of urine into the pelvis and various ionic changes. Some respond to changes in urinary flow rate. The neurones project to the spinal cord and medulla. Evidence suggests that they may be involved in reflexes affecting the cardiovascular system, in renorenal reflexes, which may be involved in physiological regulation of renal function, and also in interrenal adjustments resulting from alterations in the function of one or other of the kidneys.

An increased renal nerve activity has been implicated in cases of hypertension, and in animal models there is a relationship between sodium retention, renal sympathetic nerve activity and hypertension.

10.2 Ureters

Structure and function

The ureters connect the kidneys to the bladder, and aid the transport of urine by propagated waves of contraction which begin in the renal pelvis. The muscle contracts myogenically in response to action potentials that are initiated in the renal pelvis (Fig. 10.2) and propagate from cell to cell along the length of the ureter, which acts as a functional syncytium.

A transverse section of the ureter shows that the walls are composed of

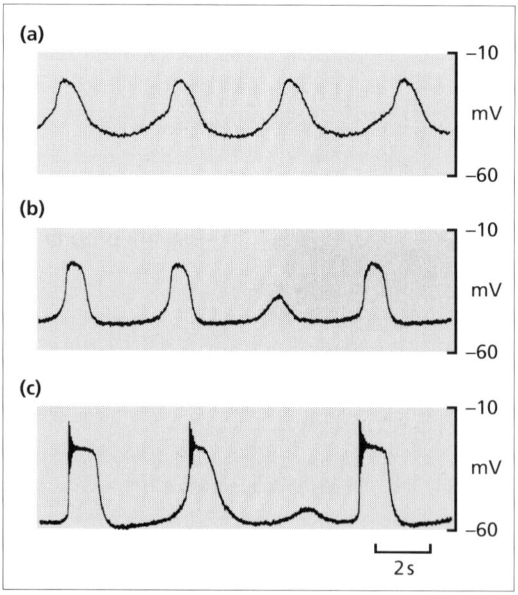

Fig. 10.2 Spontaneous action potentials recorded with microelectrodes from cells in a strip of the guinea-pig renal pelvis. Three types of cells were seen: (a) 10% were simple pacemaker cells, with small membrane potentials (−40 to −45 mV); (b) 15% were intermediate cells, had a faster rise and a plateau, and (c) 75% of the cells were driven cells, and had a larger membrane potential (−55 to −60 mV) and an initial spike and well-developed plateau component. Adapted from Zhang & Lang (1994).

an outer adventitial layer of loose fibro-elastic connective tissue, a smooth muscle layer and an inner mucosal layer composed of the lamina propria (another fibro-elastic connective tissue layer) lined with the urothelium. The smooth muscle layer is fairly uniform throughout the length of the ureter, with the smooth muscle cells tightly packed together into muscle bundles, which are interspersed with connective tissue. The muscle bundles branch and interconnect, forming a complex network. In the upper ureter, the inner bundles tend to lie longitudinally, while the outer bundles are more oblique or circular in orientation. Lower in the ureter, the bundles are almost entirely longitudinal or oblique (Fig. 10.3).

Autonomic innervation

The role of the autonomic nervous system in the control of the ureters is uncertain. In the muscle layer, nerves are present, increasing in density from the renal to the vesical end. There is histological evidence for three types of autonomic nerve – cholinergic, noradrenergic and peptidergic. However,

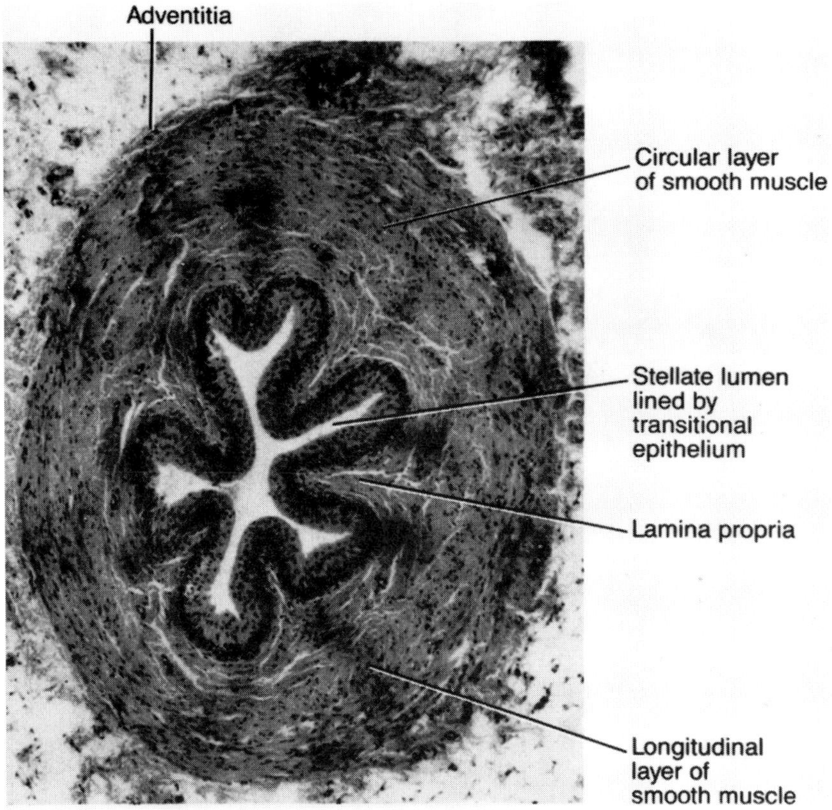

Fig. 10.3 Cross-section of a ureter. From Cormack (1987), with permission from the publisher, Lippincott-Raven.

varicose terminal axons are very rarely seen, and any synaptic sites between nerves and smooth muscle are exceedingly sparse, suggesting little nervous control of the tissue. This is supported by physiological observations which show that ureter strips mounted for tension recording (these are normally quiescent) do not respond to cholinergic or adrenergic agonists and cannot be made to contract by short electrical pulses, which are known to activate intrinsic nerves in other urinary tract smooth muscles. Phasic contractile responses can only be elicited by long depolarising current pulses, which directly activate the smooth muscle cells. Such responses are not affected by tetrodotoxin. Electrophysiological studies, however, suggest that autonomic transmitters may be able to alter the action potential shape, and have effects on the size of contraction initiated. It has been shown in the guinea-pig, for instance, that noradrenaline and histamine both prolong the action potentials and enhance the phasic contractions (Fig. 10.4). It is probable, therefore, that the autonomic nervous system plays a relatively small role in the motor activity of the ureter, but may have a modulatory effect in some circumstances.

There are extensive sensory nerves present in the lamina propria. Branches of them may innervate the smooth muscle cells and release peptides that can modulate the excitability of the smooth muscle cells. This could be important, since local inflammation could result in depolarisation of the smooth muscle cells and initiation of action potentials, which could propagate back towards the renal pelvis, causing reflux of urine from the

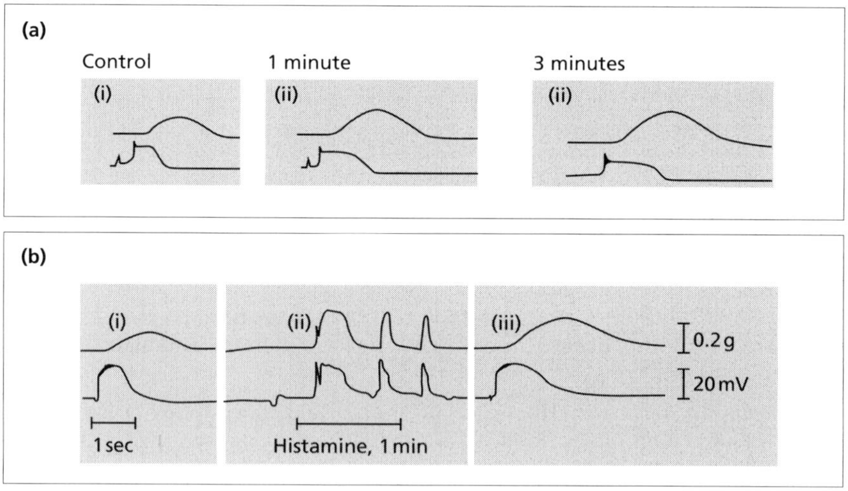

Fig. 10.4 Effects of noradrenaline (a) and histamine (b) on the electrical (lower traces) and mechanical (upper traces) activity of the guinea-pig ureter. Action potentials were evoked by current pulses. In (a) panels (ii) and (iii) noradrenaline (10^{-5} g/ml) causes prolongation of the plateau and an increase in the size of the mechanical response. In (b), application of histamine (10^{-6} m) in the middle panel causes the appearance of spontaneous action potentials and contractions. (i) Before and (ii) 1 min after washout of histamine. Adapted from Shuba (1977).

bladder – a situation that can lead to kidney infections. Sensory nerves have been shown to release CGRP, which hyperpolarises the smooth muscle cells and reduces their excitability. This effect is mediated by the opening of glibenclamide-sensitive K^+ channels.

Relevant pharmacology

It is common knowledge that obstruction of the ureters, or passage of stones down them, can lead to excruciating pain. These are the most relevant clinical problems, and pharmacological treatment is aimed at relieving the pain and reducing inflammation of the ureters. Since the pain may be very severe, pethidine may be prescribed, and non-steroidal anti-inflammatory agents such as diclofenac are useful. Current research suggests that K^+-channel-opening drugs may be able to reduce ureteric spasm. Another group of conditions in which pharmacological treatment could be relevant is diseases associated with impaired peristaltic activity, such as pelvi-ureteric junction dysfunction.

10.3 The lower urinary tract

This comprises the bladder and the urethra (Fig. 10.5). The function of these organs is to allow the storage of urine until a suitable time and place occur for its release, when it is rapidly voided in the process of micturition. The organs receive a rich parasympathetic and sympathetic innervation from the pelvic plexus, and it is this innervation that is responsible for the sequence of events occurring during micturition. Nervous activity may also help maintain low pressure in the detrusor and high pressure in the urethra during the filling phase, but evidence confirming this is scanty.

Preganglionic parasympathetic neurones leave the spinal cord in roots S2–S4, and travel in the pelvic nerves to the pelvic plexus. The postganglionic neurones are present both in the pelvic plexus and in the wall of the bladder. The sympathetic preganglionic fibres originate in T11–L2, and enter the sympathetic chain, whence they pass via the lumbar splanchnic nerves to the superior hypogastric plexus. Postganglionic, and possibly some preganglionic, fibres run in the hypogastric nerves, and also enter the pelvic plexus (Fig. 10.6).

Afferent fibres pass to the spinal cord mainly in the pelvic nerves (sacral afferents), but some also run with the sympathetic fibres (thoracolumbar afferents). The sacral afferents are essential for the micturition reflex, whereas those entering the thoracolumbar cord are activated by marked distension of the bladder, and are not necessary for micturition.

10.3.1 Bladder

The bladder is conventionally divided into the dome (detrusor muscle), the

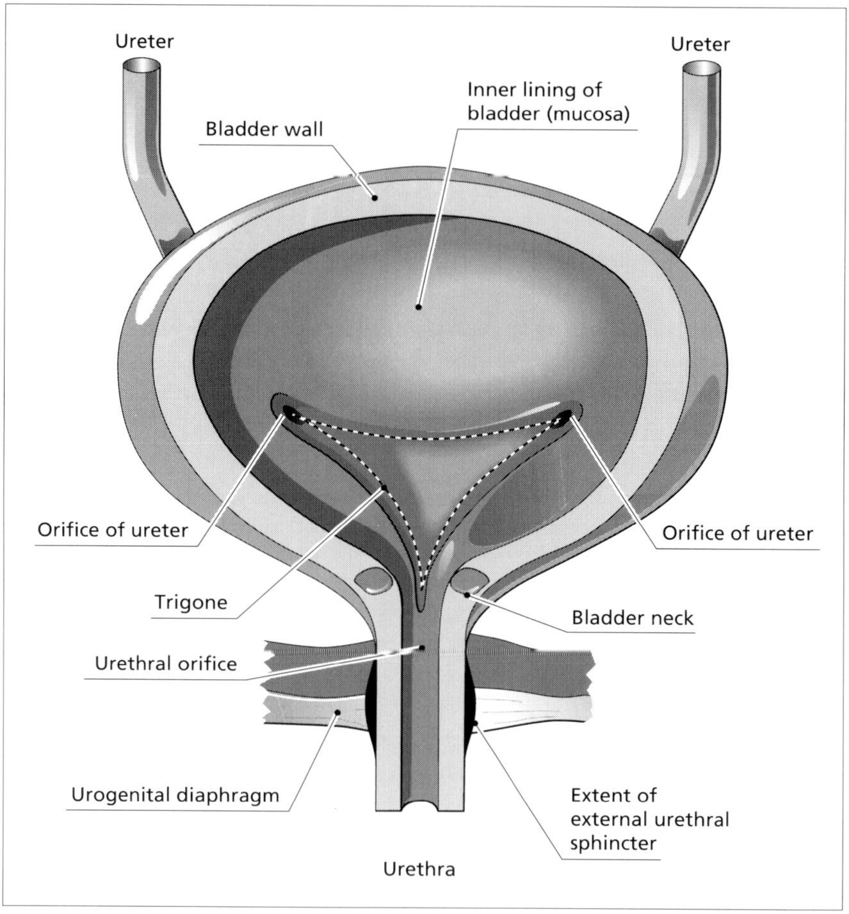

Fig. 10.5 Diagram of human lower urinary tract. The ureters enter the bladder wall and form the two outer corners of the trigone, a specialized triangular structure (dotted outline) extending from between the urethral orifices to the bladder neck. The bladder wall is made up of smooth muscle (the detrusor) and lined with urothelium. The bladder neck forms the internal urethral sphincter, and links the bladder to the urethra. The external urethral sphincter is not really a distinct structure, but is the region of the urethra that generates a high urethral pressure through a combination of smooth and striated muscle in the urethral wall. The urethra penetrates the pelvic floor through the urogenital diaphragm.

trigone and the bladder neck (Fig. 10.5). The trigone is the triangular area lying between the two orifices at which the ureters enter and the beginning of the urethra. The smooth muscles from these three areas show differences in their anatomical organisation, innervation and behaviour.

Dome

The arrangement of the smooth muscle is fairly uniform throughout the

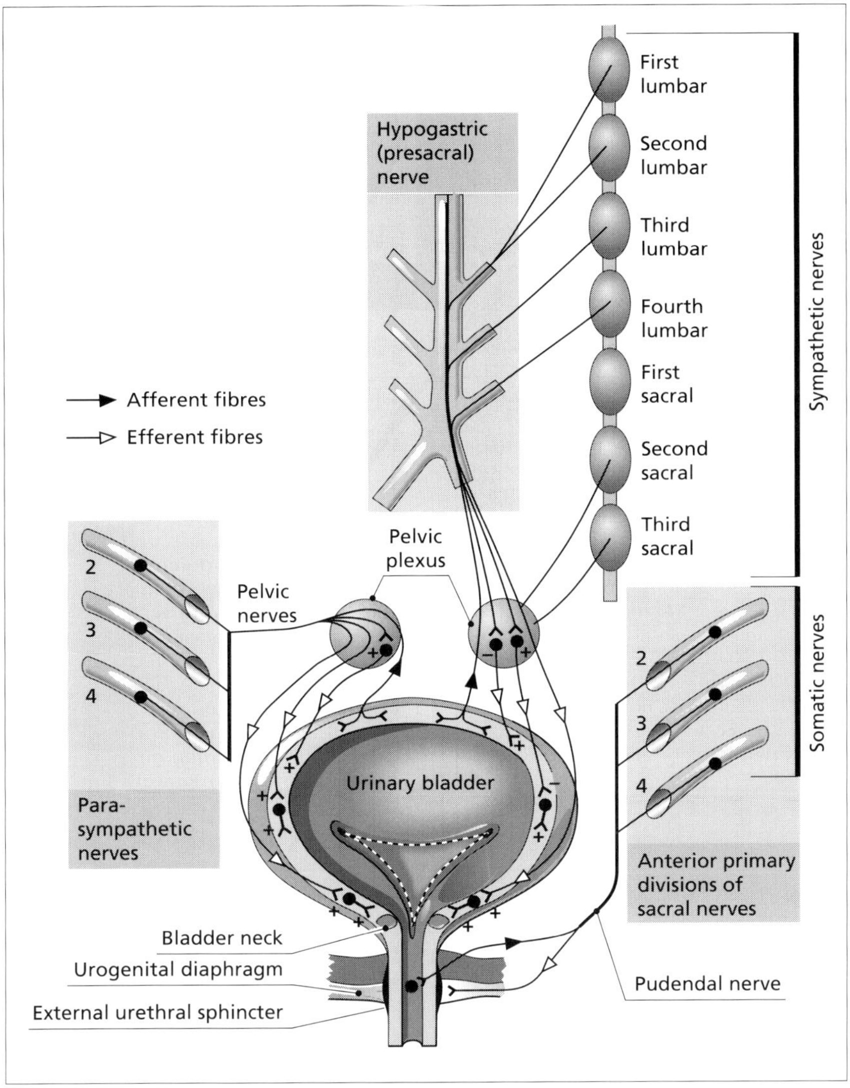

Fig. 10.6 Innervation of the lower urinary tract. Parasympathetic preganglionic fibres leave the cord in the sacral roots, and enter the pelvic plexus, where they may synapse with ganglion cells, or pass through and synapse with neurones in the bladder wall. Sympathetic innervation comes from the thoracolumbar cord, and preganglionic fibres enter the paravertebral chains, and may synapse in various of the paravertebral ganglia, or pass out and synapse with neurones in the pelvic plexus or the urethral wall. Postganglionic fibres innervate ganglia in the bladder wall, and smooth muscle in the urethra. Somatic motor nerves leave through the sacral roots and innervate the striated muscle in the urethral wall. Afferent fibres may run with any of the divisions.

dome. The individual muscle cells are grouped into well-defined muscle bundles large enough to be seen under a dissecting microscope, separated by connective tissue rich in collagen (Fig. 10.7). The muscle bundles are not arranged in any obvious orientation, but interdigitate with each other

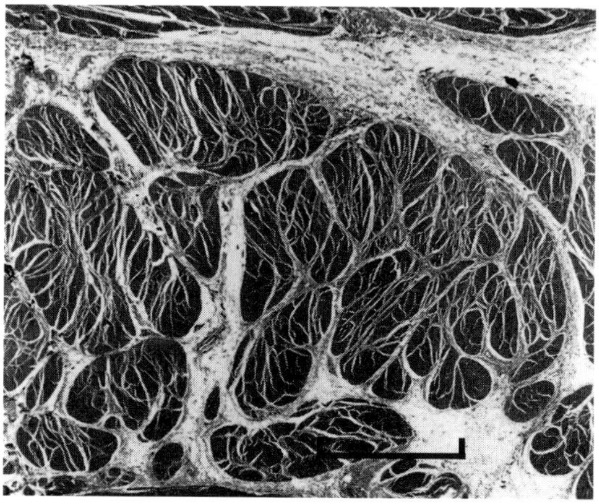

Fig. 10.7 Low magnification cross-section of muscle bundles from normal human detrusor. Note that the muscle cells are arranged into small bundles or fascicles that are grouped together into larger bundles divided from each other by connective tissue containing collagen. Scale bar: 1 mm.

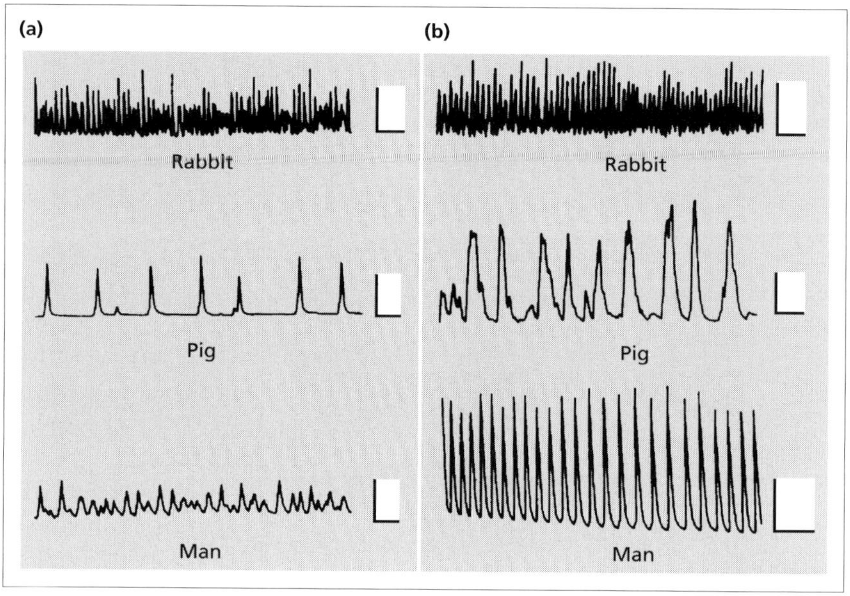

Fig. 10.8 Examples of spontaneous activity in strips dissected from the bladder dome (a) and the trigone or bladder base (b) from rabbit, pig and man. Vertical bars represent 0.25 g wt of tension, and horizontal bars 1 min. Adapted from Sibley (1984).

throughout the thickness of the wall, so that synchronous contraction can result in a decrease in intravesical volume and concomitant wall thickening during voiding. In spite of the low intravesical pressure during filling, evidence strongly suggests that the smooth muscle is spontaneously active. As shown in Fig. 10.8, isolated smooth muscle strips show rhythmic contractions that rise from and fall to a baseline that has no sustained tone. The contractions are not abolished by poisoning the nerves with tetrodotoxin, or by muscarinic receptor blockade, and the activity is myogenic. Electrical coupling probably exists between the smooth muscle cells, but this appears to

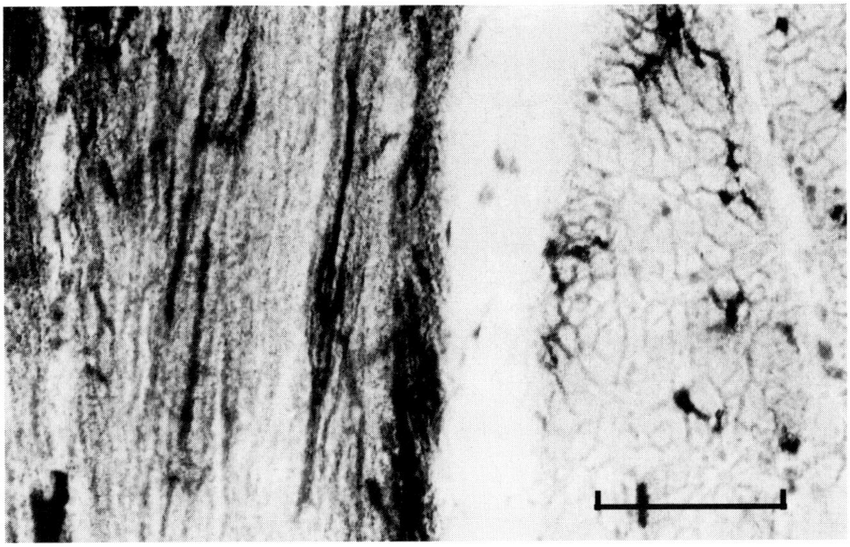

Fig. 10.9 Section of human detrusor stained to demonstrate cholinesterase-positive nerve fibres. The muscle bundle on the left is sectioned in the longitudinal direction, and on the right is in cross-section. Note extensive distribution of darkly stained nerve fibres. Scale bar: 500 μm.

be less extensive than in many other smooth muscles, so that spontaneous mechanical activity is not sufficiently synchronous throughout the detrusor to allow a build-up of intravesical pressure. The activity will, however, prevent the bladder from being floppy, and will keep its surface area–volume ratio at a minimum. This will allow an immediate build-up of intravesical pressure if the contractile activity in the cells is synchronised, as occurs in response to excitation of the parasympathetic nerves.

The smooth muscle of the detrusor is densely innervated with cholinesterase-positive nerve terminals (Fig. 10.9). Naked varicosities, with the small clear vesicles characteristic of cholinergic neurones, make close contacts with the smooth muscle cells (see Figs 4.3 and 4.4), although the frequency with which these are seen in human bladder suggests that not every cell will receive direct innervation. There is no evidence of any direct sympathetic innervation of the detrusor smooth muscle cells, although sympathetic nerves innervate vascular smooth muscle in the bladder wall. The postganglionic sympathetic fibres mainly innervate the parasympathetic ganglion cells in the pelvic plexus and the bladder wall, and reduce the excitability of these neurones via activation of α-adrenoceptors.

Activation of the sacral spinal roots, pelvic nerves and intrinsic nerves in bladder strips leads to contraction of the smooth muscle. In normal human detrusor, this excitatory input can be entirely abolished by atropine, showing that muscarinic acetylcholine receptors mediate the response. In other mammals, and possibly in some pathological conditions in the human bladder, an atropine-resistant component of the contraction is seen, which appears to be mediated by adenosine triphosphate (ATP) acting on purinergic P_{2x} receptors.

Trigone

The trigone is about the size of a large postage stamp in the human, and it consists of a superficial layer of smooth muscle under the mucosa, and a deep layer continuous with the detrusor. The muscle bundles of the superficial layer are smaller than in the detrusor. They are continuous with the smooth muscle of the proximal urethra. The deep trigone is indistinguishable from the detrusor under the dissecting microscope, and is also similar in its innervation. The superficial trigone, however, appears to receive three types of excitatory innervation: cholinergic, noradrenergic and non-adrenergic, non-cholinergic (NANC), and also an NANC inhibitory innervation (Fig. 10.10). There is at present little evidence about the role of these inputs, although it has been proposed that the trigone is important in preventing reflux of urine up the ureters during micturition.

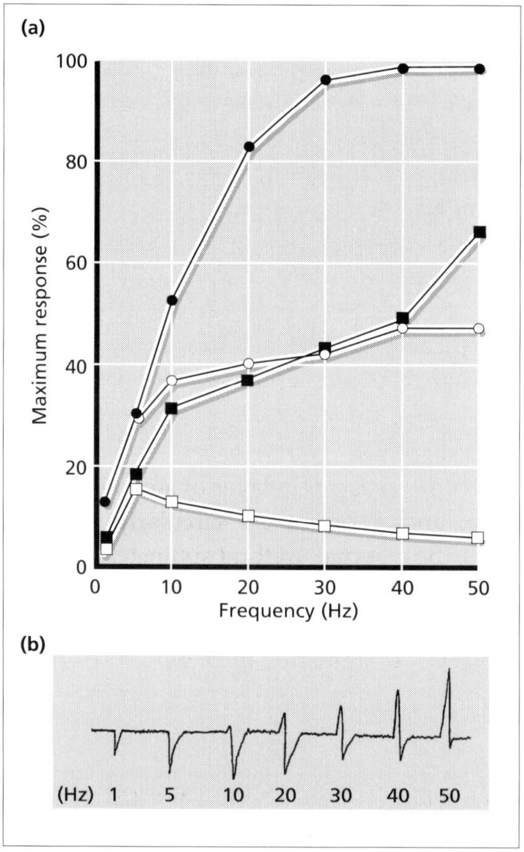

Fig. 10.10 An illustration of the complexity of the innervation of the trigone. Responses are shown of strips of human superficial trigone to transmural nerve stimulation. In (a) parameters were chosen which produced contractile responses only, whereas in (b) both contractile and relaxant responses are apparent. In (a) the filled circles show the control responses. The open circles show responses in the presence of atropine (10^{-6} M) to block the cholinergic response, the filled squares in the presence of phentolamine (10^{-6} M) to block the adrenergic response, and the open squares in the presence of both drugs. Note there is still a non-adrenergic, non-cholinergic response left. These results suggest that the trigone is innervated by at least three types of excitatory nerve and an inhibitory one.

Bladder neck

The bladder neck smooth muscle is histologically and pharmacologically distinct from the detrusor proper. Muscle bundles are much smaller, and in the male these are mainly circularly oriented, so that there is a collar of smooth muscle round the bladder neck (the internal sphincter), contraction of which probably prevents retrograde ejaculation. Cholinergic and noradrenergic nerve fibres supply this muscle and the smooth muscle of the proximal urethra. In the female, the muscle bundles extend obliquely and longitudinally from the bladder neck into the urethral wall, and there is no true internal sphincter, although the bladder neck is normally closed during filling. The innervation of the female bladder neck is largely cholinergic, with only a sparse sympathetic supply.

10.3.2 Urethra

Male

In the male, the urethra is often considered as comprising four sections, the preprostatic, the prostatic, the membranous and the penile urethra (Fig. 10.11). The preprostatic urethra is about 1.5 cm long, and extends from the bladder neck to the prostate. The smooth muscle is richly supplied with noradrenergic nerve fibres, and there is only a sparse cholinergic innervation. The prostatic urethra is about 3–4 cm long and runs through the substance of the prostate. It has a crescent-shaped cross-section due to the posteriorly positioned urethral crest, which protrudes into the lumen. The ejaculatory ducts open on the surface of this crest (called the verumontanum). On either side of the crest are the openings of the prostatic ducts. There are many mucosal glands opening around the entire circumference of the prostatic urethra. The thin smooth muscle coat of longitudinally and circularly arranged muscle bundles is continuous with the strands of smooth muscle pervading the prostate. The membranous urethra extends from the prostate to the bulb of the penis, passing through the muscles of the pelvic floor. The adventitia of the membranous urethra contains two bulbourethral glands (Cowper's glands). There is a thin layer of smooth muscle lining the membranous urethra, and a prominent circularly oriented sphincter of striated muscle fibres, the external urethral sphincter, or rhabdosphincter (Fig. 10.11). The rest of the urethra, the penile or spongy urethra, is the longest part, running through the penis to the exterior. It is surrounded by erectile tissue and has little smooth muscle in its walls.

Female

In the female, the urethra is 3–4 cm long, and runs in the adventitial coat of the anterior wall of the vagina, passing through the pelvic floor musculature (Fig. 10.12). The lumen is crescent-shaped, and lined with a mucous

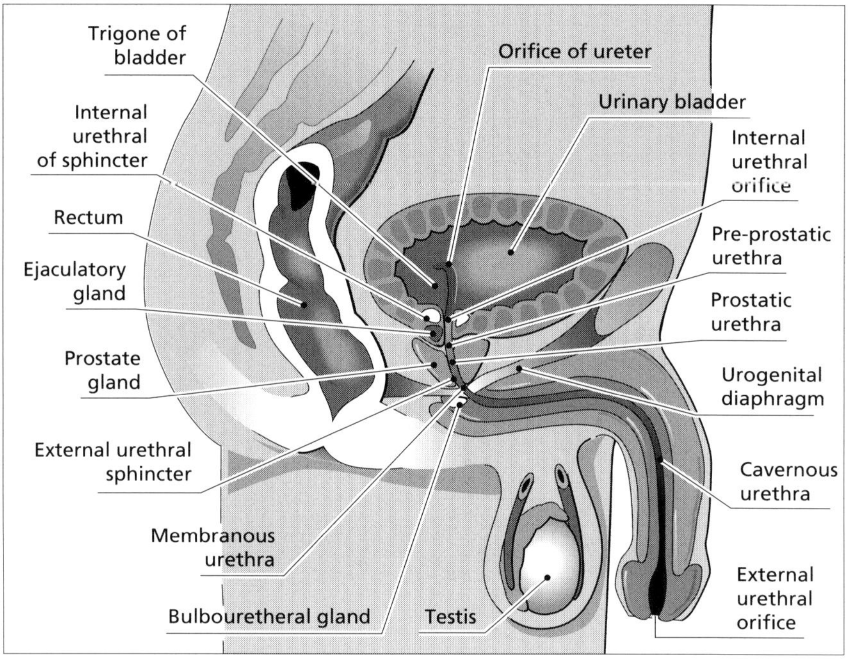

Fig. 10.11 Sagittal section of a human male. Note the four sections of the urethra: the preprostatic urethra between the bladder neck (internal urethral sphincter) and the prostate, the prostatic urethra, the membranous urethra (the site of the external sphincter mechanism) and the cavernous (penile or spongiose) urethra running through the penis.

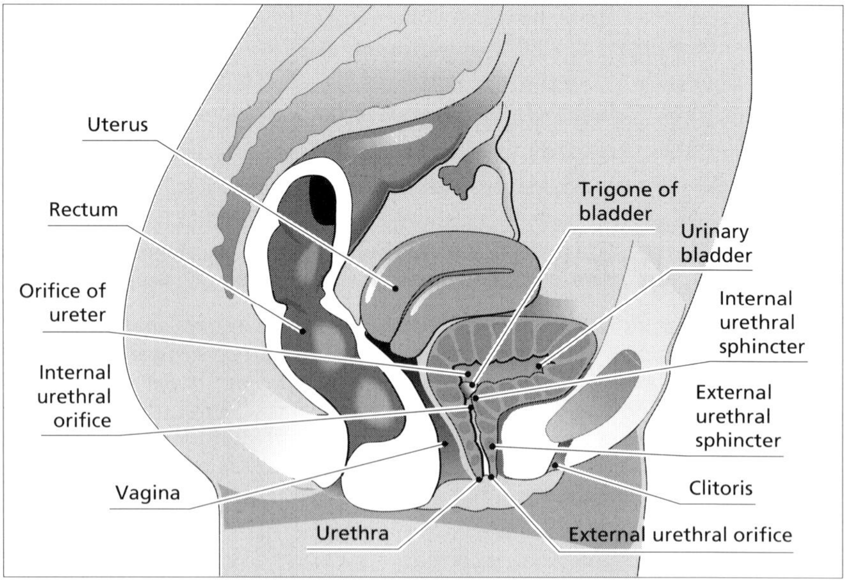

Fig. 10.12 Sagittal section of a human female. Note the comparatively short urethra.

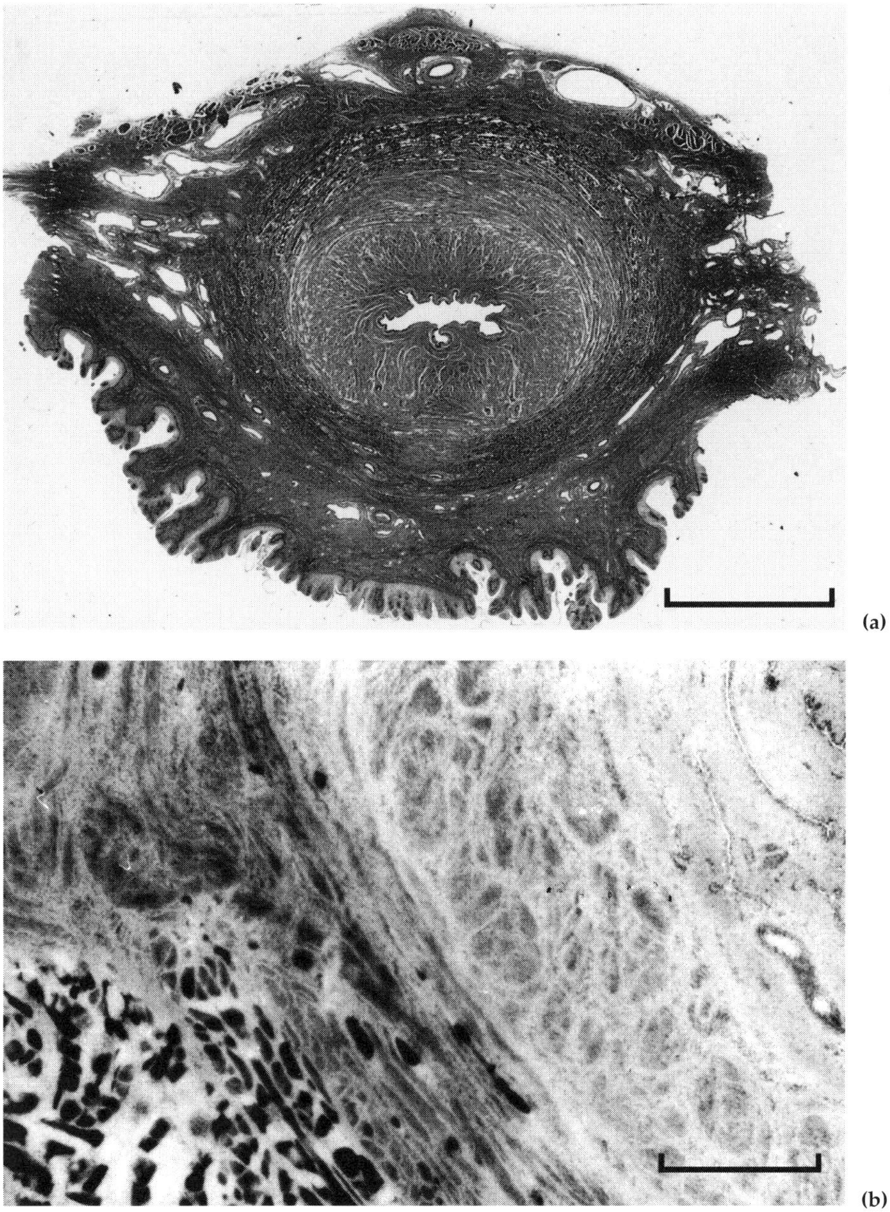

Fig. 10.13 Light microscopic sections of human female urethra. (a) Section at low power, with vaginal wall at the bottom, where the striated muscle layer is incomplete. Scale bar: 5 mm. (b) Section from a different specimen at higher power. Note from left to right, first a striated muscle layer, and inside this a circular orientated smooth muscle layer, with interspersed striated fibres. Within this is a thicker layer of longitudinal smooth muscle cut in cross-section, and then the lamina propria, with urothelium and urethral lumen showing in the top right corner. Scale bar: 1 mm.

membrane. The lamina propria of the mucosal layer contains collagen fibres, elastic fibres and elongated fibrocytes. It also contains many thin-walled veins, which when engorged may play a role in maintaining urethral closure. Behind the lamina propria, there is a smooth muscle coat, and outside it, a striated muscle layer forming the rhabdosphincter (Fig. 10.13). The smooth muscle bundles lie mainly in an oblique or longitudinal direction, with a few circularly arranged bundles near the rhabdosphincter. The smooth muscle bundles are widely separated by connective tissue containing collagen and elastin. The female urethral smooth muscle receives an extensive cholinesterase-positive (presumably parasympathetic) innervation, with some adrenergic fibres. Experimentally, strips of urethral smooth muscle can be shown to receive at least three distinct innervations: two excitatory and one inhibitory. Excitatory responses can be abolished by blocking muscarinic receptors and sympathetic nerve activity, leaving a transient inhibitory response that can be abolished by nitric oxide synthase inhibitors, suggesting that the transmitter is NO. In the pig, there is also another sustained NANC inhibitory response, but the transmitter for this sustained inhibition is unknown at present, although it could be a peptide; there is little evidence for it in the human. Very little information is available about the role of the innervation of the urethra in the micturition reflex, or in the maintenance of urethral tone during filling of the bladder.

10.3.3 Continence

As long as the pressure in the bladder (intravesical pressure) is lower than the urethral pressure, urine will be stored, and continence maintained. During micturition, the situation must be reversed. Synchronous contraction of the bladder smooth muscle must occur, with a drop in the urethral pressure, and the whole process is under voluntary control, making micturition an interesting example of the voluntary control of smooth muscles. The detrusor is a very compliant structure, and during filling with urine, the bladder can accommodate large volumes without a significant rise in intraluminal pressure. This is largely due to the intrinsic properties of the bladder wall, although there is some evidence that the activity in the parasympathetic ganglia is kept low during filling by activation of a reflex inhibitory pathway, possibly involving their sympathetic innervation. During the filling phase of the micturition cycle high pressure can be recorded in the urethra. There is evidence that the urethral smooth muscles can develop myogenic tone, and it is probable in the human that the autonomic nerves are also involved in maintaining the urethral pressure, although this has not been conclusively established. At present, many urologists believe that the high intraurethral pressure is due largely to activity of the striated muscle of the rhabdosphincter, although others believe that these muscles are mainly important in a reflex response designed to prevent leakage of urine when there is an increase in intra-abdominal pressure (and

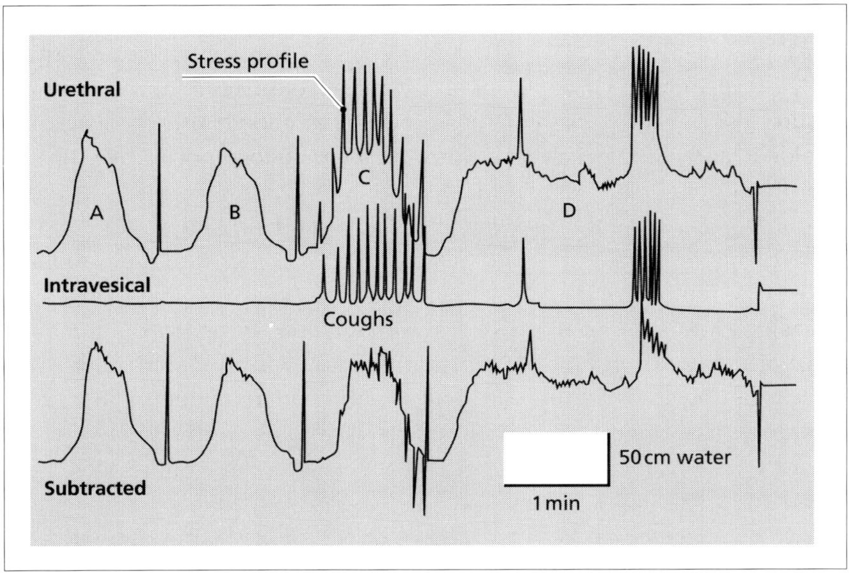

Fig. 10.14 Pressure recording in the female bladder and urethra. Upper trace, pressure recorded in the urethra, middle trace, pressure recorded in the bladder, bottom trace subtracted pressure, showing the element generated by the urethra and its surrounding structures. A, B and C are urethral pressure profiles, recorded by pulling the recording catheter through the length of the urethra from the bladder (Lt) to the external meatus (right). In C the subject was asked to cough during the recording. Coughing increases abdominal pressure, which is reflected equally in the bladder and proximal urethra, as can be seen on the left of the subtracted trace where the pressure rises are cancelled out. In the centre of the urethra, the subtracted trace shows a positive response to coughing, but as the catheter is pulled further, the negative going deflections indicate that the bladder pressure is not passively transferred to the distal urethra. In D, the catheter is kept in the maximum pressure region of the urethra, and again the patient asked to give a single, then a series of, coughs. In this region the subtracted trace shows the active response of the urethral wall. This reflex helps prevent leakage when the abdominal pressure rises.

hence the pressure in the bladder), as occurs with such events as coughing, sneezing or straining (Fig. 10.14). This striated muscle is supplied by motor nerves with their cell bodies in S2–S4, the fibres running mostly in the pudendal nerve and pelvic nerves. The striated muscle fibres are heterogeneous (particularly in the male), being a mixture of the slow-twitch and fast-twitch types (Fig. 10.15), the slow-twitch fibres being capable of sustained contraction over relatively long periods of time. The striated muscle of the pelvic floor also contains fast-twitch and slow-twitch fibres, and may be important in maintaining continence, particularly for holding the urethra in the correct position. It might also supply an additional occlusive force on the urethra.

10.3.4 Mechanisms of micturition

The bladder wall is well innervated with sensory fibres, and a subset of

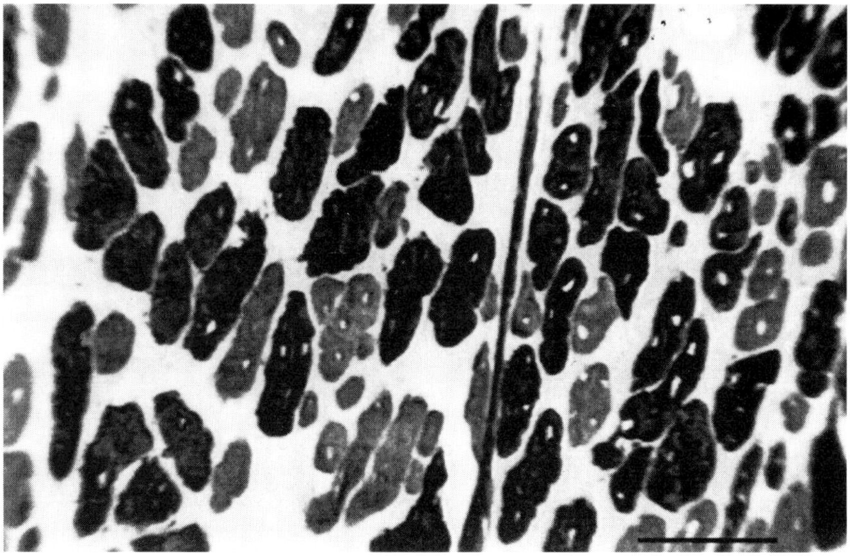

Fig. 10.15 Section of rhabdosphincter from male membranous urethra. Striated muscles stained for troponin. Note there are two populations of fibres, the larger darkly stained ones being fast-twitch, and the rest slow-twitch fibres. Scale bar: 10 μm. Figure kindly supplied by Kossen Ho.

these fibres is activated by stretching. This afferent activity is responsible for triggering both the perception of bladder fullness, and the complex mechanisms responsible for micturition. Urodynamic monitoring of normal humans, in which bladder pressure is recorded during filling, shows that the first desire to void occurs when the bladder pressure is still low, and is not associated with any transient increase in bladder pressure. This perception of bladder filling is thought to be mediated by sensory fibres that ascend in the lateral spinothalamic tracts to the frontal cortex. When the individual decides to void, the first urodynamic sign is a reduction in the urethral pressure, followed shortly by funnelling of the bladder neck and an increase in intravesical pressure (Fig. 10.16). These events have to be synchronised in order for normal voiding to occur, and it is known that micturition involves a spinopontine–spinal reflex, with a micturition centre in the pons that is essential for this co-ordination. The pontine centre is itself controlled by higher centres, allowing the voluntary control of micturition. The precise details of the efferent innervation to the various muscles triggered in micturition are still very poorly understood. In the female pig, in which the process has been studied in more detail, a high urethral pressure can occur in the absence of activity in the rhabdosphincter, and the initial fall in urethral pressure is caused by relaxation of the urethral smooth muscles. In the human, relaxation of the striated muscle of the rhabdosphincter is probably more important than in the pig. It is not known whether the funnelling of the bladder neck is caused by excitatory nerves to the smooth muscle pulling the neck open, or by activation of inhibitory

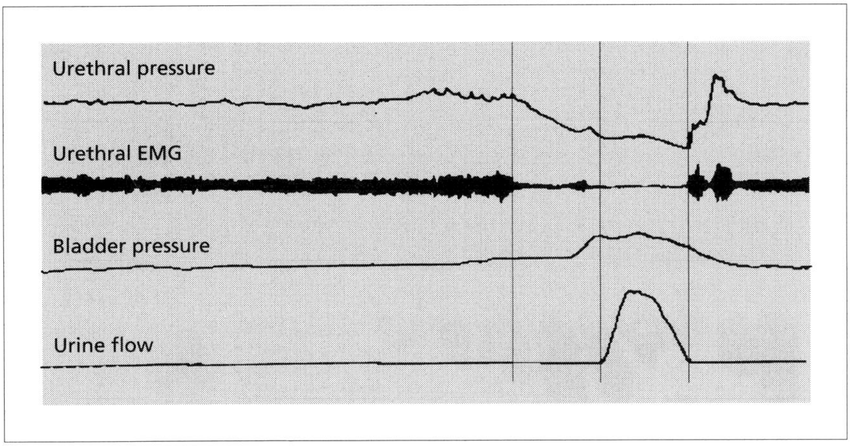

Fig. 10.16 Typical urodynamic recording from a normal subject. Maximum urethral pressure, EMG electromyogram recorded from the urethral striated muscle (rhabdosphincter), B bladder pressure (generated by the bladder wall) and urine flow. During the filling phase the bladder pressure only rises by a small amount. Towards the end of filling the EMG activity increases and there is a small increase in the urethral pressure. The first event of micturition is a drop in urethral pressure, and a reduction in the EMG activity. This precedes the detrusor contraction which raises intravesical pressure and leads to cessation of the EMG activity and urine flow. Adapted from Torrens & Morrison (1987).

innervation to the smooth muscles causing their relaxation. The transmitters and receptors involved in these events are at present still not firmly established. The contraction of the detrusor is known to be mediated by the excitatory parasympathetic innervation, with acetylcholine as the transmitter, acting through muscarinic receptors (largely of the M_3 subtype).

It is worth noting that events during micturition are very variable, even in one individual. The volume in the bladder when a desire to void is felt can vary markedly, as can the peak voiding pressure and the flow rate of the urine. Normally, voiding is to completion, and there is little if any residual urine, but this can again vary. This implies that many of the steps in the reflex are susceptible to modulation. It has been suggested that local release of peptides from the sensory nerve terminals may play a role in the sensitivity of the reflex even at the level of the smooth muscle, and modulation of the sensitivity of transmission at the autonomic ganglia and at various synaptic sites in the central nervous system is undoubtedly possible.

10.3.5 Incontinence and relevant pharmacology

Incontinence can be crudely divided into urge and stress incontinence, although many incontinent people show symptoms of both types. Urge incontinence occurs when inappropriate contraction of the bladder wall leads to a rise in pressure that overcomes the urethral closure pressure, resulting in leakage of urine. Stress incontinence occurs when the mechanisms ensuring urethral closure are unable to prevent leakage of urine when the bladder pressure rises due to increases in abdominal pressure.

Urge incontinence is associated with detrusor instability – spontaneous contraction of the bladder wall that cannot be voluntarily suppressed. This condition is associated with bladder outflow obstruction (and thus is common in men with benign prostatic hypertrophy), with neuronal injury (e.g. spinal lesions, multiple sclerosis, spina bifida) and can occur spontaneously (idiopathic instability). Treatment of urge incontinence is designed to suppress these spontaneous contractions. Underlying the contractions are changes in the properties of the smooth muscles, which become more easily excited and better coupled, allowing the spread of contractile activity throughout the bladder. There also appears to be an element of neuronal activity associated with the pressure rises, and current pharmacological treatment is largely by use of muscarinic antagonists, which may also have some ability to block smooth muscle Ca^{2+} channels, such as oxybutynin. The side-effects of muscarinic antagonists are such as to render their long-term use undesirable, and efforts are being made to develop more selective muscarinic antagonists (tolterodine and darifenacin are currently undergoing clinical trials). Another approach under investigation is to develop K^+-channel-opening drugs that are bladder-specific. Potentially, these could relax the detrusor without interfering with normal micturition.

The bladder outflow obstruction associated with prostatic hypertrophy can be treated with drugs designed to reduce smooth muscle activity in the prostate and prostatic urethra. α-Adrenoceptor antagonists such as prazosin and indoramin can be effective.

Stress incontinence is commonly seen in women, presumably because of their much shorter urethras. Stress incontinence after childbirth injuries is largely treated surgically. Other types may respond to drugs such as α-adrenoceptor agonists.

10.4 The female reproductive tract

10.4.1 Overview

The female reproductive tract contains smooth muscle in its walls, and has a secretory epithelium lining it. As one would expect, it is innervated throughout by the autonomic nervous system. Nevertheless, it is intriguing that – apart from a few obvious exceptions – the functions of the innervation are largely unknown. It has been demonstrated in the rat, for instance, that complete autonomic denervation does not preclude normal intercourse, conception, pregnancy, delivery of live pups, and their suckling. Obvious functions of the innervation pertain largely to the behavioural aspects of sexual activity – erection of the clitoris, mucous secretion in the cervix providing lubrication of the vagina and orgasm probably all have reflex components in which the autonomic innervation provides the efferent limb.

However, these activities also involve hormonal secretions, and it is not always easy to separate them. Another intriguing factor is the almost complete denervation of the uterus that occurs during pregnancy, and its reinnervation after delivery. It has been suggested that denervation, which has been particularly studied for the sympathetic innervation, is necessary to preserve the blood flow to the placenta, and protect against sympathetic vasoconstriction in the uterine wall. However, it could also simply be a consequence of the increased pressure and stretching of the uterine wall, since in animals with two uterine horns, if pregnancy occurs in only one, the denervation only occurs in the same horn. Denervation develops in a patchy fashion close to each implanted fetus as it develops. Denervation of smooth muscle in other organs can also occur in situations in which luminal pressure increases.

Immunohistochemical and functional studies of the smooth muscles and epithelia in the female genital tract show that they receive cholinergic, adrenergic and NANC innervation. The functions of the cholinergic input are not well understood, although muscarinic receptor activation normally leads to excitation of the smooth muscles. Activation of the α-adrenoceptors is excitatory on smooth muscles, and β-adrenoceptor activation inhibitory. In many parts of the tract, the relative proportions of α- and β-adrenoceptors vary with the hormonal condition. The NANC innervation is probably peptidergic, since many peptides have been identified in the nerves. Substance P and CGRP are located in sensory nerves, but these are in a class of sensorimotor nerves, which can release locally active peptides from collateral branches. Substance P causes vasodilation, but activation of non-vascular smooth muscles in the tract. Peptidergic motor nerves probably contain vasoactive intestinal polypeptide (VIP). Activation of VIP receptors leads to inhibition of both vascular and non-vascular smooth muscle cells. Another peptide that is present is neuropeptide Y (NPY), which is often – but not always – associated with sympathetic nerves, and appears to be facilitatory in its actions. Very little is at present known about the effects of the autonomic nerves on the epithelial secretions, but this is likely to be important.

10.4.2 Components of the tract and their innervation

A diagram of the human female genital tract is given in Fig. 10.17.

Ovaries

The human ovaries are covered by a layer of germinal epithelium surrounding a thick cortex that contains the follicles and corpora lutea, and a vascular medulla. The ground substance or stroma of the cortex and medulla is interstitial connective tissue containing several cell types, some of which are probably smooth muscle cells.

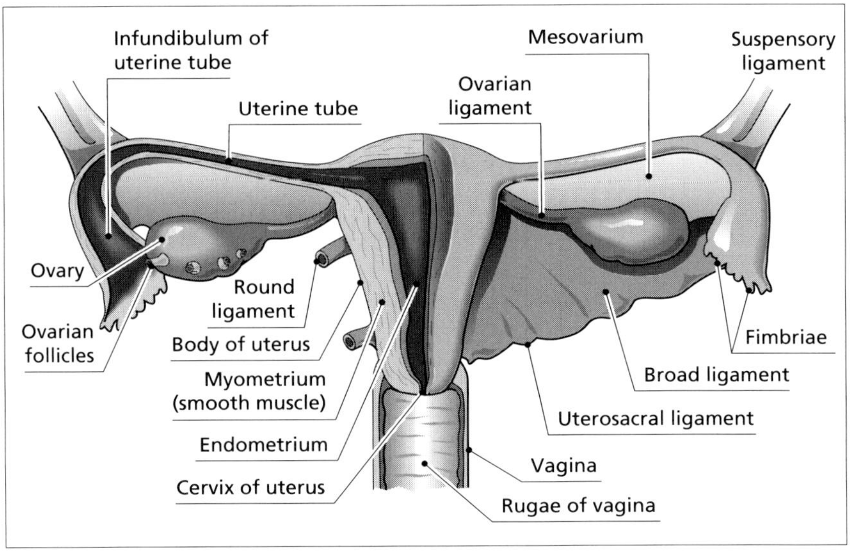

Fig. 10.17 Diagram of the human female reproductive tract. On the left the tract is shown in sagittal section.

The ovaries are innervated both by sensory nerves that project to the central nervous system and by adrenergic and cholinergic autonomic nerve fibres. Sympathetic fibres arise from the pre-aortic plexus and enter the ovaries with the ovarian arteries. Some of the parasympathetic fibres may enter the ovary along the branches of the uterine artery, distributed to the ovary by way of the broad ligament and mesovarium (the peritoneal fold surrounding the ovaries). Many of the autonomic nerves innervate the blood vessels, but there is some evidence for association with non-vascular elements in the uterus. Some 25% of the adrenergic nerves seem to be associated with the follicles. It has been demonstrated in some mammals that the ovaries undergo contractile activity, which is increased by α-adrenoceptor activation, and this probably involves activity of the smooth muscle cells in the stromal fibromuscular tissue. It is possible that the contraction of these cells may assist in the rupture of the follicles. Early work on transplanted ovaries has, however, shown them to function normally although they show no evidence of re-innervation, suggesting that intact innervation is unnecessary.

Fallopian tubes

The ovaries are linked to the uterus via the oviducts, or Fallopian tubes, which have muscular walls and complex mucosal linings. The nearest part of each tube to the ovary is called the ampulla, and opens via a flower-like expansion, the infundibulum, into the abdominal cavity. The mucosal lining of the ampulla extends into the fringe-like fimbriae lining and extending from the infundibulum, one of which, the ovarian fimbria, is attached to the inner surface of the ovary. The ampulla joins to the isthmus at the ampullary–isthmic junction, and the isthmus reaches the uterus at the uterotubal junction, with its last part, the intramural portion, running inside the wall of the uterus, entering the cavity of the uterus at the small uterine ostium. The oviducts and ovaries are suspended in peritoneal folds (the broad ligaments of the uterus) and joined to the ovaries by membranes containing smooth muscle cells, the mesotubarium and mesosalpinx.

The oviducts function to capture the released ova, and transport them to the uterus. The ova are, however, retained in the oviducts for three to four days, to increase the chances of them meeting a sperm and becoming fertilised. *In situ* observation of the human oviduct shows a great deal of contractile activity, which varies depending on the state of the menstrual cycle. The contractile activity of the smooth muscle cells in the mesotubarium and mesosalpinx alters the anatomical relationship between the oviducts and their fimbriae with the ovaries, and this may assist capture of released ova. The activity in the ampulla and isthmus of the oviducts is not synchronous, and there is no synchrony between the two oviducts. The contractions in the oviduct can run as waves along the tubes. In the ampulla, the waves most often run towards the ovaries, whereas in the isthmus the waves normally run towards the uterus. There is no structural sphincter at the ampullary–isthmic junction, although it is at this point that the egg is delayed in its passage to the uterus. It seems likely that activity in the smooth muscles provides a physiological sphincter.

Although, as has been mentioned earlier, animal experiments show that transport and fertilisation of the ovum can occur normally in denervated organs, there is nevertheless a dense innervation of the oviducts, particularly at the ampullary–isthmic junction, and it seems likely that nervous activity plays a role in controlling the smooth muscle activity. An excitatory sympathetic input reaches the tubes from the hypogastric plexus along the ovarian and uterine arteries, and forms its densest innervation at the isthmus, close to the ampullary–isthmic junction. The parasympathetic input is both from vagal fibres (which are thought to supply the lateral part of the tubes) and pelvic splanchnic nerves to the more medial parts. This is probably also excitatory to the non-vascular smooth muscle. It is not certain where the ganglia in the parasympathetic pathway are situated, but they are possibly in the paracervical ganglia. More recently, peptide-containing nerves have been demonstrated in the walls of the oviducts, apparently innervating the smooth muscle cells. The dominant peptide is VIP, and the VIPergic nerves also densely innervate the isthmus and inhibit smooth muscle activity. The concentration of VIP in the human oviduct is affected by the hormonal status. Sensory nerves run with the adrenergic input.

Uterus

The uterus in the human differs from that of many commonly used experimental animals in that it is a single triangular-shaped dorsoventrally flattened hollow organ, rather than a bicornate one. The uterus is linked to the vagina via the cervix, at the narrow end of the uterus. Moving through the cervix towards the uterus proper, the cervical cavity narrows at the internal os, and then expands into the triangular cavity of the uterus, with the Fallopian tubes entering at the two corners made by the uterine walls with the fundus of the uterus. The thick uterine walls have a thin outer serous layer, a thick muscular layer composed of smooth muscle and an internal mucous layer. The muscular layer is composed of an outer longitudinally arranged layer, a middle layer in which the muscle bundles run in all directions, and an inner layer that has both longitudinal and circularly arranged bundles. The smooth muscle shows myogenic activity, regular slow depolarisations of the cells occurring with superimposed spike activity that initiates contraction (Fig. 10.18). The contractile activity is under hormonal control, which varies during the menstrual cycle and in pregnancy. The mucosal layer, or endometrium, is highly vascular and contains uterine glands. Its thickness and structure change during the menstrual cycle, and it is of the utmost importance in the implantation and development of the placenta. The body of the uterus is innervated by cholinergic, adrenergic and peptidergic neurones, which innervate both the smooth muscle and the epithelial layers. Parasympathetic input is from the second, third and fourth sacral segments, via the pelvic plexus, and sympathetic input from the twelfth thoracic and first lumbar segments, via the hypogastric plexus, entering the uterus along the uterine arteries. The paracervical ganglia contain the cell bodies of many VIP-containing neurones, which innervate the whole of the uterus. Stimulation of the intrinsic nerves in strips of myometrial smooth muscle from non-pregnant non-parous women demonstrates excitation through muscarinic receptors (blocked by atropine) and α-adrenoceptors

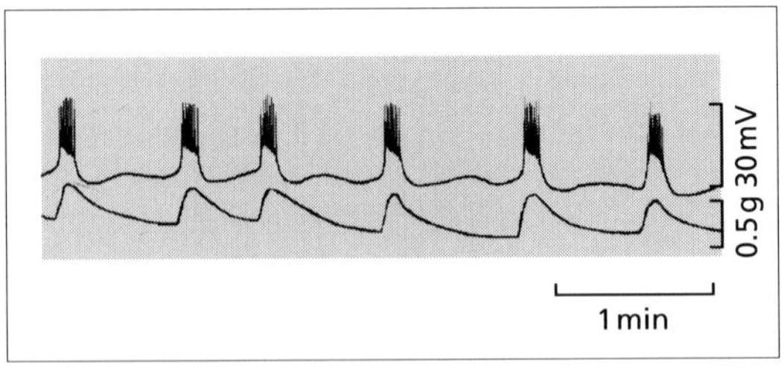

Fig. 10.18 Electrical and mechanical activity recorded from strips of smooth muscle from the guinea-pig uterus. The upper trace shows microelectrode recordings of spontaneous myogenic slow waves with superimposed spikes, and the bottom trace shows the contractile response. Trace kindly supplied by H. Parkington.

(blocked by phentolamine). There is no evidence of a nerve-mediated inhibition of activity. Exogenously applied VIP inhibits smooth muscle activity in the non-pregnant uterus, and causes vasodilation. This may have a role in menstrual bleeding. Afferent nerves leave the uterus through the hypogastric plexus.

During pregnancy, there is an almost total loss of the innervation to the body of the uterus, although the smooth muscle continues to show myogenic activity. Waves of contraction pass along the uterus at regular intervals, but these do not elevate the intrauterine pressure. The size and frequency of these waves change during pregnancy as the hormonal status changes. Towards the end of pregnancy, the smooth muscle becomes increasingly sensitive to oxytocin, which can powerfully enhance this activity, and just before delivery, there is a large increase in the number of gap junctions between the smooth muscle cells, which allows the electrical activity of the cells to be synchronised, thus initiating co-ordinated contractions of the smooth muscle that are necessary to expel the fetus.

Cervix

The innervation of the cervix is similar to that of the body of the uterus, but more dense. In contrast to the uterus, however, its innervation is preserved during pregnancy. There is a particularly high density of VIP-containing fibres, and it has been suggested that they may play a role in the relaxation of the cervix during parturition. These neurones, along with some of the noradrenergic neurones, arise in the paracervical ganglia. The cervix also contains a large number of NPY-containing nerves, some of which are probably adrenergic. The cervix has interesting functions – it facilitates the entry of sperm into the uterus around the time of ovulation, allows the escape of menstrual debris, permits passage of the fetus at delivery, but prevents entry of infectious organisms. Many of its functions depend on the quantity and characteristics of the mucus secreted from the cervical epithelium. This is probably largely controlled by the hormonal state of the body, but the dense innervation and the observation that the transmitter contents also change with the hormonal state suggest that nervous control may also play an important role.

Vagina

This extends from the cervix to the vulva. The outer wall of the vagina is covered in a connective tissue coat, which is continuous with the pelvic fascia. This coat contains striated muscle fibres near the opening of the vagina. The main vaginal wall is muscular, with a thin outer longitudinal smooth muscle layer, and an ill-defined inner circular layer, both interspersed with elastic fibres. The mucosa is thick and non-glandular. It is lined by a stratified but non-keratinised squamous epithelium, which has a high glycogen content. Lubrication of the vagina is from the secretions of the cervix, but the high glycogen content allows bacteria within the vagina to form lactic acid, which keeps the vaginal fluid acid. The vagina is a very vascular organ, and is supplied by sympathetic and parasympathetic nerves, which may be important in controlling the blood flow – the parasympathetic fibres are vasodilatory. Sensory nerves leave the vagina by way of the pudendal plexus.

External genitalia

The only part of the external genitalia in which the autonomic innervation plays an important role is the clitoris. Since the structure and mechanisms involved in the erection of the clitoris are very similar to those of the penis, they will not be dealt with here. The importance of the sensory innervation of the clitoris is, however, worth mentioning, since its activation plays a significant role in the pleasure of sex, and appears largely responsible for the initiation of female orgasm. In some societies, female 'circumcision' is practised – a misnomer, since what occurs is excision of the clitoris. This presumably helps to emphasise the subjugation of women in societies that practise it. Orgasm in the female has similarities with the ejaculatory reflex in the male, and also involves reflex activation of muscles and glands, including rhythmic activation of many of the smooth muscles, both of the reproductive tract and the urethra, as well as the striated muscles of the pelvic floor.

10.4.3 Relevant pharmacology

Little of the pharmacological treatment of the female reproductive system involves modulation of the innervation or activation and inhibition of receptors to neurotransmitters. Drugs having direct effects on uterine smooth muscle are important for the induction of abortions, for the induction and augmentation of labour and for the suppression of premature labour. Vasoconstrictor drugs are of use for the suppression of postpartum haemorrhage.

Oxytocin is used to enhance uterine contractions during labour. The sensitivity of the uterine smooth muscle to oxytocin increases during pregnancy, and is at its maximum at parturition, when oxytocin from the posterior pituitary causes regular co-ordinated contractions that sweep along the uterus without significantly increasing the intrauterine pressure (which would be dangerous, as it can reduce or block placental blood flow). Intravenous oxytocin can enhance the amplitude and frequency of the contractions, and only at very high doses is there danger of sustained contractions. Ergometrine is also a powerful stimulant of uterine contraction, and before the isolation of oxytocin was used for induction of labour. However, it produces prolonged contractions of the smooth muscle and an elevation of uterine tone. It is thus dangerous to use during parturition, but valuable to prevent postpartum bleeding. Induction of labour and abortion can also be achieved by the use of prostaglandins E and F, which are often given as vaginal pessaries. Prostaglandins are produced in the myometrium and endometrium and also have effects on the non-pregnant uterus. Dysmenorrhoea is associated with increased natural production, and can be treated with non-steroidal anti-inflammatory drugs. Activation of β_2-adrenoceptor agonists will relax uterine smooth muscle, and such drugs as salbutamol and ritodrine have been used as tocolytic agents to try to suppress premature labour.

10.5 The male reproductive tract

10.5.1 Overview

The male reproductive tract consists of the paired testes, epididymides and vasa deferentia and the penis. There are also the accessory structures of the seminal vesicles, prostate and bulbo-urethral glands (Fig. 10.19). As in the female reproductive tract, the development and function of many of these organs is very much under hormonal control. However, the precise timing of erection, emission and ejaculation required to ensure the completion of the primary function of the tract, i.e. insemination of the female, requires accurate neural control, and thus, in contrast to the female, the autonomic innervation of many of these organs is of paramount importance.

In the periods between intercourse, the sperm are produced, matured and stored in the epididymis and vas deferens, and the components of the seminal fluid are secreted and stored in the seminal vesicles and prostate. These processes are under hormonal control. For intercourse, erection is produced through a complex neuronal process using the parasympathetic nervous system as the main effector. Emission and insemination require activation of the ejaculatory reflex, which is a complicated reflex involving both somatic and autonomic effectors. To produce the seminal fluid, it uses the sympathetic nervous system to produce vigorous contraction of the smooth muscles of accessory glands and the vasa deferentia. The sequence of activation is normally that the prostate contracts first, followed by the vas deferens and then the seminal vesicles, so that the ejaculate is divided into three distinct fractions, the first rich in prostatic fluid, the middle containing most of the sperm and the last portion mainly consisting of fluid produced in the seminal vesicles. Intercourse and ejaculation also initiate rhythmic activation of the smooth muscles of the urethra and the striated muscles of the urethral sphincter, pelvic floor and anal canal.

Students will not need reminding that, in both the male and female, psychogenic stimuli and physical stimulation of the external genitalia can also lead to widespread autonomic responses not just of the reproductive tracts

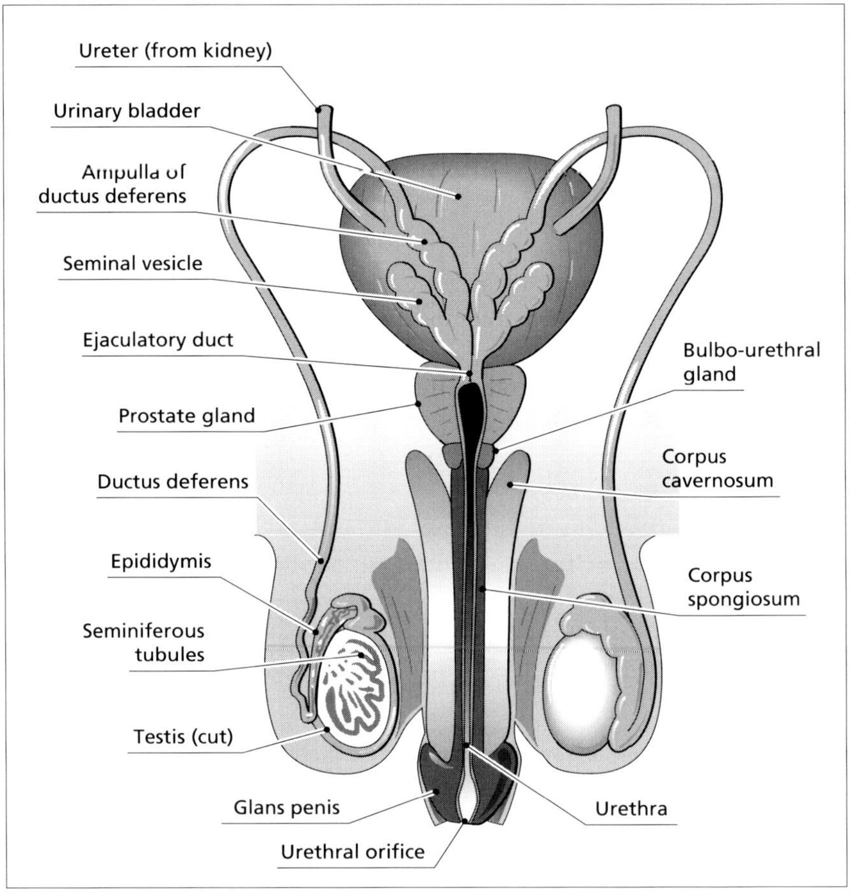

Fig. 10.19 Diagram of the human male reproductive tract.

but of the whole body, presumably to ensure efficient insemination, but also as part of the pleasurable sides of sexual activity that are necessary to ensure continuation of the species.

10.5.2 Components of the tract and their innervation

A diagram of the human male genital tract is given in Fig. 10.19.

Testes and epididymides

These are the organs of spermatogenesis. They are located outside the abdominal cavity in the scrotum, a thin-skinned pouch with a layer of smooth muscle (the dartos muscle), which on contraction in the cold or during exercise allows the testes to be pulled nearer to the body for protection or increased warmth, and when relaxed allows elongation and thus lowering of the testes away from the abdomen for cooling. Correct temperature is necessary for normal development of the sperm.

The testes are ovoid structures covered by a thick white capsule, the tunica albuginea. Inside, each testis is divided into about 250 compartments or lobes, each containing one to three highly convoluted seminiferous tubules. These tubules join a series of some 30 short collecting tubules, the straight seminiferous tubules, which converge into the rete testis, a network of spaces on the medial aspect of the testis under the epididymis. From the rete, efferent ductules enter the head of the epididymis, which is a tortuous canal in which the coils form a compact body extending from the cranial to the caudal pole of the testis.

There is smooth muscle both in the capsule of the testis and in the walls of the epididymis. In both these organs, the smooth muscles display automaticity, i.e. they appear spontaneously active. This activity in the testis may be important in transporting spermatozoa into the epididymis. Both organs are innervated by sympathetic and parasympathetic nerves, entering mainly with the testicular arteries. The main targets of these adrenergic nerves seem to be the blood vessels, although in the more distal part of the ducts some control of the smooth muscle contractile activity may be exerted by the innervation. Both cholinergic and adrenergic nerves are excitatory.

Vasa deferentia and ejaculation

Each vas deferens is a continuation of the duct of the epididymis. Initially, the vas deferens is tortuous, but it becomes straighter as it passes back along the testis and up through the spermatic cord and the inguinal canal into the pelvic cavity. Here it runs between the peritoneum and the lateral wall of the pelvis, from whence it runs backwards, downwards and medially, crossing the ureter to run behind the bladder, approaching its pair between the seminal vesicles at the base of the bladder. Here the tube swells into the wider ampulla of the vas deferens. On each side, the vas deferens then begins to penetrate into the substance of the prostate, and joins the duct from the seminal vesicle to form an ejaculatory duct. These ducts run through the prostate and open upwards into the prostatic urethra on the top of the urethral crest, close to the openings of the prostatic utricle.

The vas deferens is a thick-walled tube about 4–5 cm long. The wall contains three layers of smooth muscle cells in the human, a small inner and variable outer longitudinal layer and a middle circular layer. The lumen of the tube is very small and is lined by a mucous membrane made up of a lamina propria of connective tissue with elastic fibres and a lining epithelium.

More detail is known about the innervation and excitation of the smooth muscle of vas deferens than for any other smooth muscle-containing organ. This is probably because it is easily removed from the body with its main innervation intact, and since it lacks spontaneous electrical activity, it is relatively easy to study with electrophysiological techniques. Some further information about it is given in Chapter 4. The main excitatory innervation is via the sympathetic nervous system, although there is a sparse cholinergic innervation, more clearly seen in the circular smooth muscle layer. The smooth muscle is very densely innervated throughout its thickness by classical varicose postganglionic sympathetic nerve terminals. Many of the ganglion cell bodies lie in the hypogastric nerve close to the vas deferens. The walls of the tube are normally relaxed, and the tube is usually filled with sperm. Contraction of the smooth muscle is brought about through activation of the nerves in the ejaculatory reflex, in which a nearly simultaneous activation of the smooth muscle constricts the lumen and supposedly sweeps the spermatozoa into the urethra. In animals, the sympathetic innervation provides a dual excitatory input to the smooth muscles, the transmitters being ATP and noradrenaline. ATP, acting through P_{2x} purinoceptors, is responsible for excitatory junction potentials, which can summate to initiate action potentials that are transmitted from cell to cell in the longitudinal direction through gap junctions between the smooth muscle cells. Noradrenaline, on the other hand, results in elevation of intracellular free calcium concentration by activating α-adrenoceptors, with the probable involvement of the phosphatidylinositol pathway, but with little effect on the membrane potential. The relative importance of noradrenaline and ATP as excitatory transmitters is very species-dependent, and the purinergic component is almost absent in man. It is thought that the cholinergic nerves may also play a role in modulating the activity of the sympathetic nerves.

Seminal vesicles

These paired organs do not in fact store sperm (they are stored in the epididymis and vas deferens), but with the secretions of the prostate they produce the bulk of the seminal fluid. The seminal vesicles secrete a slightly alkaline fluid containing fructose, which is an energy source for the sperm, and a coagulating enzyme. The vesicles are in fact sacculated tubes, lined with secretory epithelium containing goblet cells. Their walls contain a longitudinal and a circular layer of smooth muscle, innervated predominantly by the sympathetic nervous system, which when activated propels the contents of the glands into the ejaculatory ducts.

Prostate

This is a partly glandular and partly fibromuscular organ situated at the base of the bladder, and surrounding the prostatic urethra. It secretes an important component of the seminal fluid. The secretion is slightly acidic and contains many important constituents, including acid phosphatase, fibrinolysin and prostaglandins. The stroma of the gland is composed of a meshwork of smooth muscle, in which the glandular tissue is embedded.

The glandular tissue is composed of follicles that open into elongated canals, which join to form the thirty or so collecting ducts on each side. The collecting ducts drain the prostatic secretions into the urethra via the prostatic sinuses, which lie on either side of the urethral crest. The prostate is innervated by both the sympathetic and parasympathetic nervous systems, but the main activation of the smooth muscle in the ejaculatory reflex is brought about through the sympathetic innervation and α-adrenoceptor activation.

Bulbo-urethral glands

These glands lie, one on each side, between the lower part of the prostate and the bulb of the penis. Their ducts enter the bulb of the penis and run down either side of the urethra, opening in the posterior floor of the spongy urethra. They are mucus-secreting glands and contribute a small amount to the seminal fluid. The arrangement of all of these accessory glands is shown in Fig. 10.19.

Penis and erection

The penis contains three longitudinally arranged erectile bodies that run from the base to the tip of the organ (Fig. 10.20). They are the paired corpora cavernosa on the dorsal aspect of the penis, and the ventral corpus spongiosum. The corpora cavernosa begin as the crus penis, attached to the bony pelvis where the pubis and ischium join, and extend the length of the shaft of the penis. The corpus spongiosum starts as the bulb of the penis, and contains the urethra. Distally, it expands into the glans penis, which carries the exit of the urethra (external urethral meatus). These three erectile bodies are covered by a tough fibrous envelope, the tunica albuginea. Outside this is the superficial fascia and the thin, loosely fitting skin. The erectile tissue itself consists of numerous trabeculae arising from the inner surface of the tunica, and dividing the bodies into cavernous spaces, giving them a sponge-like form. The trabeculae contain fibrous tissue, elastin and smooth muscle cells, and in them run nerves and blood vessels. The deep arteries of the penis and the urethral arteries supply the erectile tissue either directly or through the convoluted helicine arteries, and end in a capillary network that opens into the cavernous spaces. These spaces are lined throughout by endothelium, and drain into a series of emissary veins that leave the erectile tissue through the tunica and drain either into the circumflex veins or directly into the deep dorsal vein of the penis.

Erection is brought about by relaxation of the smooth muscle in the trabeculae, allowing filling of the cavernous spaces with blood, combined with relaxation of the smooth muscle of the incoming arteries, allowing the intracavernosal pressure to rise to values close to the mean arterial pressure, conferring considerable rigidity to the erect penis. This high pressure requires

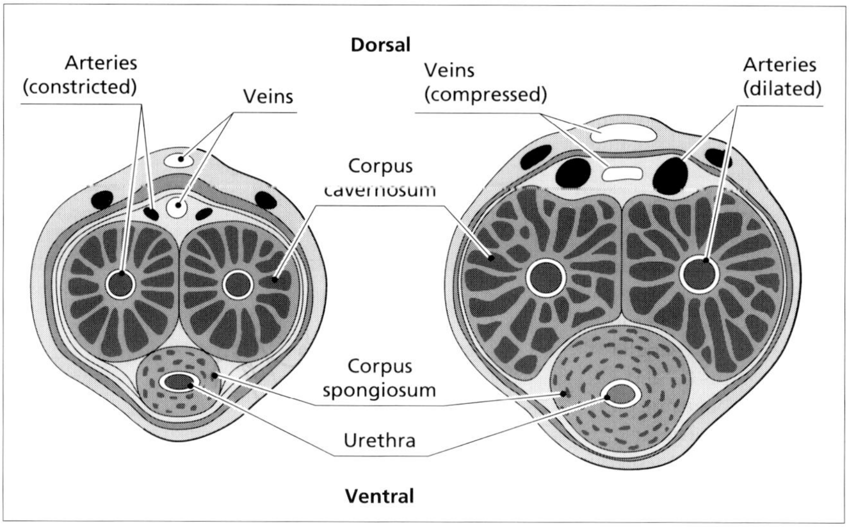

Fig. 10.20 Diagrammatic cross-section of the penis. (Left) flaccid, (right) erect.

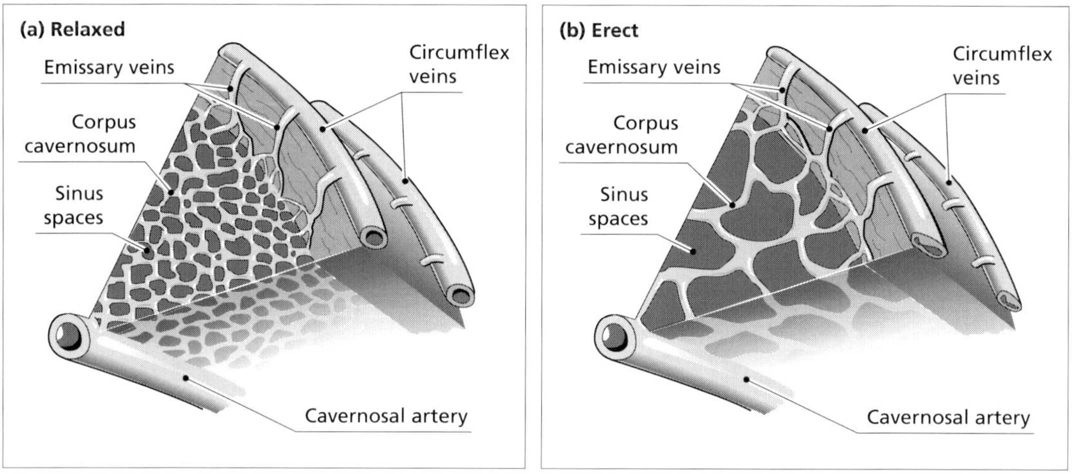

Fig. 10.21 Wedge segments of the penis to show relationship between the cavernosal arteries, sinuses and circumflex veins in the relaxed (a) and erect (b) penis. The distance from the centre to the outside of the erect penis in (b) would be much greater than actually shown.

both relaxation of the arteries and an increase in resistance of the venous vessels draining the spaces. The latter is brought about by compression of the emissary veins due to the expanding cavernosal spaces pressing on them as they pass through the fibrous tunica albuginea (Fig. 10.21). Detumescence requires constriction of the smooth muscle in the trabeculae, and their continued constriction is necessary to maintain a flaccid penis.

The changes in tone in the various smooth muscles leading to erection

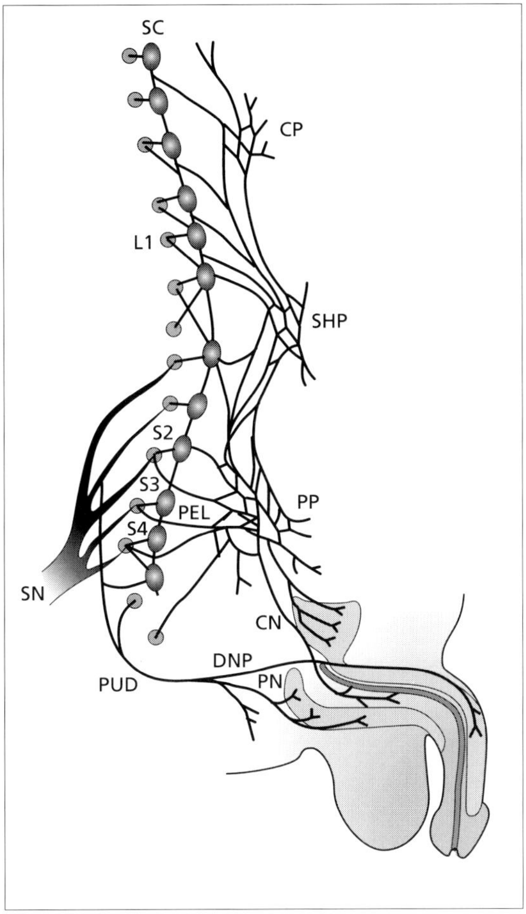

Fig. 10.22 Diagram of the innervation of the penis. The sympathetic outflow arises from segments T9 to L2 of the spinal cord (SC) and runs to the prevertebral ganglia (coeliac plexus CP and superior hypogastric plexus SHP) via the splanchnic nerves, and from thence via the hypogastric nerves to the pelvic plexus (PP). Parasympathetic input comes from segments S2 to S4 of the sacral cord, and travels to the pelvic plexus via the pelvic nerves (PEL). The autonomic nerves then travel to the penis in the cavernous nerves (CN). The sensory output from the penis travels in the perineal nerves (PN) and the dorsal nerve of the penis (DNP) to the pudendal nerve (PUD), which enters the cord through the S2–S4 roots. (SN) sciatic nerve.

and detumescence are entirely neural in origin. The penis is innervated by parasympathetic, sympathetic and somatic nerves. Both sympathetic (from T9 to L2) and parasympathetic (S2–S4) inputs converge at the level of the pelvic plexus (Fig. 10.22), and the innervation to the erectile tissues runs into the penis in the cavernous nerves, which contain preganglionic and postganglionic autonomic axons, sensory nerves and also the cell bodies of many postganglionic neurones. Several different potential transmitters and modulatory peptides have been shown in nerves in the penis, and clearly the processes of erection and detumescence are complex. Erection probably involves reduction in the effectiveness of the constrictor innervation to the arteries and trabecular smooth muscle, as well as activation of inhibitory nerves. Experiments on isolated segments of the corpus cavernosum demonstrate the presence of an excitatory adrenergic innervation and an NANC inhibitory innervation. Tone in the arteries, which controls the amount of blood flowing into the cavernous bodies in the flaccid penis, is clearly due to ongoing sympathetic activity, working through noradrenaline release and α-adrenoceptors. Vasodilation and an increase in tumescence can be brought about by α-receptor blockers, although they will not reliably produce full erection. Erections can, however, be abruptly terminated by injection of α-agonists into the cavernosal bodies. Stimulation of the parasympathetic sacral outflow can induce full erections, suggesting that it is this system that is responsible for relaxation of the trabecular smooth muscles, as well as relaxation of the arterial muscles. Currently, the evidence strongly suggests that the NANC inhibitory transmitter to the trabecular smooth muscle is NO, although VIP is also present with inhibitory effects, and may play some role. The nerve-mediated relaxations are inhibited by drugs that block nitric oxide synthase and by substances that can scavenge NO from the extracellular fluid. Postganglionic cholinergic nerves are present in the penis, both innervating the arteries and the trabeculae, but they are relatively sparse, and far less common than adrenergic fibres. Although acetylcholine can cause some dilation of the blood vessels and relaxation of the trabecular smooth muscle, it appears to be acting by the release of endothelium-derived relaxing factor (EDRF, nitric oxide) from the endothelium. Acetylcholine released from nerves probably plays a role in modulating transmitter release – possibly facilitating the NANC transmitter release and inhibiting noradrenaline release from adrenergic nerve fibres.

10.5.3 Relevant pharmacology

Pharmacological induction of erection in impotent men can be brought about by intracavernosal injection of the potent smooth muscle-relaxing drug papaverine, or by mixtures of papaverine and the α-receptor blocker phentolamine, or by injection of prostaglandin E1, which is also a powerful relaxant of the erectile smooth muscle. The use of phenoxybenzamine (another α-receptor blocker) has been largely discontinued, since although it can produce long-lasting erections, these are often painful and damaging. More recently oral ingestion of a specific phosphodiesterase-5 inhibitor (Viagra) has gained popularity by enhancing erections to psychogenic stimuli. This drug works by reducing breakdown of cGmP, the second messenger mediating the relaxant effects of NO.

Bladder outflow obstruction due to benign prostatic hyperplasia may be treated with α-receptor blocking agents such as finasteride, since it is thought that activity in the smooth muscle cells in the stroma of the gland may contribute to the obstruction.

Further reading

Kidney

Di Bona, G.F. & Kopp, U.C. (1997) Neural control of renal function. *Physiol Rev* **77**, 75–197.
Stella, A. & Zanchetti, A. (1991) Functional role of renal afferents. *Physiol Rev* **71**, 659.

Lower urinary tract

Torrens, M. & Morrison, J.F.B. (eds) (1987) *The Physiology of the Lower Urinary Tract.* Springer-Verlag, London.

Female reproductive tract

Greep, R.O. (ed) (1975) *Handbook of Physiology. Endocrinology,* Vol. 2. *Female Reproductive System.* American Physiological Society, Washington DC.

Male reproductive tract

Andersson, K.E. & Wagner, G. (1995) Physiology of penile erection. *Physiol Rev* **75**, 191–236.

Hamilton, D.W. & Greep, R.O. (eds) (1975) *Handbook of Physiology. Endocrinology,* Vol. 5. *Male Reproductive System.* American Physiological Society, Washington DC.

References

Cormack, D.H. (1987) *Ham's Histology*. Lippincott-Raven, Philadephia.

Shuba, M. (1977) Mechanisms of excitatory action of catecholamines and histamine on smooth muscle cells of guinea-pig ureter. *J Physiol* **264**, 853–64.

Sibley, G.N.A. (1984) A comparison of spontaneous and nerve-mediated activity in bladder muscle from man, pig and rabbit. *J Physiol* **354,** 431–43.

Zhang, Y. & Lang, R.J. (1994) Effects of intrinsic prostaglandins on the spontaneous contractile and electrical activity of the proximal renal pelvis of the guinea-pig. *Br J Pharmacol.* **113**, 431–38.

Index

Page numbers in *italics* refer to figures, those in **bold** refer to tables